International Boehringer Mannheim Symposia

The Heart in Hypertension

Editor
B.E. Strauer

With 187 Figures and 55 Tables

Springer-Verlag Berlin Heidelberg New York 1981

Prof. Dr. Bodo Eckehard Strauer
Medizinische Klinik I
der Universität München
Klinikum Großhadern
Marchioninistraße 15
D-8000 München 70

ISBN 3-540-10496-8 Springer-Verlag Berlin Heidelberg New York
ISBN 0-387-10496-8 Springer-Verlag New York Heidelberg Berlin

Library of Congress Cataloging in Publication Data. Main entry under title: The Heart in hypertension. (International Boehringer Mannheim symposia) "International symposium München, Germany, June 13-16, 1979." Bibliography: p. Includes index. 1. Heart--Hypertrophy--Congresses. 2. Hypertension--Complications and sequelae--Congresses. I. Strauer, Bodo Eckehard. II. Series. [DNLM: 1. Hypertension--Physiopathology--Congresses. 2. Heart--Physiopathology--Congresses. WG 340 H436 1979] RC685.H9H42 616.1'2 80-28500

Typesetting: Schreibsatz-Service Weihrauch, Würzburg,
Offsetprinting, and Binding: Beltz Offsetdruck, Hemsbach/Bergstr.
2127/3321-543210

Table of Contents

Participants

Alpert, N., Prof. Dr.
Department of Physiology and Biophysics, University of Vermont, Given Building, Burlington/Vermont 05401, USA

Behrenbeck, D.W., Prof. Dr.
Med. Universitätsklinik III — Kardiologie —, Joseph-Stelzmann-Straße 9, D-5000 Köln 41, Federal Republic of Germany

Bleifeld, W., Prof. Dr.
Abteilung für Kardiologie, II. Medizinische Klinik des Universitätskrankenhauses Eppendorf, Martinistraße 52, D-2000 Hamburg 20, Federal Republic of Germany

Blömer, H., Prof. Dr.
I. Medizinische Klinik der Technischen Universität München, Klinikum rechts der Isar, Ismaninger Straße 22, D-8000 München 80, Federal Republic of Germany

Bock, K.D., Prof. Dr.
Universitätsklinikum Essen, Medizinische Klinik und Poliklinik, Hufelandstraße 55, D-4300 Essen, Federal Republic of Germany

Büll, U., Prof. Dr.
Nuklearmedizinische Abteilung der Radiologischen Klinik, Klinikum Großhadern, Marchioninistraße 15, D-8000 München 70, Federal Republic of Germany

Bürger, S.B., Dr.
Medizinische Klinik I der Universität München, Klinikum Großhadern, Marchioninistraße 15, D-8000 München 70, Federal Republic of Germany

Cohn, J., Prof. Dr.
Department of Medicine, Cardiovascular Division, University of Minnesota Medical School, 420 Delaware Street S.E., Minneapolis, Minnesota 55455, USA

Doering, W., Dr.
II. Medizinische Abteilung des Städtischen Krankenhauses München-Schwabing, Kölner Platz 1, D-8000 München 40, Federal Republic of Germany

Frohlich, E.D., Prof. Dr.
Alton Ochsner Medical Foundation, Education and Research, 1516 Jefferson Highway, New Orleans, Louisiana 70121, USA

Girndt, J., Priv. Doz. Dr.
Medizinische Klinik und Poliklinik der Universität Göttingen, Robert-Koch-Straße 40, D-3400 Göttingen, Federal Republic of Germany

Grobecker, H., Prof. Dr.
Lehrstuhl für Phamakologie, der Universität Regensburg, Universitätsstraße 31, D-8400 Regensburg, Federal Republic of Germany

Gross, F., Prof. Dr.
Pharmakologisches Institut der Universität Heidelberg, Im Neuenheimer Feld 366, D-6900 Heidelberg, Federal Republic of Germany

Günther, K.H., Prof. Dr.
Kardiologische Abteilung der II. Medizinischen Universitätsklinik der Charite, Schumannstraße 20/21, DDR-104 Berlin, German Democratic Republic

Hanrath, P., Priv. Doz. Dr.
Abteilung für Kardiologie, II. Medizinische Klinik des Universitätskrankenhauses Eppendorf, Martinistraße 52, D-2000 Hamburg 20, Federal Republic of Germany

Hort, W., Prof. Dr.
Pathologisches Institut der Universität Düsseldorf, Moorenstraße 5, D-4000 Düsseldorf, Federal Republic of Germany

Jacob, R., Prof. Dr.
Physiologisches Institut der Universität Tübingen, Lehrstuhl II, Gmelinstraße 5, D-7400 Tübingen, Federal Republic of Germany

Just, H., Prof. Dr.
Abteilung Innere Medizin III, Medizinische Universitätsklinik, Hugstetter Straße 55, D-7800 Freiburg/Br., Federal Republic of Germany

Kannel, W.B., Prof. Dr.
National Heart Institute, Heart Disease Epidemiology Study, 118 Lincoln Street, Framingham, Mass. 01701, USA

Karliner, J.S., Prof. Dr.
Clinical Cardiology Section, 225 West Dickinson Street, San Diego, California 92103, USA

Kaufmann, W., Prof. Dr.
Medizinische Klinik und Poliklinik der Universität Köln, Ostmerheimer Straße 200, D-5000 Köln 91, Federal Republic of Germany

Kment, A., Dr.
Medizinische Klinik I der Universität München, Klinikum Großhadern, Marchioninistraße 15, D-8000 München 70, Federal Republic of Germany

Kochsiek, K., Prof. Dr.
Medizinische Klinik der Universität, D-8700 Würzburg, Luitpoldkrankenhaus, Federal Republic of Germany

Linzbach, J., Prof. Dr.
Pathologisches Institut der Universität Göttingen, Neues Klinikum, Robert-Koch-Straße 40, D-3400 Göttingen, Federal Republic of Germany

Mayr, G.W., Dr.
Medizinische Klinik der Universität München, Klinikum Großhadern, Marchioninistraße 15, D-8000 München 70, Federal Republic of Germany

Opherk, D., Dr.
Medizinische Klinik der Universität Heidelberg, Abteilung Innere Medizin III, Bergheimer Straße 58, D-6900 Heidelberg 1, Federal Republic of Germany

Pfeffer, M.A., Dr.
Harvard Medical School, Peter Bent Brigham Hospital, Huntington Ave., Boston, Massachusetts, USA

Rahlf, G., Priv. Doz. Dr.
Pathologisches Institut der Universität Göttingen, Robert-Koch-Straße 40, D-3400 Göttingen, Federal Republic of Germany

Riecker, G., Prof. Dr.
Medizinische Klinik I der Universität München, Klinikum Großhadern, Marchioninistraße 15, D-8000 München 70, Federal Republic of Germany

Schneider, A., Dr.
Medizinische Klinik I der Universität München, Klinikum Großhadern, Marchioninistraße 15, D-8000 München 70, Federal Republic of Germany

Swynghedauw, B., Prof. Dr.
Unite de Recherches sur le Metabolisme du coeur et des Vaisseaux — U 127, Batiment I.N.S.E.R.M., Hopital Lariboisiere, 41, Boulevard de la Chapelle, 75010 Paris, France

Strauer, B.E., Prof. Dr.
Medizinische Klinik I der Universität München, Klinikum Großhadern, Marchioninistraße 15, D-8000 München 70, Federal Republic of Germany

Tarazi, R., Prof. Dr.
Cleveland Clinic, 9500 Euclid Ave., Cleveland, Ohio 44106, USA

Weber, K.T., Prof.
Hospital of the University of Pennsylvania, 3600 Spruce Street, Philadelphia, Pennsylvania 19124, USA

Introduction

Hypertensive heart disease is one of the most frequent diseases in man. It is estimated that there are six to eight million hypertensive patients in the Federal Republic of Germany today. This corresponds with an incidence of 10%—15% in the whole population. Approximately between three and four million show organic cardiac manifestations of hypertension. Of all deaths occurring before the age of 65, 30%—40% are attributable to hypertension, and the total mortality from hypertension is about 20%—25%. Recent epidemiological and clinical studies have revealed similar figures for other countries, such as the United States and Japan.

Hypertensive hypertrophy and cardiac failure are found to be many times more frequent than cardiac hypertrophy and failure of any other origin. Despite the apparent clinical and social importance of the biological system "blood pressure and the heart", data on cardiac performance, on systemic and coronary haemodynamics and on the morphological, biochemical and contractile properties of ventricular heart muscle in both experimental and clinical hypertension are rare. This is the reason and stimulus for having organized this symposium, which is the first one concerning this topic.

Hypertensive hypertrophy, as will be shown in the course of the symposium, may be quite different from myocardial hypertrophy due to ventricular overload in aortic stenosis, hypertrophic obstructive cardiomyopathy, aortic coarctation or other forms of left ventricular pressure load. The specific hypertensive history, as evidenced by the amount of mechanical, hormonal, and neural factors imposed to the heart, seems to have similarities with other types of left ventricular overload, however, may characteristically diverge from them. Accordingly, the diagnostic and therapeutic consequences may differ and may specifically guide our diagnostic and therapeutic management in hypertensive hypertrophy and failure.

One of the main reasons for our limited knowledge concerning heart function in arterial hypertension refers to a methodological problem. Invasive cardiac studies in arterial hypertension, which would be necessary to obtain data on cardiac performance, are not justified in patients if only an extension of our knowledge about heart function is desired. Accordingly, most of our data on hypertensive heart disease stem from patients having been investigated because of secondary hypertensive cardiac lesions, such as angina, cardiac enlargement, cardiac arrhythmias and others. Repeated investigations which would be necessary, for example, for the evaluation of progression and of regression of hypertensive heart disease, cannot be obtained systematically. Therefore, noninvasive techniques (echocardiography, calibrated apexcardiography, radionuclide ventriculography, cardiac computer tomography etc.) should be increasingly utilized for acute as well as for long-term studies in hypertensive heart disease.

For the above-mentioned reasons, that is due to (1) the epidemiological and social significance of heart function in arterial hypertension, (2) the importance of diagnostic and therapeutic management of hypertensive heart disease and (3) the need of further data on cardiac performance in hypertension, we felt it necessary and useful to present recent results and to search for a better understanding of the cardiac consequences of high blood pressure disease.

This book represents the proceedings of the symposium held in June 13—16, 1979 in München (Germany). Accordingly five sessions, each containing two sections, have been grouped:

1. Cardiac performance in experimental hypertension.
2. Cardiac mechanochemistry and morphology in various forms of hypertensive heart disease.
3. Cardiac function and metabolism in clinical hypertension.
4. Central haemodynamics, regional wall mechanics and ventricular relaxation in clinical hypertension.
5. Therapy of hypertensive heart disease.

The encouraging advice and cooperation of all chairmen in planning and performing the scientific sessions is gratefully acknowledged. I am very much indebted to the participants and to the organizing committee for all the effort in preparing and realizing both the meeting and the proceedings.

Finally, I would like to express our gratefulness to Boehringer GmbH, Mannheim, and especially to Dr. H. Kienzl, for supporting the entire process of this symposium in a generous and unselfish way.

I hope that this symposium as well as the proceedings will represent a stimulus for new ideas in pathophysiology and in diagnostics and will ultimately increase our therapeutic success in hypertensive heart disease.

München, December 1980 B. E. Strauer

Session A: Cardiac Performance in Experimental Hypertension

Chairmen: F. Gross/Heidelberg (FRG), R.C. Tarazi/Cleveland (USA)

Part I: Pathogenesis of Experimental Hypertension; Ventricular Function and Myocardial Contractility

Experimental Hypertension and Its Significance for Clinical Hypertension

F. Gross

Methods to Induce High Blood Pressure in Experimental Animals

Animal models which simulate human diseases are useful for two reasons: (1) to study the pathogenesis of the disorder and (2) to investigate means by which the pathological state can be controlled. Hypertension is one of the few human diseases that can be reproduced in experimental animals, and, as in man, high blood pressure may be the primary manifestation of a genetic disorder or the consequence of some other pathological event. Hence, we may distinguish also in animals between primary and secondary hypertension just as is done in cases of human hypertension.

Each type of experimental hypertension should be:

1. simple to elicit;
2. easily and uniformly reproducible;
3. comparable to some form of the human disease; and
4. producible in small laboratory animals, preferably rats.

Although, at the beginning, most studies on experimental hypertension were done in dogs, the rat is the preferred animal species today. Rabbits are only rarely used and develop merely a moderate increase in blood pressure after renal artery stenosis. Corticosteroid hypertension has been studied occasionally in monkeys and quite recently in pigs.

Experimental hypertension can be subdivided into hereditary (primary) hypertension and the renal, endocrine, neurogenic, and dietary forms (secondary hypertension). Various forms of experimental hypertension can be connected with some types of clinical hypertension, whereas others, such as adrenal regeneration hypertension, have no equivalent in human pathology (Table 1). In the past years, hereditary hypertension has been studied more intensely than the different types of secondary hypertension, and various strains have been bred in several laboratories. Most strains have been derived from the Wistar Kyoto rats [20] and, quite recently, from its stroke-prone substrain, in which the incidence of strokes rose to 80% [21]. Other strains with hereditary hypertension have been selected in New Zealand [25], in the United States [3], and in West Germany [22]. In contrast to the increased sensitivity of the cerebrovascular system to high blood pressure which is found

Table 1. Comparable forms of experimental and clinical hypertension[a]

Experimental	Clinical
Spontaneous hypertension of rats (SHR)	Essential hypertension (?)
Renal artery stenosis (rat, rabbit, dog)	Renal artery stenosis
Renal infarction (rat, rabbit)	Renal infarction
Perinephritis (wrapping, figure-of-8-ligature) (rat, dog)	
Overdosage of glucocorticoids (rat)	Cushing's syndrome
Overdosage of mineralocorticoids (rat, pig)	Primary aldosteronism (adenoma, hyperplasia)
	Overproduction of DOC
	Overdosage of licorice
Overdosage of salt (rat)	Chronic high salt intake
Subtotal nephrectomy (rat)	Various forms of renal damage
	Loss of nephrons

a [9]

in stroke-prone rats, no comparable predilection for characteristic lesions has been observed in other vascular beds, such as the coronary or renal circulation. It remains to be demonstrated whether the high incidence of cerebrovascular lesions is the consequence of high blood pressure only or whether hereditary structural changes are, at least in part, also responsible.

The heredity of high blood pressure in these strains of rats is probably of multifactorial origin. In most cases, a salt dependence and an increased sensitivity to other hypertensinogenic factors could be observed. For the Okamoto strain, a reduced capacity of the kidney to excrete a sodium load has been described, and, in addition, the sympathetic tone is increased [4]. Similarly, a delayed renal excretion of sodium has been reported for the Dahl strain [27] and the Milano strain [1].

Variable findings have been reported on salt appetite and salt intake of spontaneously hypertensive rats. While some authors observed salt appetite and an increased preference for saline solution in rats of the Okamoto-Aoki strain [18], others reported that stroke-prone, spontaneously hypertensive rats (Okamoto strain) drank less of a 2% saline solution than Wistar-Kyoto control rats when water and saline were offered simultaneously [4]. Young hypertensive rats had a lower fluid intake than old rats, which drank more water, but less saline than normotensive controls.

Although hereditary hypertension in rats is in some way comparable to primary hypertension in humans, no data are available that would permit the definition of the genetic deviations responsible for the human disease. Furthermore, little is known of the factors which influence the course of the disease, except for the noxious effect of salt and of "emotional stress", the latter being poorly defined. Several types of renal hypertension in rats and dogs are still used in numerous laboratories for the studies on the pathogenesis of this type of secondary hypertension as well as for the evaluation of antihypertensive drugs.

Although the renin-angiotensin system may be of some pathogenic significance in the initial phase of renal hypertension, this is no longer the case during the chronic phase. Furthermore, in some types of experimental renal artery stenosis (e.g., after unilteral nephrectomy or after bilateral stenosis), the renin-angiotensin system is not stimulated initially, but the blood pressure increases even more rapidly than after unilateral renal artery stenosis in the presence of an intact kidney [11]. In the latter type, a renin dependence of the high blood pressure may occur as a consequence of pressure-induced natriuresis, which results in a stimulation of the renin-angiotensin-aldosterone system. This situation can be characterized as a secondary hyperaldosteronism, which also occurs in the malignant phase of the human disease [10]. The fact that renal hypertension may develop without an increased activity of the renin-angiotensin system or even when the system is suppressed demonstrates that factors other than the renin-angiotensin system are involved in the pathogenesis of this type of the disease. However, little is known about those factors.

Mineralocorticoid hypertension, especially that induced by high doses of desoxycorticosterone (DOC), is a salt-dependent form of high blood pressure. Salt can be offered either in the food or in the drinking fluid, the latter usually being a 1% saline solution. Reduction of renal mass by unilateral nephrectomy favors the development of this type of hypertension. The most suitable experimental animal is the rat, while in dogs only a mild increase in blood pressure is seen, simultaneously with marked polydipsia and polyuria. Recently, sustained hypertension has been induced by DOCA in pigs [26]. Desoxycorticosterone is mostly given in the form of the acetate (DOCA), more rarely in the longer acting trimethylacetate ester. Aldosterone also causes hypertension, if it is administered in doses that are five to ten times lower than those of DOC; it, too, has been used in the form of the acetate. The more rapid metabolization of aldosterone makes it less suitable than DOC as a hypertension-induced corticosteroid. In mineralo-corticoid hypertension, as in human primary hyperaldosteronism, sodium is retained and total body potassium is reduced. The intravascular volume is increased in the first phase, but may be decreased later on, when sustained hypertensive levels have been reached and a pressure-induced saluresis occurs. Severe vascular lesions and cardiac hypertrophy as well as renovascular lesions, which may eventually result in nephrosclerosis, are frequently seen. Hypertension with severe renal damage has also been obtained in monkeys after high doses of 2α-methyl-9α-fluorocortisol or the corresponding 9α-chloro derivative [23].

High blood pressure elicited by DOC may become sustained after some time, when the steroid is no longer administered nor additional salt is given. This type of hypertension has been characterized as metacorticoid hypertension and is probably caused by irreversible changes in the resistance vessels. It has been claimed that metacorticoid hypertension could be an experimental equivalent to essential hypertension in man, but this is of course not justified in view of the primarily different pathogenesis of the two types of hypertension [7].

In contrast to mineralocorticoid hypertension, hypertension caused by high doses of glucocorticoids, such as cortisol, cortisone, or prednisone, is independent of high salt intake [15]. The pressure values reached are definitely lower than those obtained in mineralocorticoid hypertension, and the pressure is less stable, falling towards normal after the administration of glucocorticoids has been stopped. The catabolic effect of the glucocorticoids is responsible for the fact that the animals do not gain weight or even lose weight, and the decrease in resistance favors the manifestation of infections. Hence, this procedure, i.e., inducing a type of experimental hypertension which to a certain degree corresponds to that seen in hypercorticism or Cushing's syndrome, is not suitable to elicit high blood pressure.

An intermediate position takes 9α-fluorocortisol, which causes hypertension independent of additional salt supply [14]. As an experimental model, this type of hypertension does not offer any advantage.

Adrenal regeneration hypertension in rats has found wide interest and for some time has been a standard model in the United States. It is a sodium-dependent form of hypertension, which is caused by taking out one adrenal and leaving only the capsule of the other [24]. Subtotal adrenalectomy is followed by a marked regeneration of adrenocortical tissue, and simultaneously the blood pressure rises. Originally, it was claimed that the adrenal tissue had to be removed in juvenile rats, but later on similar results were obtained in adult rats. As drinking fluid, a 1% saline solution should be given. The reproductibility of this type of hypertension is not as good as that of mineralocorticoid hypertension, and therefore the method does not offer any advantage. Attempts have been made to find a special corticosteroid, which might be responsible for the increase in blood pressure during and after adrenal regeneration, but the results of those studies have not provided evidence for such a secretory product of the adrenal gland [6, 19]. The sodium dependence of various forms of experimental hypertension is summarized in Table 2.

Various forms of neurogenic hypertension have been described, but none of them has become widely accepted as a standard model. In dogs, the denervation of the carotid sinus and other baroreceptor areas has been a recommended procedure, but the increase in blood pressure obtained in this way is not very marked and is unstable [8]. After several weeks, the blood pressure returns to normal. In rats, the denervation of sino-aortic baroreceptor areas may be followed by a marked and sustained elevation of blood pressure, comparable to that obtained in renal or DOCA hypertension [16, 17].

An audiogenic hypertension has been described in wild rats that had been exposed to various sounds and noises for several weeks up to several months. Other types of "stress", such as electric stimuli, socioecological changes, and

Table 2. Experimental hypertension

Sodium-dependent	Sodium-independent
Overdosage of mineralocorticoids	Overdosage of glucocorticoids
Adrenal regeneration	Renal artery stenosis
Spontaneous hypertension (Okamoto strain, Dahl strain, Smirk strain)	Wrapping of the kidneys
Subtotal nephrectomy	

emotional stimuli, have been applied, but in all cases the results were similar, and the degree and stability of hypertension were not comparable to those of other types of hypertension. In mice, a blood-pressure increase could also be elicited by psychosocial or socioecological changes [12, 13]. These observations are of interest from the pathophysiologic point of view, since they demonstrate that under certain conditions psychic factors may have an influence on the development of hypertension.

This short and incomplete review only gives some examples of those types of experimental hypertension that are most often used for the evaluation of antihypertensive agents.

Experimental Hypertension as a Tool for the Evaluation of Antihypertensive Drugs

For the assessment of the antihypertensive action of drugs, various types of experimental hypertension have been increasingly used during the past years, especially since rats with hereditary hypertension have been available in most laboratories. Today, each new drug with an antihypertensive potential will be studied in at least one, if not several forms of experimental hypertension before it undergoes clinical trials. However, it has to be kept in mind that all the antihypertensives now available either have been found and tested in normotensive animals or have shown their effect on high blood pressure only during their clinical use in man. Of course, the blood-pressure lowering effect may be more pronounced in a hypertensive than in a normotensive animal; however, according to their mode of action, some drugs may affect the blood pressure in certain types of experimental hypertension only and not in others. Saluretics, for instance, have no effect in renal hypertension, but are active in mineralocorticoid or plainly salt-induced hypertension. Beta-adrenoceptor blocking drugs lower the blood pressure neither in renal nor in mineralocorticoid hypertension, but may show some effect in spontaneously hypertensive rats, especially at a stage when sympathetic activity is high. On the other hand, it is evident that drugs which interfere with the renin-angiotensin system, such as angiotensin II antagonists or converting enzyme inhibitors, can only show an action in renin-dependent forms of experimental hypertension or under conditions in which the renin-angiotensin system contributes to the maintenance of normal blood pressure, as for example during sodium depletion.

All drugs which lower high blood pressure by acting on the efferent sympathetic nervous system at various levels have also in acute blood-pressure lowering effect in normotensive animals. This effect is less pronounced for the centrally acting drugs α-methyldopa or clonidine than for the ganglionic blockers or the drugs which interfere with the storage and liberation of noradrenaline at adrenergic nerve terminals, such as reserpine or guanethidine and various of the latter's analogues. Similarly, all vasodilators acting directly on the vascular smooth muscle, such as hydralazine and its derivatives, sodium nitroprusside, minoxidil, and others, can easily be characterized on the basis of their acute blood-pressure lowering effect in anesthetized normotensive animals, mainly dogs and cats. Alpha-adrenoceptor blocking drugs, such as prazosin, but also phentolamine, have an acute hypotensive effect in normotensive animals of various species.

Several attempts have been made to develop a method for the assessment of the antihypertensive potential of a new drug in animals, preferably rats, with one type of experimental hypertension, but no procedure has been found that would offer a better chance than would the investigation of the compound in normotensive animals. On the basis of such studies it should be relatively easy to characterize the mode of action of the new compound and to allocate it to one of the groups of already-known drugs. However, it has to be admitted that even for drugs that have been already in use for the treatment of high blood pressure for many years, the mechanism of action is unknown. This is the case for most vasodilators, but also for the β-adrenoceptor blocking agents and for the saluretics; the mechanism involved in the lowering of high blood pressure has not yet been elucidated in any of these cases. Of course, such an allocation of new drugs to one of the available groups is not possible, if a drug with a mechanism of action is discovered that is not similar to any one of those already known. In such a case, erroneous attributions may be made, as has been the case for prazosin, which was originally characterized as a vasodilator, without considering its main activity, namely to block α-adrenoceptors. The various types of drug interferences with the efferent sympathetic system are well known today, but it cannot be excluded that there are other possibilities than those which take place by affecting the peripheral sympathetic tone. The situation for the vasodilators is more complex, since much less is known about their mechanism of action than about that of the substances acting on the efferent sympathetic system. By means of conventional testing methods further drugs with antihypertensive activities will be discovered, but no fundamentally new type of drug may be anticipated. This does not exclude the possibility that some of the new drugs differ with respect to their mechanism of action from those already available, but it is difficult to predict whether such a difference will be of therapeutic significance.

Experimental Hypertension as a Tool for the Control of High Blood Pressure

In contrast to what has been said for the discovery of new antihypertensive drugs, studies on the control of high blood pressure have to be done in animals with experimental hypertension. Today, different strains of rats with genetic hypertension are available, and in most laboratories "therapeutic" studies are carried out on this type of experimental hypertension. Occasionally, renal hypertension and mineralocorticoid hypertension are also used as models. In the assessment of the antihypertensive activity, it is essential to make sure that the drug is administered according to a fixed schedule which corresponds to its duration of action. Similarly, the blood pressure has to be measured at various intervals after the administration of the drug. Hence, it is necessary to prepare a protocol for such a study, which has to be strictly adhered to and monitored. If the blood pressure is measured once daily, within a few hours after a single daily administration, it may be found to be reduced, but it may return to high values within the period remaining until the next dose is administered. Such variations in pressure may escape observation, unless the blood pressure is measured again just before the administration of the dose on the following day.

Relatively few studies have been published on the effects of long-term control of experimental hypertension by antihypertensive drugs [5]. In rats with spontaneous hypertension, it is possible to administer drugs, at an early phase, in order to prevent the increase in blood pressure or, after hypertension has been established, in order to obtain a therapeutic effect. Complications of high blood pressure, mainly vascular damage, can be abolished or at least delayed by an effective control of hypertension. However, it is difficult to draw direct conclusions from such experiments to the situation in hypertensive patiens. Even if it is considered that a treatment period of six months corresponds to about one quarter of the total life span of a rat, the duration of the disease and of the treatment as well as the hemodynamic consequences of high blood pressure and the vascular lesions occurring in various organs cannot be directly compared with the pathophysiologic changes in hypertensive patients. Hence, nothing more than suggestive evidence may be expected from animal experiments. However, it can be demonstrated beyond any doubt that a reduced increase in blood pressure prevents the development of vascular lesions, and that after the lowering of an already established hypertension vascular lesions may be diminished or may even disappear [2]. These experimental data have clearly shown the significance of the blood pressure for the induction of vascular damage, particularly in certain vascular beds, such as the brain, the heart, the kidneys, and the splanchnic area. Furthermore, it could be demonstrated that even severe vascular lesions are reversible, at least to a certain degree. Hence, experimental data strongly support the view that high blood pressure should be effectively controlled to prevent vascular lesions, to favor their repair, or to inhibit their further progress. In this respect, not specific effect of any antihypertensive drug has been demonstrated. It is only the reduction of blood pressure which is responsible for relieving vascular lesions; it does not matter by which means the high blood pressure is controlled.

Conclusions

In conclusion it may be stated that the various models of experimental hypertension are useful tools for the study of the pathophysiology of sustained hypertension in animals and in particular of the damaging effect that high blood pressure may have on various vascular beds. Sustained experimental hypertension, especially primary or hereditary hypertension of rats, can be controlled by various antihypertensive drugs or by dietary methods, such as sodium deprivation. These studies prove that the prevention of blood-pressure increase as well as the lowering of an already established hypertension are effective in reducing or precluding vascular lesions and impaired organ function. Experimental hypertension may be of some help in evaluating the antihypertensive potential of new drugs, but in most cases their blood-pressure lowering action will already be discovered by pharmacologic studies in normotensive animals.

References

1. Bianchi G, Baer PG, Fox U, Duzzi L, Pagetti D, Giovannetti AM (1975) Changes in renin, water balance, and sodium balance during development of high blood pressure in genetically hypertensive rats. Circ Res [Suppl I] 36 : 153—161
2. Byrom FB (1969) The hypertensive vascular crisis. An experimental study. Heinemann, London
3. Dahl LK, Heine M, Tassinari L (1962) Effects of chronic excess salt ingestion. Evidence that genetic factors play an important role in susceptibility to experimental hypertension. J Exp Med 115 : 1173—1190
4. Dietz R, Schömig A, Haebara H, Mann JFE, Rascher W, Lüth JB, Grünherz N, Gross F (1978) Studies on the pathogenesis of spontaneous hypertension of rats. Circ Res [Suppl 1] 43 : 98—106
5. Freis ED, Ragan D, Pillsbury H III, Mathews M (1972) Alteration of the course of hypertension in the spontaneously hypertensive rat. Circ Res 31 : 1—7
6. Gaunt R, Melby JC, Dale SL, Grekin RJ, Brown RD (1973) Adrenal regeneration hypertension. In: Scow RO (ed) Endocrinology. Proceedings of the Fourth International Congress of Endocrinology 1972. Excerpta Medica, Amsterdam, pp 740—745
7. Green DM (1953) Experimental hypertension. Ann Intern Med 39 : 333—344
8. Grimson KS (1941) The sympathetic nervous system in neurogenic and renal hypertension; experimental correlation and clinical consideration. Arch Surg 43 : 284—305
9. Gross F (1977) Antihypertensive drugs. In: Gross F (ed) Antihypertensive agents. Springer, Berlin Heidelberg New York (Handbook of experimental pharmacology, new series, vol 39), pp 1—11

10. Gross F, Dietz R, Mast GJ, Szokol M (1975) Salt loss as a possible mechanism eliciting an acute malignant phase in renal hypertensive rats. Clin Exp Pharmacol Physiol 2 : 323—333
11. Gross F, Dietz R, Lüth JB, Mann JFE (1977) Welche Rolle spielt das Renin-Angiotensin-System in der Pathogenese des Hochdruckes? Verh Dtsch Ges Kreislaufforsch 43 : 177—187
12. Henry JP, Cassel JC (1969) Psychosocial factors in essential hypertension. Recent epidemiologic and experimental evidence. Am J Epidemiol 90 : 171—200
13. Henry JP, Meehan JP, Stephens PM (1967) The use of psychosocial stimuli to induce prolonged systolic hypertension in mice. Psychosom Med 29 : 408—432
14. Hepp R, Garbade K, Oster P, Gross F (1974) Arterial hypertension induced by 9α-fluorocortisol in rats. Acta Endocrinol (Copenh) 75 : 539—549
15. Knowlton AI, Loeb EN, Stoerk HC, White JP, Heffernan JF (1952) Induction of arterial hypertension in normal and adrenalectomized rats given cortisone acetate. J Exp Med 96 : 187—205
16. Krieger EM (1964) Neurogenic hypertension in the rat. Circ Res 15 : 511—521
17. Krieger EM (1967) Effect of sinoaortic denervation on cardiac output. Am J Physiol 213 : 139—142
18. McConnell SD, Henkin RI (1973) NaCl preference in spontaneously hypertensive rats: Age and blood pressure effects. Am J Physiol 225 : 624—627
19. Melby JC, Dale SL, Grekin RJ, Gaunt R, Wilson TE (1972) 18-Hydroxy-ll-deoxycorticosterone (18-OH-DOC) secretion in experimental and human hypertension. Recent Prog Horm Res 28 : 287—351
20. Okamoto K, Aoki K (1963) Development of a strain of spontaneously hypertensive rats. Jpn Circ J 27 : 282—293
21. Okamoto K, Yamori Y, Nagaoka A (1973) Establishment of the stroke-prone spontaneously hypertensive rat (SHR). Circ Res [Suppl I] 34/35 : 143—153
22. Samizadeh A, Losse H, Wessel F (1977) Einfluß von Kochsalz und Beta-sympathikolytika auf den Blutdruckverlauf der erblichen spontanen Hypertonie der Ratte (SH-Rattenstamm Münster). Med Welt 28 : 2050—2054
23. Selye H, Bois P (1957) The hormonal production of nephrosclerosis and periarteriitis nodosa in the primate. Br Med J I : 183—186
24. Skelton FR (1959) Adrenal regeneration and adrenal-regeneration hypertension. Physiol Rev 39 : 162—182
25. Smirk FH, Hall WH (1958) Inherited hypertension in rats. Nature 182 : 727—728
26. Terris JM, Berecek KH, Cohen EL, Stanley JC, Whitehouse WM Jr, Bohr DF (1976) Deoxycorticosterone hypertension in the pig. Clin Sci Mol Med [Suppl 3] 51 : 303—305
27. Tobian L, Lange J, Azar S, Iwai J, Koop D, Coffee K, Johnson MA (1978) Reduction of natriuretic capacity and renin release in isolated, blood-perfused kidneys of Dahl hypertensionprone rats. Circ Res 43 : 92—98

Left Ventricular Hypertrophy in Chronic Pressure Load Due to Spontaneous Essential Hypertension
I. Left Ventricular Function, Left Ventricular Geometry, and Wall Stress[1]

S.B. Bürger and B.E. Strauer

Essential hypertension represents the most frequent form of left ventricular pressure overload and hypertrophy in man. Previous studies in patients with essential hypertension have shown normal left ventricular function at rest and during exercise as long as coronary artery disease, regional wall motion abnormalities, or left ventricular dilatation are absent [17, 18]. In contrast, most experimental findings have demonstrated reduced myocardial contractility in pressure hypertrophy due to pulmonary artery banding [7, 16], aortic constriction [4, 9], or experimental renal hypertension [1, 9]. In contrast to the rapid onset of pressure overload due to outflow tract banding, spontaneously hypertensive rats (SHR), originally developed by Okamoto and Aoki [12], represent a model for slowly proceeding left ventricular pressure overload and in this way most closely resemble left ventricular pressure overload and hypertrophy in essential hypertension in man. Accordingly, the course of development of hypertensive hypertrophy can be systematically investigated by this experimental model.

Previous studies of Pfeffer [13] concerning left ventricular function in SHR have shown normal peak cardiac output per left ventricular weight in younger SHR and reduced peak cardiac output in 52—90-week-old SHR. Hallbäck-Nordlander investigated left ventricular hypertrophy in SHR using an isolated heart preparation [6, 11]. Since the data in patients with essential hypertension have shown a close dependence of left ventricular function on left ventricular geometry and wall stress [18], we designed our research to examine left ventricular function in various age groups of SHR with special reference to left ventricular geometry and wall stress.

Methods

Experiments were performed on 96 male 5—85 week-old SHR and on 88 age-matched normotensive Wistar Kyoto inbred rats (NR) from the same progenitor strain. The rats were housed in plastic cages (maximal five rats per cage) and fed with standard rat chow (Altromin) and tap water ad libitum. Before the be-

1 Supported by Deutsche Forschungsgemeinschaft

ginning of the experiment, systolic blood pressure and heart rate were measured by the tail cuff method. Afterwards, in light ether anesthesia (ether drip apparatus) the left femoral artery and vein were canulled and the centrally placed catheters were connected to Statham pressure transducers (P 23 Db). After intratracheal intubation, artificial ventilation (Harvard's rodents respirator), parasternal thoracotomy by cauterization, and incision of the pericardium, an 1,5—5-mm electromagnetic flow probe according to the aortic diameter was placed around the ascending aorta (flowmeter Recomed RM 302/2327, Fa. Hellige, Germany). Pressure measurements in the left ventricle were usually done by direct puncture of the left ventricle at the apex with fluid filled PE 60—160 metal cannulas using Statham pressure transducers.

In additional control experiments catheter tip manometers were used or the left ventricles were cannulated along the right carotid arteries with bent metal cannulas (closed chest). Since the results were comparable when regarding the difference between SHR and NR, only the data derived by direct left ventricle (LV) puncture were used for statistical evaluations. Aortic pressure, LV pressure and its first time derivative, phasic aortic flow and its first time derivative, LV end-diastolic pressure, i.e., LV pressure using high amplification, and integrated mean aortic flow were registered simultaneously (recording system Fa. Hellige, UV recording system Fa. Honeywell) (Fig. 1). Paper speed was usually 1,50 and 250 mm/sec, 2000 or 4000 mm/sec for the UV recording system.

Ventricular function studies included resting values, aortic clamping, rapid volume load (infusion of dextran or blood at a speed of 40 ml/min. kg until reaching peak cardiac output), aortic clamping after volume load, and in a few cases further volume load or rapid volume loss (10 ml/kg) with immediately following aortic clamping. Aortic clamping usually lasted 5—10 beats. After clamping, all parameters were evaluated beat by beat. For Fig. 7 and Fig. 8 the beats with highest systolic pressure were used; the left side of Fig. 12 represents the first beats after clamping, the right side of Fig. 12 and Fig. 13 the beats with highest systolic wall stress after clamping. For Fig. 14 isovolumic wall stress was determined at various extents of volume load beat by beat until maximum value of systolic wall stress. Postextrasystolic beats were usually not evaluated. After pressure and flow measurements cardiac arrest was performed, and diastolic pressure-volume relationships of the left ventricles and the weights of the left ventricles, including septum, and of the right ventricles were determined. For each rat three to five pressure-volume relations were performed and the mean value was used for further evaluations. Rats showing differences in pressure-volume relations of more than 10% were rejected. Left ventricular diastolic dimensions were calculated from end-diastolic pressure, diastolic pressure-volume relations, and LV weight, using a spherical LV model. For comparison LV dimensions were determined by direct measurements on the diastolically fixed hearts. As the values from diastolic pressure-volume relations showed better reproductibility than the directly measured LV dimension, only the former were used for statistical evaluations.

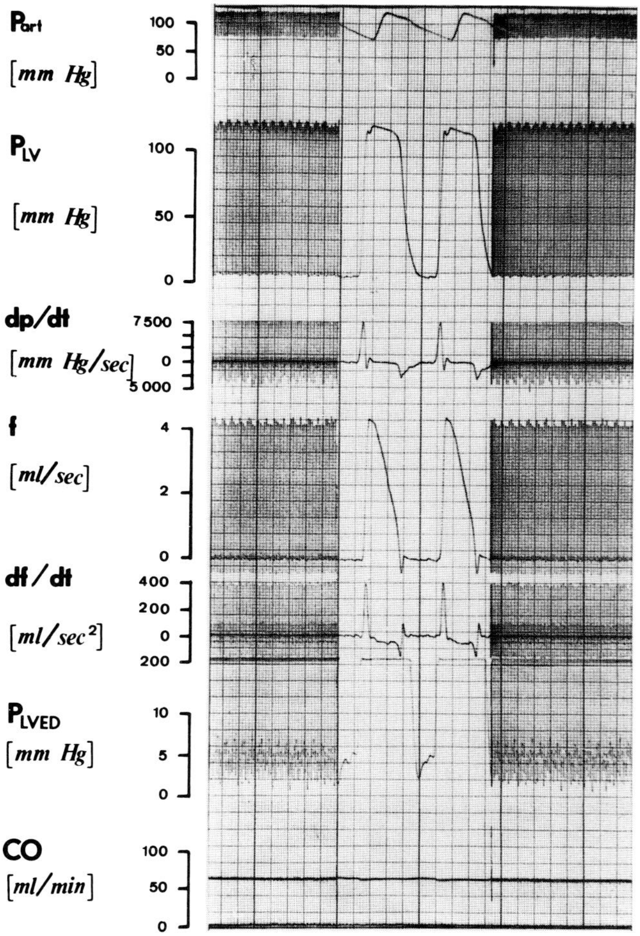

Fig. 1. Recording of hemodynamic measurements of a normotensive rat. P_{art} = arterial pressure; P_{LV} = left ventricular pressure; dp/dt = first time derivative of left ventricular pressure; f = phasic aortic flow; df/dt = first time derivative of aortic flow; P_{LVED} = left ventricular end-diastolic pressure, i.e., left ventricular pressure using high amplification; CO = integrated mean aortic flow (cardiac output)

Systolic wall stress was usually calculated from peak systolic LV pressure and diastolic LV dimensions, using a thin-walled spherical model according to the formula: systolic wall stress = $(P_{LV} - P_{LVED}) \cdot r_i / 2\,d$ (PL_V = LV systolic pressure, P_{LVED} = LV end-diastolic pressure, r_i = internal radius and d = diameter of the LV wall, i.e., wall thickness) [3, 8]. For comparison the mean values are also given in table 1 of the wall stresses, calculated using an ellipsoidal model [2, 14, 15], and of the wall stresses at the endocardium and at the mid-wall, using a thick-walled ventricular model [21]. Isovolumic wall stress in Fig. 14 includes diastolic wall stress, i.e., isovolumic systolic pressure was used for calculation of wall stress instead of $(P_{LV} - P_{LVED})$.

Table 1. Left ventricular wall thickness, internal radius, wall thickness to radius ratio, and systolic wall stress using different left ventricular models in three age groups of SHR and 34 age-matched NR[a]

	NR 20—60 weeks (n = 34)	SHR 20 weeks (n = 18)	SHR 40 weeks (n = 25)	SHR 60 weeks (n = 12)
Wall thickness (d)	1.78± 0.16	2.41± 0.18	2.62± 0.18	2.48± 0.20
Internal radius (r)	4.45± 0.30	3.65± 0.22	3.84± 0.18	4.44± 0.45
d/r	0.40± 0.04	0.67± 0.06	0.69± 0.07	0.56± 0.09
SWS	165 ±19	163 ±19	171 ±26	216 ±48
SWS_{Ell}	235 ±26	236 ±27	244 ±42	306 ±76
SWS_{thE}	180 ±18	198 ±19	210 ±27	249 ±49
SWS_{thM}	137 ±17	119 ±17	124 ±22	164 ±43
SWS_{max}	404 ±25 (n = 8)	495 ±56 (n = 6)	447 ±37 (n = 16)	400 ±37 (n = 8)

[a] d/r = wall thickness to radius ratio; SWS = systolic wall stress using a thin walled spherical left ventricular model; SWS_{Ell} = systolic wall stress using an ellipsoidal model assuming minor axis equal to half major axis; SWS_{thE} = systolic wall stress at the endocardium using a thick walled model; SWS_{thM} = systolic wall stress at the mid wall using a thick walled model; SWS_{max} = maximum value of systolic wall stress after volume load plus aortic clamping (number of animals for this column was lower and is separately given for each group). All values express mean values ± SD

Results

Arterial Pressure and Left Ventricular Hypertrophy

Arterial pressure was elevated in SHR, even in the youngest animals (4 weeks old) investigated.

The hypertensive animals had marked left ventricular hypertrophy in comparison to controls from the 5—7th week of age, with an increase in left ventricular to body weight ratio (Fig. 2) and thus a steeper course of the regression line between left ventricular weight and body weight (Fig. 3). The left ventricular to right ventricular weight ratio was likewise augmented (Fig. 2).

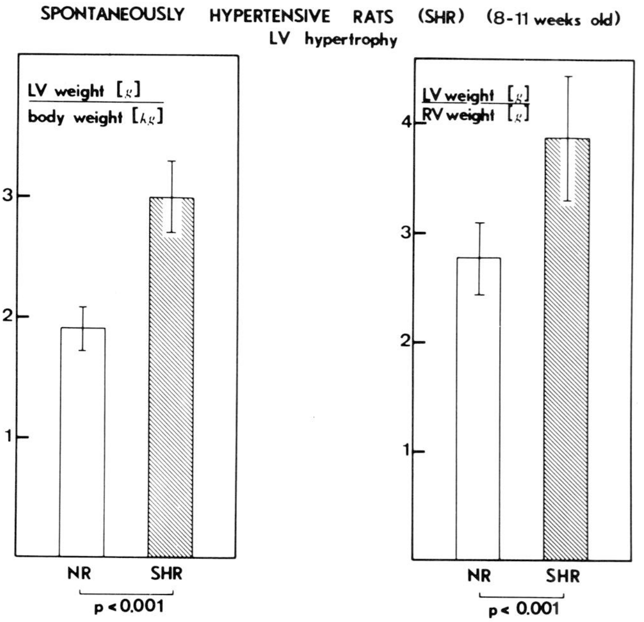

Fig. 2. Left ventricular to body weight ratio and left ventricular to right ventricular weight ratio in 8–11-week-old SHR and age-matched NR; n = 20 for each group

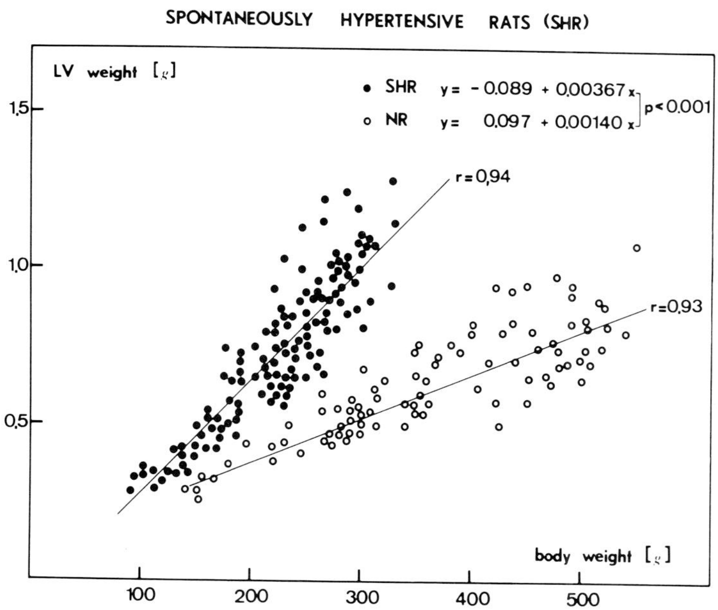

Fig. 3. Relationship between left ventricular weight and body weight in SHR (●) and NR (○)

Age Dependence of Left Ventricular Geometry and Wall Stress

Left ventricular wall thickness was increased in SHR in comparison to NR, while internal radius was decreased in the hypertensive animals up to the 40th week of age and rose in later age groups (Fig. 4). The wall thickness to radius ratio was significantly augmented in the younger SHR and tended to be numerically normalized between the 60th and 80th week of age by an increase

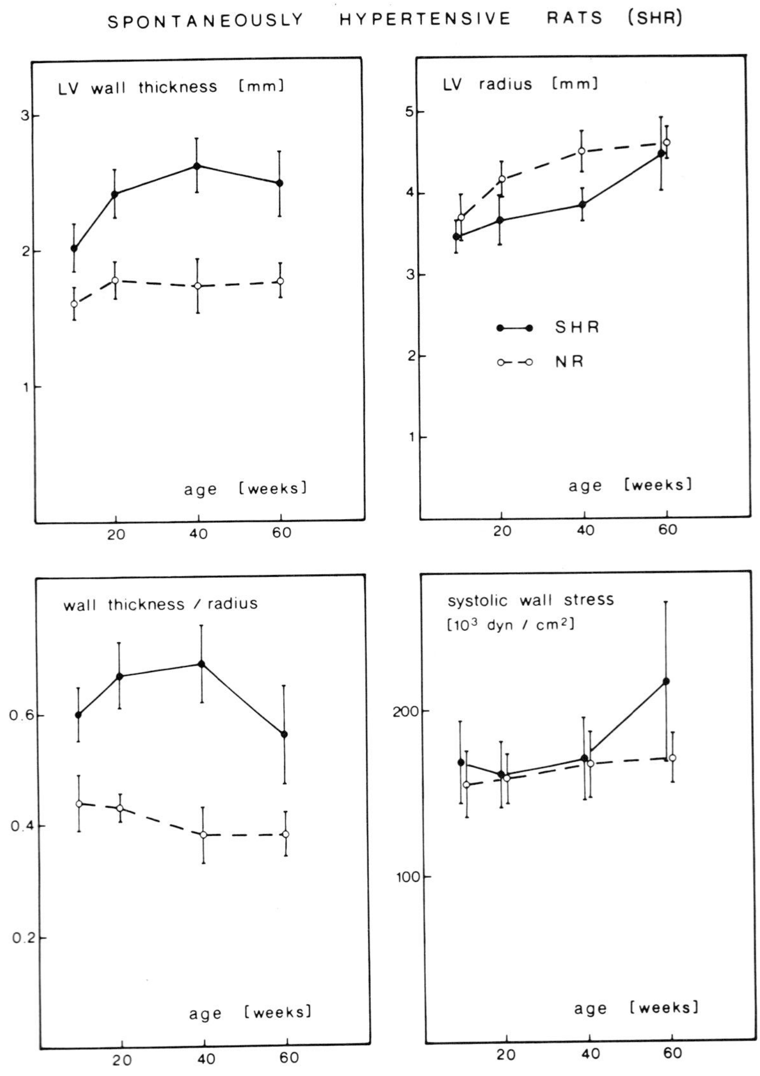

Fig. 4. Left ventricular wall thickness, left ventricular radius, wall thickness to radius ratio and systolic wall stress in 4 age groups of SHR (●—●) and NR (○—○), mean values ± SD

in LV radius. As a result of the elevated wall thickness to radius ratio, systolic wall stress was normal in the younger age groups of SHR and rose with increase in left ventricular radius and decrease in wall thickness to radius ratio. Table 1 summarizes wall stress values in NR and three age groups of SHR using different left ventricular models.

Left Ventricular Dynamics at Rest and During Stress Tests in the Younger Age Groups of SHR

Left ventricular function in the early stages of hypertrophy up to the 40th week of age was characterized by normal values for pumping parameters and isovolumic velocity indexes.

Acute Alterations in Volume Load

Rapid volume load and acute volume loss resulted in comparable responses in the younger SHR and NR (Fig. 5). There was a linear relation between stroke volume and end-diastolic volume under these conditions for 15-week-old SHR and NR (Fig. 6). Since the slope of this regression represents ejection fraction, this fact indicates identical ejection fraction in SHR and in NR under these volume loading and unloading conditions. As further shown in the figure, the

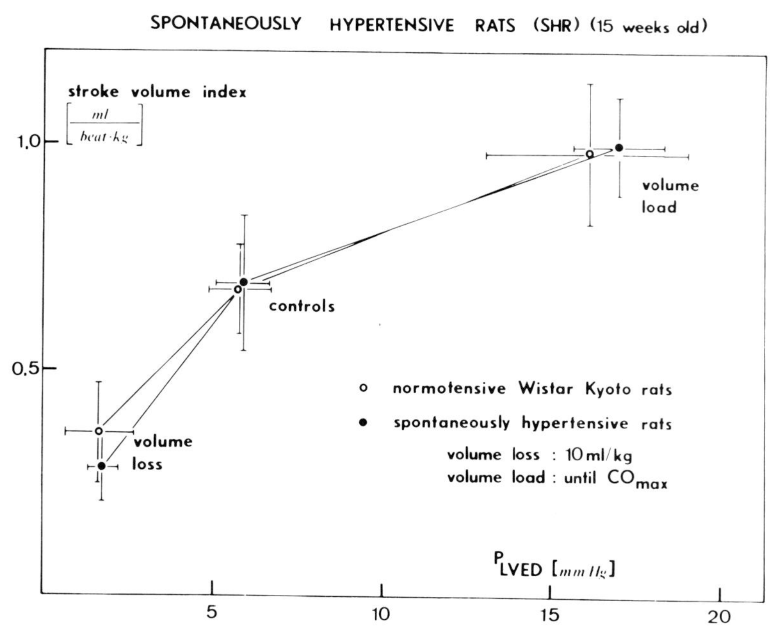

Fig. 5. Relation between stroke volume index and end-diastolic pressure at rest, after volume load and volume loss in 15-week-old SHR and NR, mean values ± SD of five rats each group

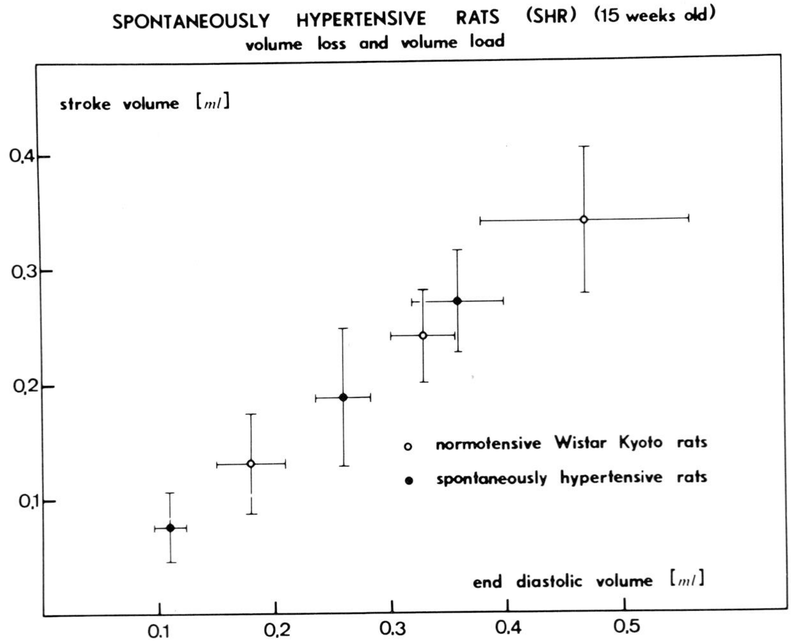

Fig. 6. Relation between stroke volume and end-diastolic volume at rest, after volume load and volume loss in 15-week-old SHR and NR, mean value ± SD of five rats each group

ejection fraction was independent of left ventricular preload in hearts with normal left ventricular function over a wide range of physiological end-diastolic volume values.

Acute Pressure Load

Acute pressure load by aortic clamping resulted in an increase in systolic pressure by the same amount in the younger SHR and in NR (Fig. 7). Maximum pressure generation after aortic clamping per gram LV mass was augmented in this age group of SHR by 35% in comparison to age matched NR.

Systolic Wall Stress After Acute Alterations in Pressure and Volume Load

Figure 8 demonstrates the relationship between wall thickness ro radius ratio (y-axis) and developed systolic pressure (x-axis). Points of identical wall stress are on straight lines through the origin. Preload and afterload were varied over a wide range. Control values showed normal systolic wall stress in younger SHR, despite the high systolic pressure, as a result of the increase in the wall thickness to radius ratio. Maximum pressure load by aortic clamping combined with volume

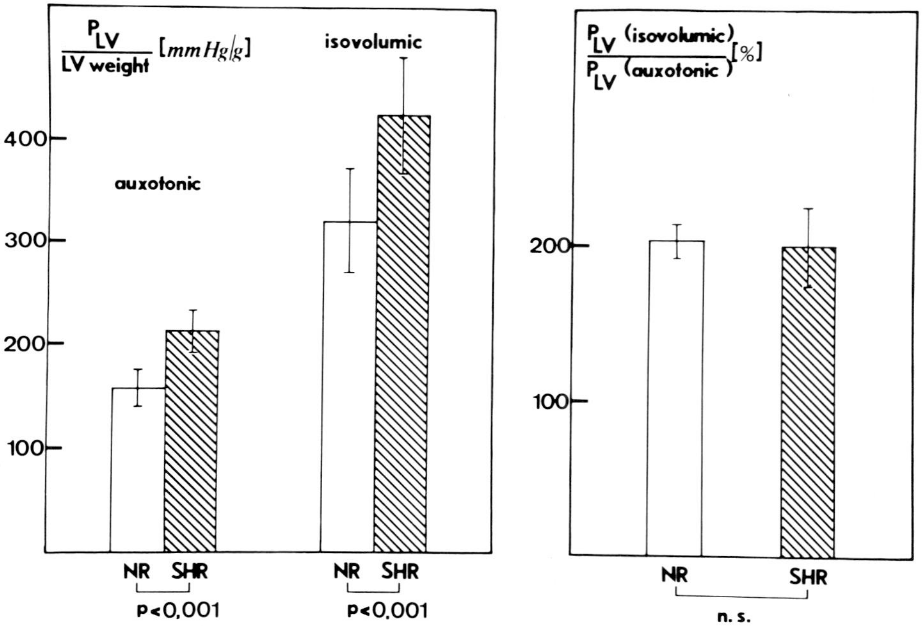

Fig. 7. Left ventricular pressure development per left ventricular weight before (*auxotonic*) and after aortic clamping (*isovolumic*) and increase in left ventricular pressure after clamping, expressed as percentage, in 15-week-old SHR and NR, ten rats each group, mean values ± SD

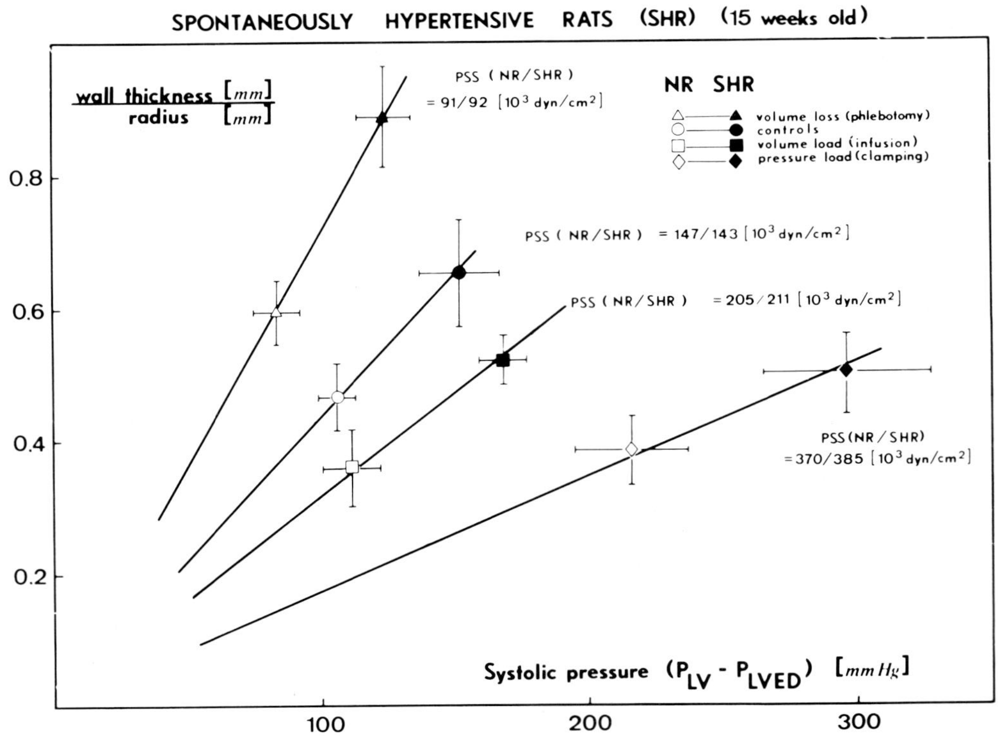

Fig. 8. Relationship between wall thickness to radius ratio and systolic pressure ($P_{LV} - P_{LVED}$) in 15-week-old SHR (*solid symbols*) and NR (*opened symbols*). Points of identical wall stress are on straight lines through the origin. Systolic wall stress (*PSS*) was varied by aortic clamping (*rhombuses*), volume load (*squares*) and volume loss (*triangles*) from 91/92 to 370/385 (10^3 dyn/cm^2). Note that systolic wall stress was nearly identical in SHR and in NR under all tested conditions, i.e., SHR and NR lay nearly on straight lines through the origin. Mean values ± SD, five rats each group

load by spontaneous filling of the LV chamber resulted in both groups in an elevation of systolic pressure by 100% and an increase in diastolic ventricular volume along with a decrease in wall thickness to radius ratio and hence an increase in wall stress. On the other hand, volume loss led to decreased systolic pressure, decreased diastolic volume, increased wall thickness to radius ratio, and hence to decreased systolic wall stress. Conversely, volume load resulted in an increase in systolic wall stress by a decrease in wall thickness to radius ratio. The alterations in systolic pressure, wall thickness to radius radio, and systolic wall stress paralleled in both groups; wall stress was nearly identical in SHR and in NR under all tested conditions while varying systolic wall stress by at least 400%.

Age Dependence of Left Ventricular Function

Figure 9 shows left ventricular function in SHR which are 15 and 60 weeks old, with all values expressed as a percentage of the normotensive controls. In the younger age group of 15-week-old SHR all LV function parameters were normal. On the other hand, in the second age group of 60-week-old SHR there was a decrease in ejection fraction (EF), maximum flow velocity (f_{max}), and isovolumic velocity indices ($dp/dt_{max}/P$, V_{max}), while systolic and diastolic wall stress increased.

Relation Between Left Ventricular Function, Wall Stress and the Degree of Left Ventricular Hypertrophy

There was a close relation between ejection fraction and systolic wall stress (Fig. 10). Ejection fraction decreased with increase in wall stress.

A non-linear and inverse relationship was found between systolic wall stress and the wall thickness to radius ratio or left ventricular mass to end-diastolic volume ratio (Fig. 11). At comparable systolic pressure wall stress decreased with increase in mass to volume ratio, thus resulting in normal or even reduced wall stress values in compensated SHR, in spite of the high pressure load. Conversely, decrease in mass to volume ratio resulted in an increase in systolic wall stress.

Since left ventricular function was closely related to systolic wall stress, left ventricular function in SHR was normal as long as the increase in the ratio of left ventricular mass to end-diastolic volume was appropriate in proportion to pressure load, keeping systolic wall stress normal. On the contrary, decrease in mass to volume ratio due to an increase in end-diastolic volume out of proportion to left ventricular mass and pressure load or due to a lack of increase in left ventricular mass resulted in an increase in systolic wall stress and was thus related to reduced left ventricular function.

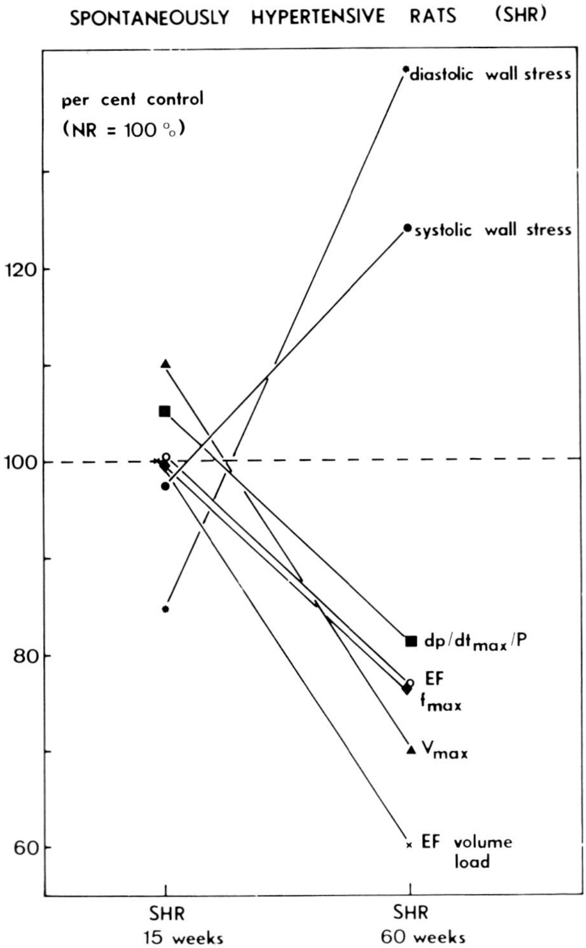

Fig. 9. Left ventricular function parameters in 15- and 60-week-old SHR, all values expressed as percentage of age matched normotensive controls. *EF* = ejection fraction; f_{max} = maximum aortic flow velocity; $dp/dt_{max}/P$ = ratio of the maximum rate of rise of left ventricular pressure and its corresponding isovolumic pressure; v_{max} = maximum velocity of shortening extrapolated from isovolumic IP-V_{CE}-curves

Maximum Value of Systolic Wall Stress and Systolic Stress Reserve

After aortic clamping, systolic wall stress increased by about 100% in compensated SHR as well as in NR, when considering the first beat after clamping, i.e., comparable preloading conditions (Fig. 12, left side). In SHR with high initial wall stress the increase in wall stress after aortic clamping was reduced.

Maximum value of systolic wall stress, except for alterations in inotropic state, was reached by rapid volume load plus aortic clamping. The right side of Fig. 12

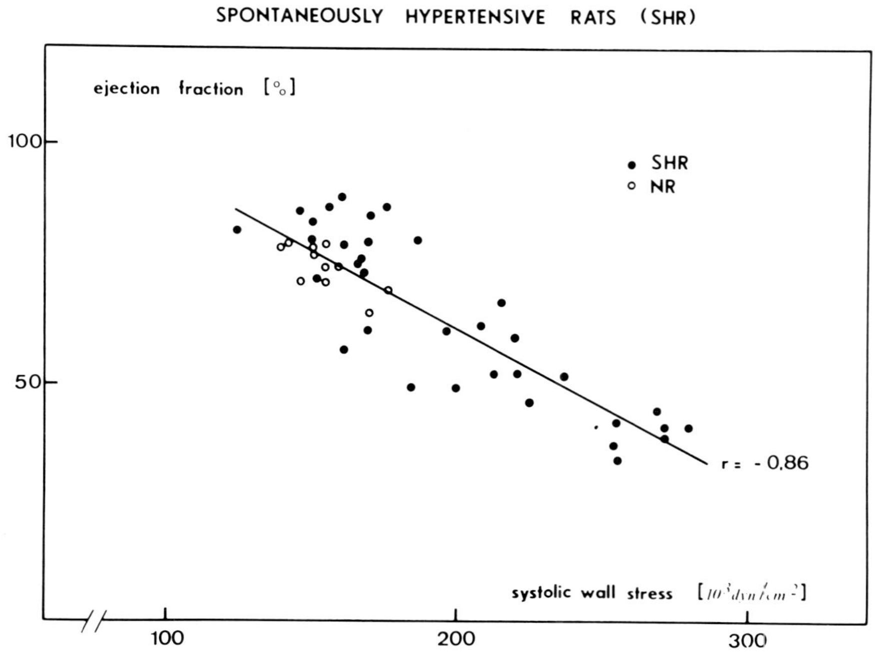

Fig. 10. Relationship between ejection fraction and systolic wall stress in SHR (●) and NR (○)

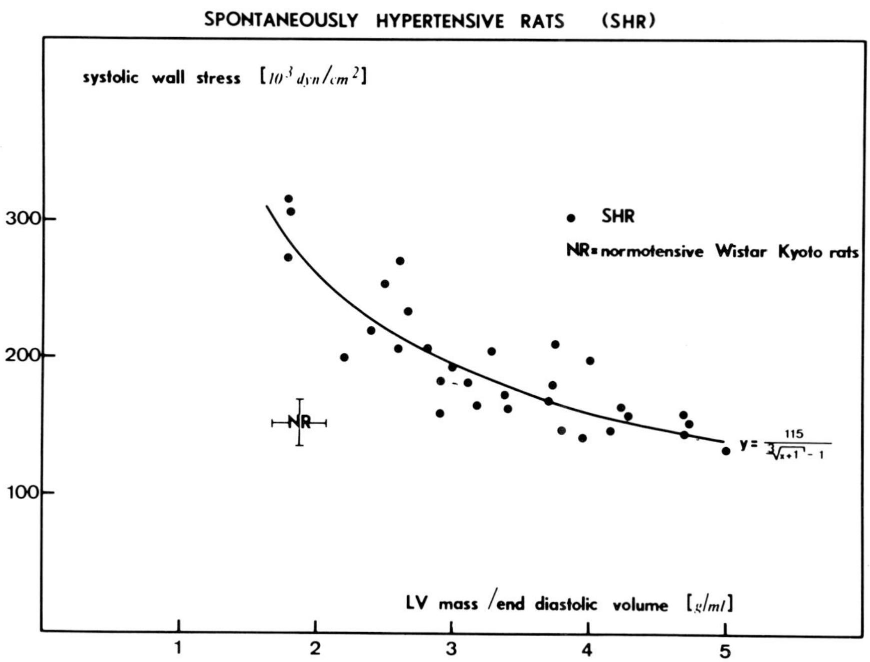

Fig. 11. Relationship between systolic wall stress and left ventricular mass to end-diastolic volume ratio in SHR. *NR* = normotensive controls, mean value ± SD

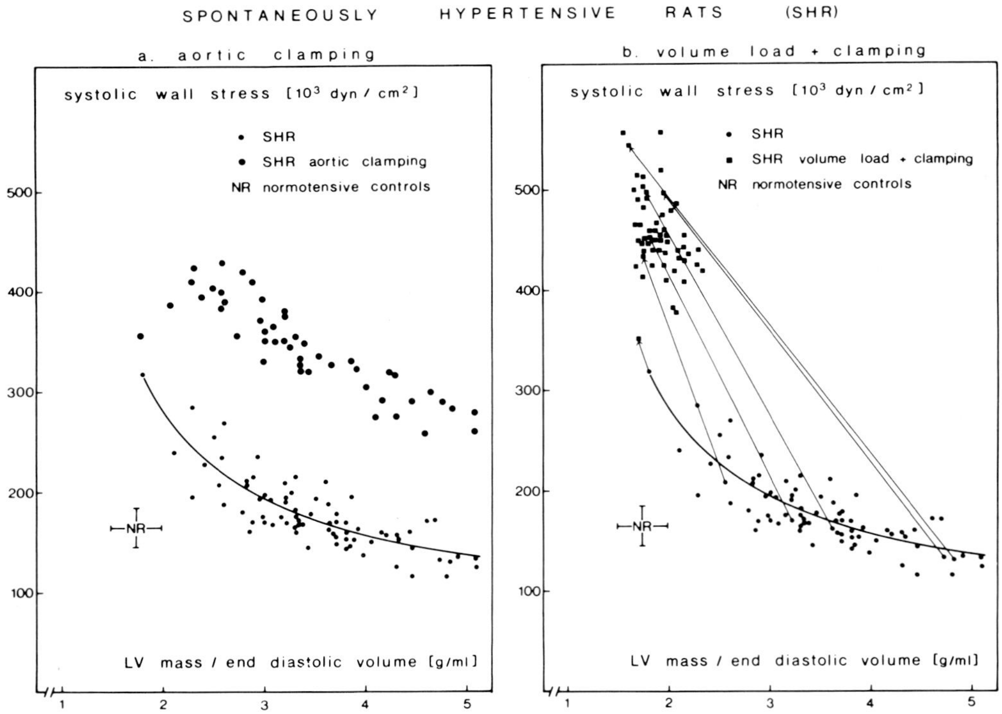

Fig. 12 (a) Relationship between systolic wall stress and left ventricular mass to end-diastolic volume ratio in SHR at rest (•) and after aortic clamping (●). (b) Systolic wall stress at rest and maximum value of systolic wall stress after volume load plus clamping is shown. *Arrows* in (b) connect wall stress values at rest and maximum wall stress values of six single rats. Note that increase in wall stress after volume load plus clamping was greatest in SHR with low initial wall stress and was reduced in SHR with high initial wall stress. *NR* = normotensive controls at rest demonstrates in a similar diagram as shown before the relation between systolic wall stress and mass to volume ratio at rest (points) and after volume load plus clamping (squares). Maximum value of systolic wall stress reached about 400—550 $\cdot 10^3$ dyn/cm^2 in SHR and was slightly higher in compensated SHR than in NR (Table 1). As the arrows in Fig. 12b show, the highest increase in systolic wall stress after volume load plus clamping was found in the hypertensive animals with low initial wall stress, while the increase in wall stress was lowest in SHR with highest initial wall stress. Thus the systolic stress reserve, which may be defined as the ratio between maximum value of systolic wall stress and initial wall stress [18], was highest in SHR with low initial wall stress and was reduced in high stress hypertrophy (Fig. 13).

Preliminary results in 10—40-week-old SHR and in NR showed an increase in maximum value of systolic wall stress by positive inotropic interventions (infusion of norepinephrine, 1—5 μg/kg · min, post extrasystolic beats) and a reduction of maximum value of systolic wall stress by propranolol (1—10 mg/kg i.v.). Since systolic wall stress before clamping was less influenced by these procedures, systolic stress reserve could be elevated by positive inotropic interventions and reduced by negative inotropism in compensated SHR as well as in NR.

Isovolumic Stress-Volume-Relationship

Figure 14 demonstrates the relationship between isovolumic systolic wall stress and end-diastolic volume index at initial end-diastolic volume, after various extents of volume load and, in a few rats, volume loss. As shown in the figure, the slope of the linear part of this regression was equal in 10—40-week-old SHR and in NR. Decompensated 60-week-old SHR were below the normal regression, and the values of the single rat showed a decreased slope of the isovolumic stress-volume relation. Some of the 60 week-old SHR with normal left ventricular function and normal initial wall stress lay within the normal range. One 10-week-old SHR with excessive high systolic pressure at rest, high systolic wall stress before clamping, and subnormal ejection fraction lay within the normal range as well.

Discussion

Experimental and clinical results concerning myocardial performance in hypertrophy due to pressure overload are controversial. In contrast to reduced myocardial function in pressure overload due to outflow tract banding [4, 7, 9, 16], our results have shown normal pumping parameters and isovolumic velocity indexes in SHR up to the 40th week of age at rest and during stress tests. The results correspond well to the data of Pfeffer [13], who could show normal peak cardiac output per left ventricular weight in SHR, with the exception of the very old animals. Likewise, left ventricular function in patients with es-

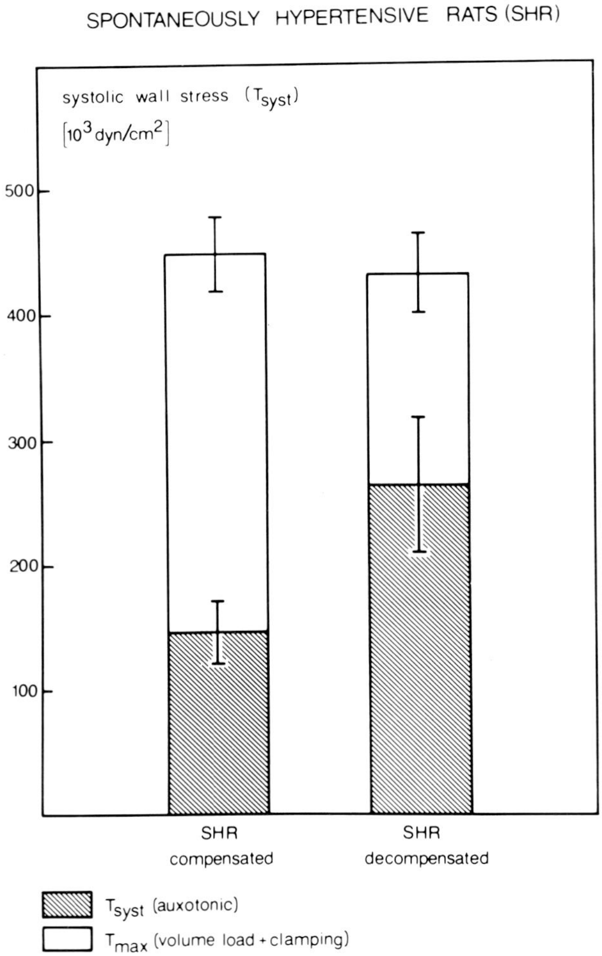

Fig. 13. Mean values ± SD of maximum values of systolic wall stress after volume load plus clamping (*opened bars*) and initial wall stress (*hatched bars*) in all compensated SHR with normal initial wall stress (*left side*) and all decompensated SHR with initial high wall stress (*right side*). Note that maximum value of systolic wall stress is even higher in SHR with low initial wall stress than in SHR with initial high wall stress, resulting in higher systolic stress reserve in SHR with normal systolic wall stress at rest than in SHR with initial high wall stress

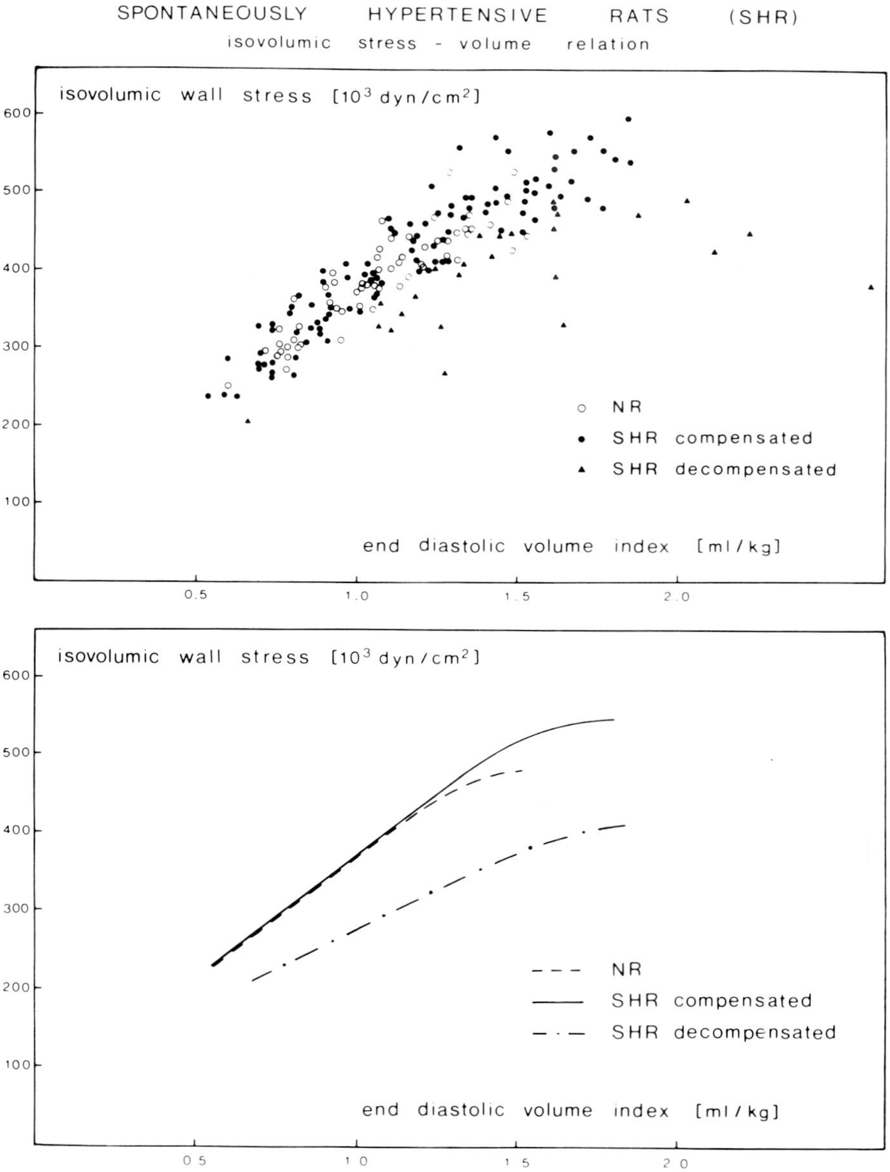

Fig. 14. Relationship between isovolumic systolic wall stress and end-diastolic volume index in 10–40-week-old SHR (●), decompensated 60 week old SHR (▲) and NR (○). End-diastolic volume was varied by rapid volume load before aortic clamping or spontaneous filling of the left ventricle during clamping and in a few rats by rapid volume loss at the end of the experiment with immediately following aortic clamping (four compensated SHR and NR, all decompensated SHR with excessive high end-diastolic volume at rest). *Lower part* = schematic diagram for the different groups

sential hypertension is normal as long as coronary artery disease, regional wall motion abnormalities, or left ventricular dilatation are absent [17, 9].

Dynamics of the left ventricular wall in pressure overload hypertrophy seem to depend on the extent and velocity of the onset of pressure overload and on the corresponding course of left ventricular hypertrophy. Increase in systolic pressure does not imply increased pressure load per cross-sectional area of the contractile element. If left ventricular mass increases in proportion to pressure load, the force per unit of cross-sectional area, i.e., systolic wall stress, remains normal [10], thus resulting in normal afterload per unit myocardium in spite of the high systolic pressure.

Determinations of systolic wall stress in the small and irregularly formed hearts of SHR are limited. We used three left ventricular models: a thin-walled spherical model [3, 8], a thick-walled model [21], and an ellipsoidal model assuming an equality of the minor axis and the half major axis [2, 14, 15]. Since simultaneous pressure and volume measurements were not possible in our procedure, peak systolic pressure and diastolic dimensions were used for calculations of systolic wall stress. Systolic wall stress values, therefore, only represent approximate values for comparison of the different groups and for evaluation of qualitative changes in stress response of the LVs under different loading conditions.

Considering these methodical limitations, systolic wall stress was normal in the early stages of hypertrophy in SHR up to the 40th week of age, in spite of the high pressure load as a result of an increase in wall thickness to radius ratio (or the ratio of left ventricular mass to end-diastolic volume) in proportion to pressure load. Even during various loading and unloading conditions with alterations of systolic wall stress by about 400%, identical wall stress values were found in the younger SHR and in NR. According to these results, left ventricular hypertrophy in the younger age groups of SHR may be termed as appropriate.

Systolic wall stress was a primary determinant of left ventricular function. Left ventricular function in SHR was normal as long as systolic wall stress was normal, while ejection fraction decreased with increase in systolic wall stress. Since systolic wall stress represents a good parameter for the left ventricular afterload, these results indicate an afterload-dependent decrease in left ventricular function in the decompensating hypertensive heart disease.

According to the law of Laplace, systolic wall stress is determined by systolic pressure, wall thickness, and radius. Figure 15 shows schematically the interrelationships between systolic wall stress (y-axis), the ratio of left ventricular mass to end-diastolic volume (Fig. 15a) or wall thickness to radius ratio (Fig. 15b, x-axis) and systolic pressure (isobars). The figure elucidates the role of left ventricular mass (or wall thickness), end-diastolic volume (or radius), and systolic pressure as determinants of systolic wall stress:

1. Increase in left ventricular mass at equal end-diastolic volume and comparable systolic pressure results in a lowering of wall stress by a rise in mass to volume ratio. Thus an increase in mass to volume ratio in proportion to pressure load results in normal systolic wall stress, even at high pressure load.

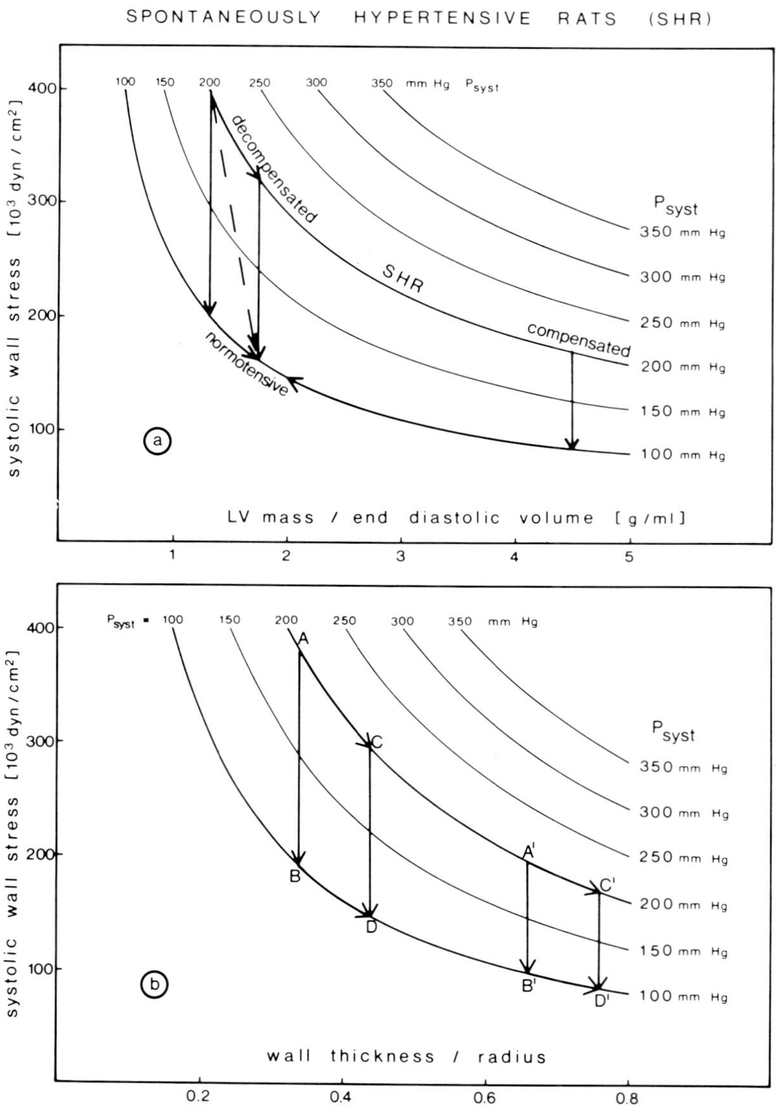

Fig. 15. Schematic diagram of the relationship between systolic wall stress (*y-axis*), left ventricular mass to end-diastolic volume ratio (a) or wall thickness to radius ratio (b) (*x-axis*) and systolic pressure (isobars), using a simplified thin-walled spherical left ventricular model. For details see text

2. Inverse augmentation of end-diastolic volume at constant left ventricular mass and comparable systolic pressure leads to an increase in wall stress by a decrease in the mass to volume ratio.

3. At constant mass to volume ratio, elevation of systolic pressure results in an elevation of systolic wall stress, and lowering of systolic pressure results in a lowering of wall stress.

Because left ventricular function was closely related to systolic wall stress, the interrelationships between systolic pressure, mass to volume ratio, and systolic wall stress enable a quantification and diagnostic classification of the degree or appropriateness of left ventricular hypertrophy:

1. Appropriate hypertrophy, i.e., increase in mass to volume ratio in proportion to pressure load with normal systolic wall stress, is accompanied by normal left ventricular function and thus corresponds to the compensated stage of hypertrophy. From the theoretical point of view, the normotensive normal state is reached in these animals by lowering of pressure and regression of hypertrophy (arrows in Fig. 15a).

2. On the other hand, inappropriate high stress hypertrophy is characterized by an increase in left ventricular volume out of proportion to left ventricular mass and pressure load or by a lack of increase in left ventricular mass. Wall stress is increased and left ventricular function is impaired, both of which correspond to the decompensated stage of hypertrophy. Therapeutically antihypertensive drugs, which per se reduce wall stress, as well as lowering of end-diastolic volume or positive inotropic agents are desirable.

As shown in the figure, the decrease in wall stress following an identical fall in pressure is higher at low mass to volume ratio (or low wall thickness to radius ratio) (see A→B, Fig. 15b) and only moderate at high mass to volume ratio (or high wall thickness to radius ratio) (see A'→B', Fig. 15b).

As further shown in Fig. 15b, an increase in wall thickness to radius ratio, for instance by a decrease in left ventricular radius (or decrease in end-diastolic volume), results in a marked fall in systolic wall stress at low wall thickness to radius ratio (see A→C, Fig. 15b), i.e., in decompensated high stress hypertrophy, and only in a slight decrease in systolic wall stress at high wall thickness to radius ratio (see A'→C', Fig. 15b).

As could be shown previously in patients with essential hypertension, not only left ventricular function but also myocardial oxygen consumption is determined by systolic wall stress [17, 18, 20]. Acute or chronic alterations of systolic wall stress by alterations of its determinants, therefore, not only influence left ventricular function but also myocardial oxygen demand.

For further characterization of left ventricular dynamics in SHR, isovolumic stress-volume relationships were examined. The maximal force-length relation and, likewise the stress-volume relation of the isovolumetrically beating heart is contractile state dependent and its slope describes myocardial contractility (see Session C, Weber et al.). In our experiments the slope of the linear part of the isovolumic stress-volume relation was identical in the younger SHR and in NR and was decreased only in decompensated 60-week-old SHR, indicating normal contractile state of the left ventricle in the early stages of hypertrophy in SHR and depressed contractile state only in decompensated 60-week-old SHR.

Systolic wall stress at rest was influenced by instantaneous variations of systolic pressure and end-diastolic volume, ejection fraction by variations of systolic pressure, and hence, systolic wall stress. In contrast, the slope of the linear part of the isovolumic stress-volume relation was rather independent from loading conditions, while it was influenced by alterations in inotropic state, for instance norepinephrine, post-extrasystolic potentiation, or propranolol. The independence of the slope of the isovolumic stress-volume relation from loading conditions may be the reason why one 10-week-old SHR — though revealing increased systolic wall stress and subnormal ejection fraction at rest as a result of an excessive high systolic pressure at the time of the experiment — lay within the normal range of isovolumic stress-volume relation. According to the age of the rat, normal left ventricular function ought to be expected and myocardial compliance was normal (see Session A, Bürger and Strauer, II).

Maximum value of systolic wall stress after volume load plus aortic clamping was highest in the younger SHR, slightly lower in NR, and lowest in decompensated 60—80-week-old SHR, corresponding well to the maximum isometric tension development of isolated left ventricular papillary muscles (see Session A, Bürger and Strauer, II). According to preliminary results in a small number of 10—40-week-old SHR and NR, maximum value of systolic wall stress could be varied by inotropic interventions: it was increased by positive inotropic interventions (norepinephrine, post-extrasystolic potentiation) and decreased by propranolol.

The ratio between maximum value of systolic wall stress and systolic wall stress at rest may be termed as systolic stress reserve [18] and may be considered an equivalent for the functional reserve of the heart. Systolic stress reserve was greatest in hearts with low initial wall stress and was reduced in high stress hypertrophy. Systolic stress reserve could be influenced by alterations of maximum value of systolic wall stress (by positive and negative inotropic interventions) and by alterations of initial wall stress (by alterations of its determinants: systolic pressure, wall thickness, and radius).

The results concerning systolic stress reserve parallel the data concerning coronary reserve in patients with essential hypertension [17, 18]: coronary reserve was highest in patients with low systolic wall stress and was reduced in high stress hypertrophy, with a good correlation between increase in wall stress and decrease in coronary reserve.

The interrelationship between systolic pressure, left ventricular wall thickness to radius ratio or left ventricular mass to end-diastolic volume ratio, and systolic wall stress, i.e. the appropriateness of left ventricular hypertrophy, thus influences not only left ventricular function but also myocardial oxygen demand and left ventricular functional, metabolic, and coronary reserve.

Summary

1. Left ventricular pumping parameters and velocity indexes were normal in SHR in comparison to NR at rest and during stress tests up to the 40th week of age and tended to be depressed in later age groups.

2. Systolic wall stress was normal in SHR up to the 40th week of age as a result of an increase in the ratio of left ventricular mass to end-diastolic volume or in the wall thickness to radius ratio. In later age groups mass to volume ratio tended to be numerically normalized by an increase in end-diastolic volume or a lack of increase in left ventricular mass: systolic wall stress increased.

3. Systolic wall stress was a primary determinant of left ventricular function: left ventricular function was normal as long as systolic wall stress was normal and decreased with increase in systolic wall stress. Since systolic wall stress is determined by systolic pressure and the ratio of wall thickness to radius, left ventricular function in SHR also depended on the interrelationships between systolic pressure and wall thickness to radius ratio, i.e., on the appropriateness of left ventricular hypertrophy.

4. Maximum value of systolic wall stress after volume load plus aortic clamping reached about 450—550 $\cdot 10^3$ dyn/cm^2 in the younger age groups of SHR and was slightly lower in normotensive controls, corresponding well to the maximum isometric tension development of isolated left ventricular papillary muscles. Maximum value of systolic wall stress tended to be reduced in 60—80-week-old SHR.

5. Systolic stress reserve, defined as the ratio of maximum value of systolic wall stress and systolic wall stress at rest, was highest in SHR with low initial wall stress and was reduced in high stress hypertrophy.

6. The slope of the linear part of the isovolumic stress volume relation was equal in the younger age groups of SHR and in NR. Decompensated 60—80-week-old SHR lay below the normal range with decreased slope of the regression. This fact indicates normal contractile state in 10—40-week-old SHR and depressed contractility only in the latest age group of SHR.

7. The results are discussed with special reference to the appropriateness of hypertrophy and its influence on left ventricular function, myocardial oxygen demand and left ventricular functional, and metabolic and coronary reserve.

References

1. Averill DB, Ferrario CM, Tarazi RC, Sen S, Bajbus R (1976) Cardiac performance in rats with renal hypertension. Circ Res 38 : 280
2. Aziz KU, van Grondelle A, Paul MH, Muster AJ (1977) Echocardiographic assessment of the relation between left ventricular wall and cavity dimensions and peak systolic pressure in children with mild aortic stenosis. Am J Cardiol 40 : 775

3. Badeer HS (1963) Contractile tension of the myocardium. Am Heart J 66 : 432
4. Bing OHL, Matsushita S, Fanburg BL, Levine HJ (1971) Mechanical properties of rat cardiac muscle during experimental hypertrophy. Circ Res 28 : 234
5. Ford EF (1976) Heart size. Circ Res 39 : 297
6. Hallbäck M, Isaksson O, Noresson E (1975) Consequences of myocardial structural adaptation on left ventricular compliance and the Frank-Starling relationship in spontaneously hypertensive rats. Acta Physiol scand 94 : 259
7. Hamrell BB, Alpert NR (1977) The mechanical characteristics of hypertrophied rabbit cardiac muscle in the absence of congestive heart failure. The contractile and series elastic element. Circ Res 40 : 20
8. Hood WP Jr (1971) Dynamics of hypertrophy in the left ventricular wall of man in: NR Alpert (ed) Cardiac hypertrophy. Academic Press, New York London pp 445—452
9. Jacob R, Ebrecht G, Kämmereit A, Medugorac I, Wendt-Galitelli MF (1977) Myocardial function in different models of cardiac hypertrophy. An attempt at correlating mechanical, biochemical and morphological parameters. Basis Res Cardiol 72 : 160
10. Meerson FZ (1969) The myocardium in hyperfunction, hypertrophy and heart failure. Circ Res [Suppl II] 24/25: II—1
11. Noresson E, Ricksten S-E, Hallbäck-Nordlander M, Thoren P (to be published) Performance of the hypertrophied left ventricle in spontaneously hypertensive rat. Effects of changes in preload and afterload. Acta Physiol Scand
12. Okamoto K, Aoki K (1963) Development of a strain of spontaneously hypertensive rats. Japn Circ J 27 : 282
13. Pfeffer MA, Pfeffer JM, Frohlich ED (1976) Pumping ability of the hypertrophying left ventricle of the spontaneously hypertensive rat. Circ Res 38 : 423
14. Pombo JF, Troy BL, Russell RO (1971) Left ventricular volumes and ejection fraction by echocardiography. Circulation 43 : 480
15. Sandler H, Dodge HT (1963) Left ventricular tension and stress in man. Circ Res 13 : 91
16. Spann JF Jr, Buccino RA, Sonnenblick EH, Braunwald E (1967) Contractile state of cardiac muscle obtained from cats with experimentally produced ventricular hypertrophy and heart failure. Circ Res 21 : 341
17. Strauer BE (1978) Das Hochdruckherz I—III. Z Kardiol 67 : 375, 452, 513
18. Strauer BE (1979) Das Hochdruckherz. Springer, Berlin Heidelberg New York
19. Strauer BE, Bürger S (1978) Das Hochdruckherz V. Z Kardiol 67 : 653
20. Strauer BE, Beer K, Heitlinger K, Höfling B (1977) Left ventricular systolic wall stress as a primary determinant of myocardial oxygen consumption: Comparative studies in patients with normal left ventricular function, with pressure and volume overload and with coronary heart disease. Basic Res Cartiol 72 : 306
21. Wong YK, Rautaharju PM (1968). Stress distribution within the left ventricular wall approximated as a thick ellipsoidal shell. Am Heart J 75 : 649

Left Ventricular Hypertrophy in Chronic Pressure Load Due to Spontaneous Essential Hypertension
II. Contractility of the Isolated Left Ventricular Myocardium and Left Ventricular Stiffness[1]

S.B. Bürger and B.E. Strauer

Left ventricular function in the younger age groups of spontaneously hypertensive rats (SHR) is normal in comparison to age-matched normotensive controls, when regarding the anesthesized animal [5, 27, see Session A, Bürger and Strauer I]. In order to exclude effects of anesthesia, catecholamines, or autonomus nervous regulations, contractility of the isolated left ventricular myocardium was investigated in left ventricular papillary muscle preparations. For further characterization of the hypertrophied left ventricle in SHR diastolic properties of the left ventricle were examined with respect to (1) left ventricular chamber stiffness, which defines distensibility characteristics of the intact left ventricular chamber, and (2) myocardial stiffness, which defines the intrinsic stiffness of isolated myocardium, i.e., the myocardial material properties [9, 25, 26].

Methods

Mechanics of isolated left ventricular papillary muscles in isotonic, isometric, and isotonic afterloaded contractions at a temperature of 32—34^0 C and a stimulation frequency of 20/min were performed on 71 male, 8—80-week-old SHR, strain Okamoto [24], and on 80 normotensive Wistar Kyoto inbred rats (NR) out of the same progenitor strain. Methods have been described previously in detail [33]. Preload was varied from 50—1000 (—1500) mg and for statistical evaluations the preloed according to L_{max} was used. The following tracings have been recorded stimultaneously (Fig. 1): stimulus artefact, muscle shortening (Δl), first time derivative of muscle shortening (dl/dt), tension development (T), and first time derivative of tension development (dT/dt). Isotonic shortening and corresponding shortening velocity were related to initial muscle length while tension development was related to the cross-sectional area of the muscle. Muscles not showing constant mechanical values during the test period and muscles showing premature contractions were rejected. Before and after the force velocity relations, several length-tension relations were determined for each muscle.

Diastolic pressure volume relations of the arrested left ventricles were performed after the hemodynamic measurements as described previously (see Session A,

1 Supported by Deutsche Forschungsgemeinschaft

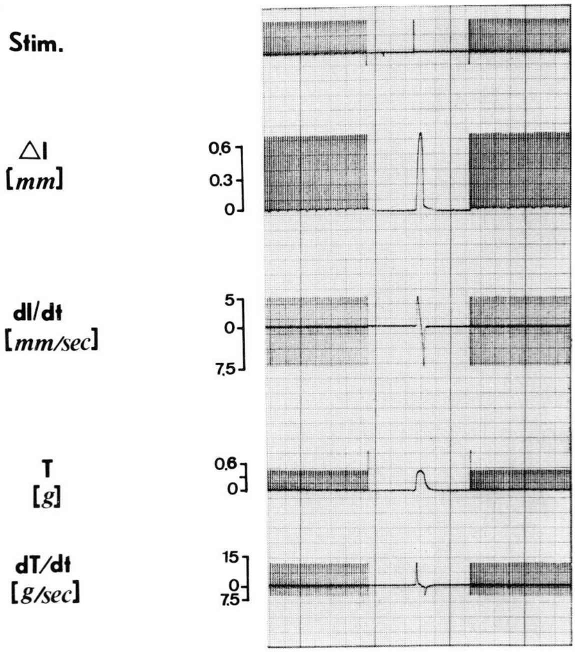

Fig. 1. Recording of papillary muscle mechanics. *Stim* = stimulus artefact : Δl = muscle shortening; *dl/dt* = first time derivative of muscle shortening; *T* = tension development; *dT/dt* = first time derivative of tension development

Bürger und Strauer, I). For each rat the mean value of 3—5 pressure-volume relations was used for further evaluation. Rats showing differences in pressure-volume relations of more than 10% were rejected. At intervals of 2 mm Hg the slope of a tangent to the exponential pressure-volume relation was determined and the tangent slope dP/dV was plotted versus filling pressure (P). Only the linear part of this relation (dP/dV versus P) was used for further evaluation. Stiffness-stress relationships were determined according to the formula of Mirsky [20]. Stiffness and stress were calculated for each rat at intervals of 2 mm Hg from the pressure-volume relations, the dP/dV versus P relations, and the weights of the left ventricles using a spherical ventricular model. Stiffness-stress relations were linear except for low stress values. Only the linear part of the relation was used for statistical evaluation and for determination of stiffness constant K, i.e., the slope of the stiffness-stress relationship. Rats showing non-linear stiffness-stress relations were rejected. Ejection fraction and systolic wall stress in Figs. 7 and 8 were determined as described previously (see Session A, Bürger and Strauer, II).

Results

Myocardial Muscle Mechanics

Mechanics of isolated left ventricular papillary muscles in isotonic contractions (Fig. 2) showed normal values for extent of shortening (Δ l), shortening velocity

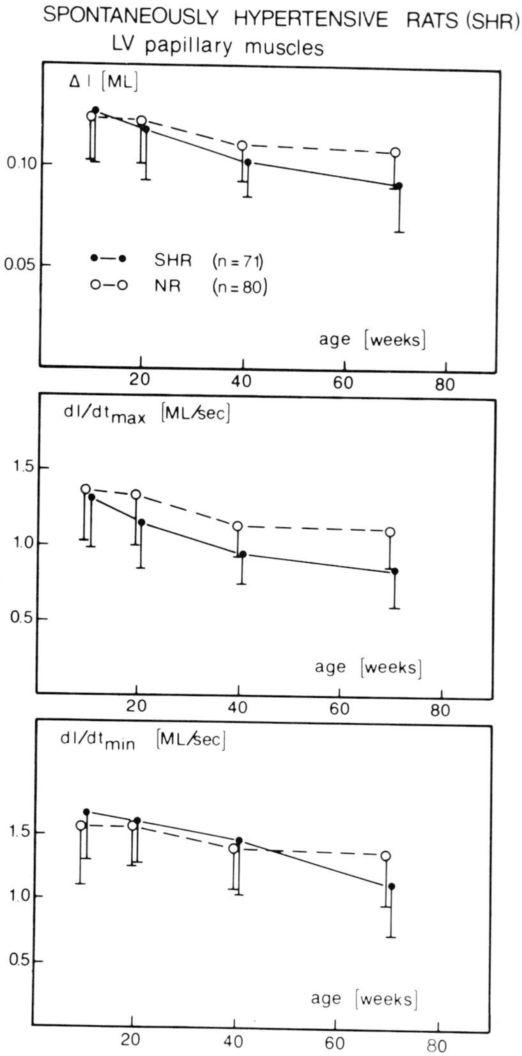

Fig. 2. Mechanics of isolated left ventricular papillary muscles in isotonic contractions. Δl = muscle shortening, dl/dt_{max} = shortening velocity, dl/dt_{min} = relaxation velocity, x ± SD

(dl/dt_{max}), and relaxation velocity (dl/dt_{min}) in 10-week-old SHR in comparison to age-matched NR. There was no significant difference in these parameters between hypertensive and normotensive animals up to the 20th—30th week of age. A slight decrease in shortening velocity in SHR at 20—30 weeks of age was not statistically significant. In the further course of left ventricular hypertrophy, isotonic shortening velocity tended to be depressed in SHR in comparison to age-matched NR with a low level of significance at 40 weeks of age ($p < 0.02$) and significant reduction at 60—80 weeks of age ($p < 0.0005$). Extent of shorten ing and relaxation velocity tended to decrease in SHR in comparison to NR at 60—80 weeks of age. In SHR as well as in NR there was an age dependent decrease in contraction velocity (Table 1).

In isometric contractions (Fig. 3) maximum isometric tension development (P_o) was even higher in SHR up to the 40th week of age and tended to decrease in 60—80-week-old SHR. The time course of isometric velocity parameters was similar to the isotonic data. Time to peak tension was normal in the younger SHR and was prolonged in 60—80-week-old SHR.

Force-velocity relations of isotonic afterloaded contractions showed normal velocity and even elevated tension development in 8—11-week-old SHR in comparison to age-matched NR (Fig. 4). On the contrary force-velocity relations in 60—80-week-old SHR were shifted to reduced velocity values and slightly reduced tension development (Fig. 5).

Increase in calcium concentration from 5 mEq to 6.5 mEq or 9.5 mEq respectively resulted in an increase in shortening velocity and in maximum tension development in SHR as well as in NR. The increase in contraction parameters following an identical rise in calcium concentration was equal in NR and in the younger age groups of SHR.

Left Ventricular Stiffness

Diastolic pressure-volume relations of the intact left ventricles showed a steeper course even in the younger SHR in comparison to age-matched NR. The slope of a tangent to the exponential pressure-volume curve (dP/dV) was higher at each filling pressure in SHR in comparison to NR, indicating elevated chamber stiffness even in the younger age groups of SHR parallel to left ventricular hypertrophy.

In contrast, when taking into account geometric factors, i.e., left ventricular mass to volume ratio and wall thickness and radius, (according to the formula of Mirsky [20]), midwall elastic stiffness to stress relationships showed an identical course in the younger age groups of SHR and in age-matched NR (Fig. 6). The regression line was steeper only in 60—80-week-old SHR. Accordingly, the slope of this regression, i.e. midwall elastic stiffness constant K or tangent modulus, was normal in the younger age groups of SHR in comparison to NR and increased in later age groups in correspondence with the increase in systolic wall stress and decrease in ejection fraction.

Comparable to these data, stress-strain relations of isolated left ventricular papillary muscles showed an identical course in the younger age groups of SHR and in NR and tended to a steeper course only in 60—80-week-old SHR.

Sufficient correlation was found between myocardial stiffness constant K and ejection fraction (Fig. 7) or between stiffness constant K and systolic wall stress (Fig. 8). Ejection fraction decreased with increase in myocardial stiffness constant, while increase in stiffness constant was related to an increase in systolic

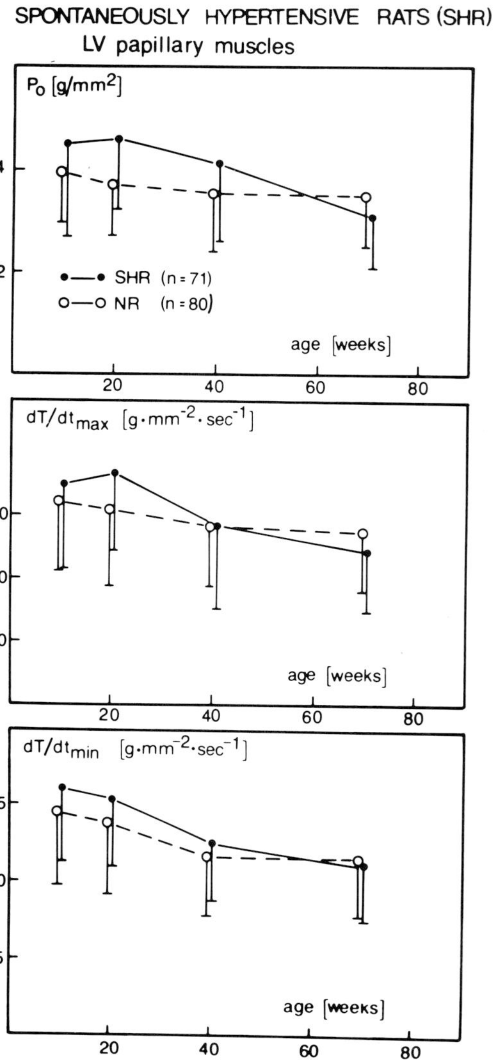

Fig. 3. Mechanics of isolated left ventricular papillary muscles in isometric contractions. P_O = maximum isometric tension development, dT/dt_{max} = maximum rate of tension development, dT/dt_{min} = maximum isometric relaxation velocity, x ± SD

wall stress. One 10-week-old SHR with excessive high systolic pressure at the time of the experiment, high systolic wall stress, and subnormal ejection fraction lay outside the range of the regression. As reported previously (see Bürger aud Strauer, I), the slope of the relation between isovolumic systolic wall stress and end-diastolic volume index was normal in this rat.

Table 1. Left ventricular papillary muscle mechanics in four age groups of spontaneously hypertensive rats (SHR) and age-matched normotensive controls (NR). Mean values ± SD. Each age group of SHR was compared to age matched NR (Δ% SHR/NR). Additionally each age group of SHR and of NR was compared to the youngest age group of the same strain, i.e., SHR to 8-11-week-old SHR, NR to 8-11-week-old NR (Δ% vs. 8—11). Statistical analysis were performed according to Student's T-test

		8—11 weeks NR n=24	8—11 weeks SHR n=21	Δ % SHR/ NR	15—25 weeks NR n=20	15—25 weeks SHR n=13	Δ % SHR/ NR	35—45 weeks NR n=17	35—45 weeks SHR n=13	Δ % SHR/ NR	60—80 weeks NR n=19	60—80 weeks SHR n=24	Δ % SHR/ NR
Muscle	x	0.124	0.126		0.122	0.117		0.111	0.101		0.109	0.091	
shortening	± SD	±0.021	±0.032	+2%	±0.021	±0.025	—4%	±0.017	±0.017	—9%	±0.027	±0.024	—17%
[ML]	Δ% vs.8-11				—2%	—7%		—10%	—20%[e]		—12%	—28%[c]	
Shortening	x	1.370	1.306		1.332	1.147		1.138	0.955		1.113	0.849	
velocity	± SD	±0.039	±0.329	—5%	±0.353	±0.295	—14%	±0.189	±0.198	—16%[b]	±0.255	±0.254	—17%[a]
[ML/sec]	Δ% vs.8-11				—3%	—12%		—17%[c]	—27%[c]		—19%[c]	—35%[c]	
Isotonic	x	1.535	1.672		1.546	1.598		1.385	1.458		1.370	1.117	
relaxation velocity	± SD	±0.480	±0.485	+9%	±0.287	±0.315	+3%	±0.301	±0.423	+5%	±0.409	±0.408	—18%
[ML/sec]	Δ% vs.8-11				+1%	+4%		—10%	—13%		—11%	—33%[c]	
Maximum isometric	x	3.91	4.50		3.70	4.60		3.54	4.10		3.52	3.12	
tension development	± SD	±1.03	±1.80	+15%	±1.07	±1.41	+24%	±1.35	±1.50	+16%	±1.00	±0.92	—11%
[g·mm^{-2}]	Δ% vs.8-11				—5%	+2%		—9%	—9%		—10%	—31%[d]	

Maximum rate of tension develop- ment	x	31.8	34.9		30.9	36.6		28.2	28.2		27.9	24.0	
	± SD	±10.1	±13.4	+1%	±11.6	±12.2	+18%	±9.9	±12.9	±0%	±2.6	±8.5	−14%
[g·mm^{-2} · sec^{-1}]	Δ% vs.8-11				−3%	+5%		−11%	−19%		−12%	−31%[d]	
Isometric relaxation velocity	x	14.5	16.1		13.9	15.4		11.7	12.5		11.7	11.2	
	± SD	±4.9	±4.8	+11%	±4.8	±4.4	+11%	±3.8	±3.6	+17%	±3.3	±3.4	−4%
[g·mm^{-2} · sec^{-1}]	Δ% vs.8-11				−4%	−4%		−19%	−22%[f]		−19%	−30%[c]	

[a] $P < 0.005$ vs. age-matched NR

[b] $P < 0.02$ vs. age-matched NR

[c] $P < 0.001$ vs. 8-11-week-old rats of the same strain

[d] $P < 0.005$ vs. 8-11-week-old rats of the same strain

[e] $P < 0.01$ vs. 8-11-week-old rats of the same strain

[f] $P < 0.02$ vs. 8-11-week-old rats of the same strain

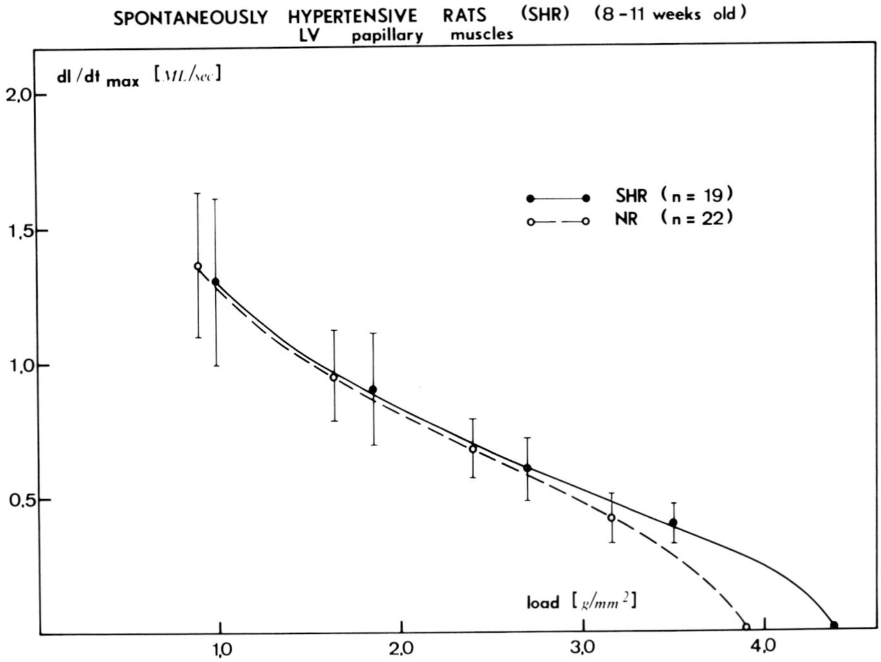

Fig. 4. Force velocity relations of isotonic afterloaded contractions in 8—11-week-old SHR (●——●) and NR (○- -○). dl/dt_{max} = isotonic shortening velocity, x ± SD

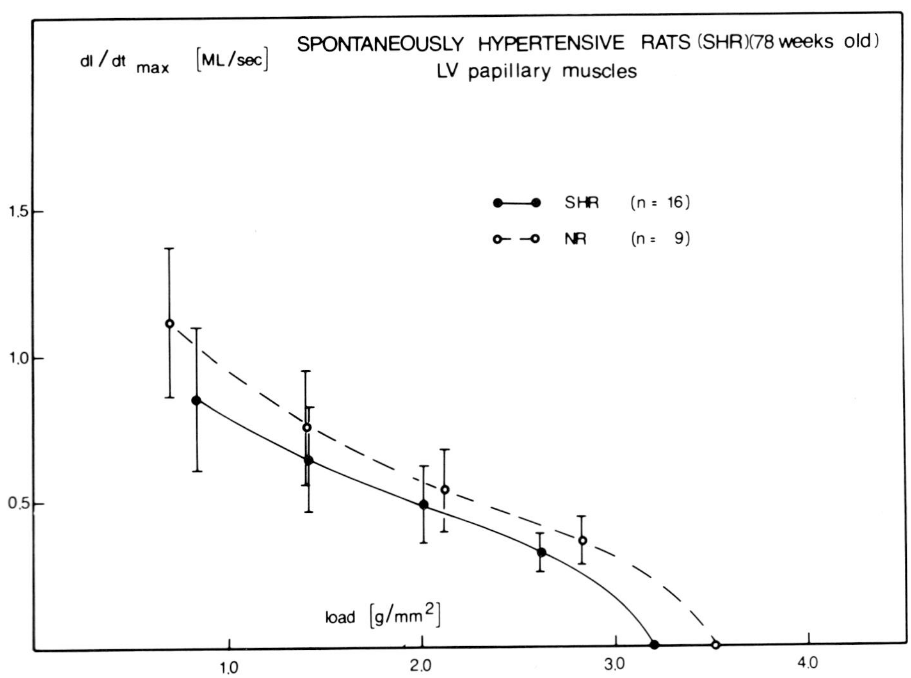

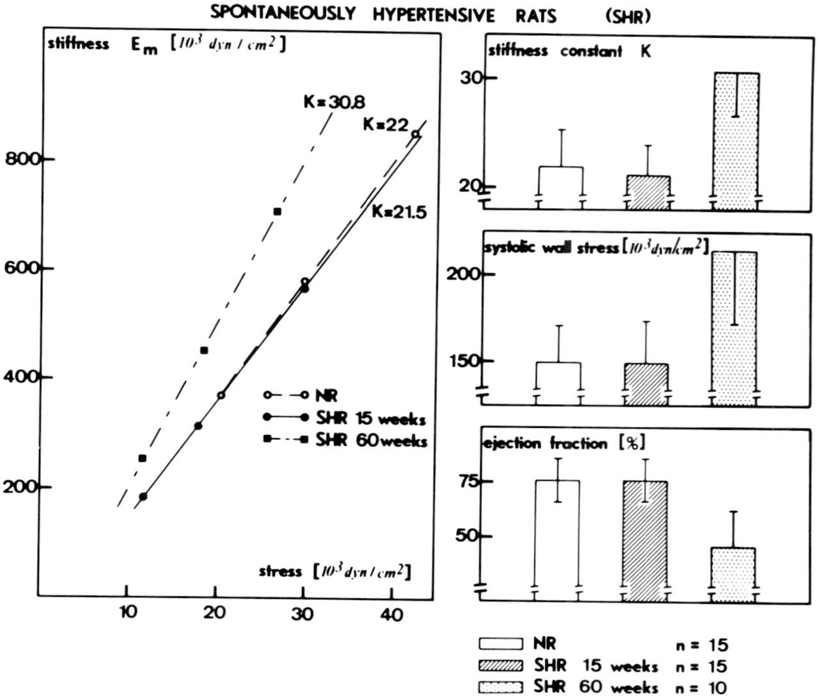

Fig. 6. Stiffness-stress relationships from intact left ventricles according to Mirsky [20] of 15-week-old SHR (●), 60-week-old SHR (■), and normotensive controls (o). Each line represents the mean value of the linear parts of the stiffness stress relations of 15/10/15 animals. Stiffness constant K (or tangent modulus) represents the slope of this regression $LVMM$ = left ventricular muscle mass; V = left ventricular volume; r_i = internal radius; r_e = external radius, P = filling pressure. Midwall elastic stiffness $E_m = d^6{}_m/d\epsilon_m \sim 3 \cdot [1 + (LVMM/V)\, r_i^2 / (r_e^2 + r_i^2)] \cdot [1 + (V/P)\,(dP/dV)] \cdot 6_m$ (Mirsky)

◂ Fig. 5. Force-velocity relations of isotonic afterloaded contractions in 60—80-week-old SHR (●——●) and NR (○– –○). dl/dt_{max} = isotonic shortening velocity, x ± SD

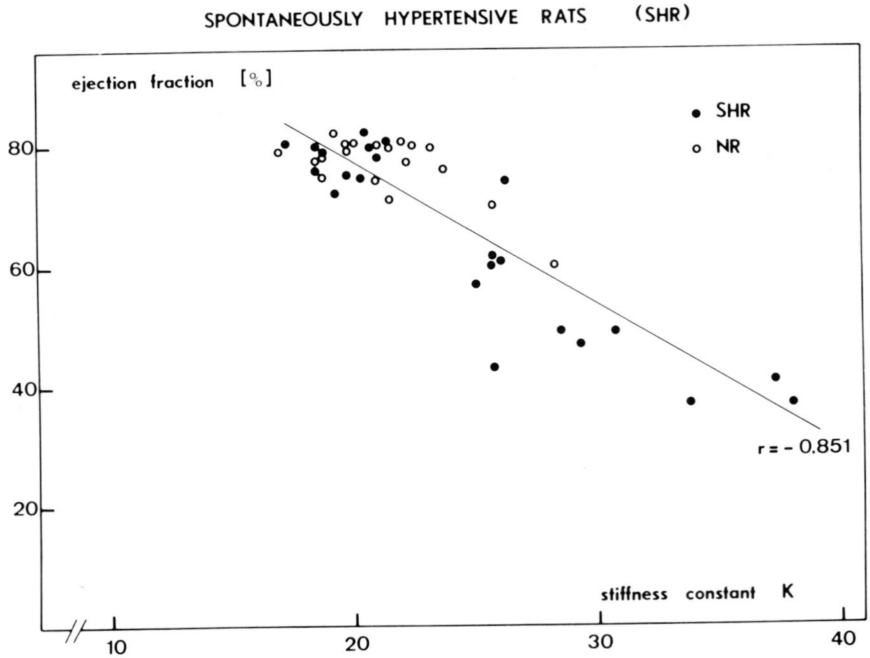

Fig. 7. Relation between ejection fraction and myocardial stiffness constant K (or tangent modulus, i.e. the slope of the stiffness stress relationship) [20]. $K = dE_m/d^6{}_m \cdot E_m = d^6{}_m/d\epsilon_m \sim 3 \cdot [1 + (LVMM/V)\, r_i^2/(r_e^2 + r_i^2)] \cdot [1 + (V/P)(dP/dV)] \cdot \sigma_m$ (Mirsky)

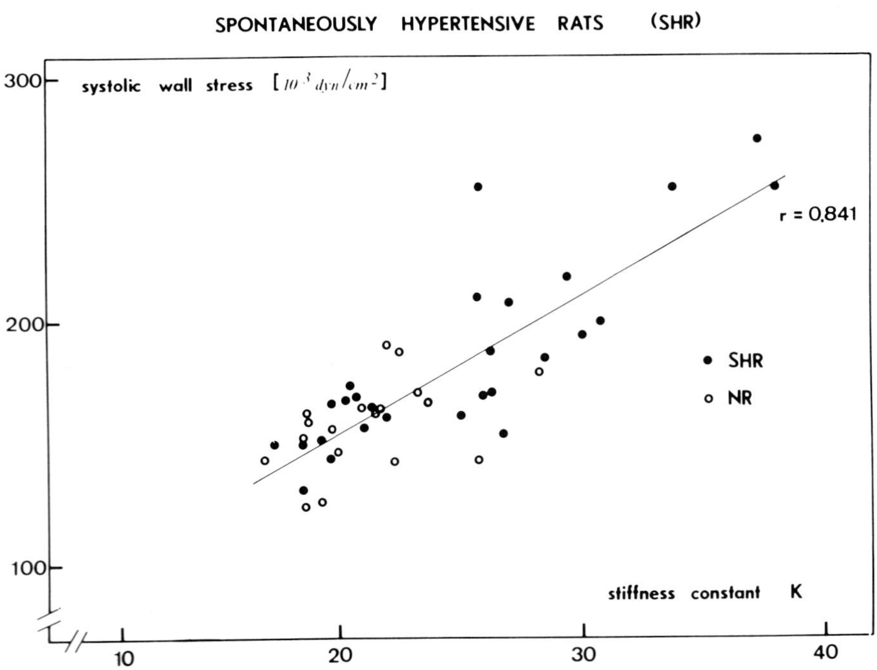

Discussion

Left ventricular hypertrophy in SHR represents one of the best models for left ventricular hypertrophy in essential hypertension in man. While determinations of the duration of hypertension and of the time course of left ventricular hypertrophy are difficult in patients with essential hypertension, SHR allow investigations of left ventricular hypertrophy as dependent on age and thus the duration of hypertension.

Myocardial Muscle Mechanics

In the younger age groups of SHR up to the 30th week of age, mechanics of isolated left ventricular papillary muscles in isotonic, isometric, and isotonic afterloaded contractions showed normal contraction and relaxation parameters in comparison to age-matched normotensive controls at various preloading and afterloading conditions. Force-velocity relations showed normal contraction velocity and even slightly increased tension development in these animals. Alterations in calcium concentration did not reveal differences between the younger SHR and NR. Consequently myocardial contractility in the younger SHR has to be characterized as normal.

The results correspond to the data of Heller [16], who reported normal tension development, velocity of tension development, and time to peak tension in isometric contractions of papillary muscles from SHR up to the 50th week of age. Left ventricular hypertrophy in SHR thus differs from other types of pressure hypertrophy, where reduced myocardial contractility has been reported even at early stages of hypertrophy [4, 15, 17, 3]. As could be shown by our results, pressure hypertrophy does not per se include reduced myocardial contractility. While outflow tract banding results in a rapid rise in systolic pressure with rapid increase in systolic wall stress and thus excessive increase in myocardial oxygen demand, the slow increase in systolic pressure in SHR and the corresponding increase in left ventricular hypertrophy even at a very early age result in normal pressure load per unit of myocardium, i.e., in normal systolic wall stress. The appropriateness of hypertrophy in proportion to pressure load, i.e., systolic wall stress, may at least partially account for the difference between outflow tract banding and spontaneous essential hypertension. Additionally, effects of catecholamines, autonomous nervous regulations, and genetic factors have to be considered.

◂ Fig. 8. Relation between systolic wall stress and myocardial stiffness constant K (or tangent modulus, i.e. the slope of the stiffness stress relationship) [20]. $K = dE_m/d^6{}_m$. $E_m = d^6{}_m/d\epsilon_m \sim 3 \cdot [1 + (LVMM/V)\, r_i^2/(r_e^2 + r_i^2)] \cdot [1 + (V/P)(dP/dV)] \cdot \sigma_m$ (Mirsky)

In the further course of left ventricular hypertrophy, first isotonic shortening velocity tended to decrease at about 40—60 weeks of age, while maximum isometric tension development was still even increased. As could be shown by Mayr (see Session B, Mayr et. al), the decrease in isotonic shortening velocity was paralleled by a decrease in myosin ATPase activity in these hearts, while our results concerning maximum isometric tension development corresponded to the myosin content of the hearts. At about 40—60 weeks of age mechanical as well as biochemical data in SHR are comparable to the results which Jacob [17] obtained in renal hypertensive rats 8 weeks after renal artery coarctation.
In the very old 60—80-week-old SHR all contraction and relaxation parameters tended to be diminished, resulting in a shift of force-velocity relations to reduced velocity values and slightly reduced tension development. Decrease in relaxation parameters did not precede decrease in contraction velocity in our experiments. The decrease in all contraction parameters in 60—80-week-old SHR corresponds to the increase in systolic wall stress, decrease in ejection fraction, and decrease in the slope of the isovolumic stress-volume relation in 60—80-week-old SHR reported earlier in this publication (see Session A, Bürger and Strauer, I).

Left Ventricular Stiffness

Technical and conceptual limitations of stiffness determinations in experiment and in man have been discussed in detail by many authors [3, 6, 8—14, 18—23, 25, 26, 28—30, 34—36]. In our experiments diastolic pressure-volume relations of the entire left ventricles were performed on the arrested hearts over a wide range of filling volumes, the pericardium was removed in all cases, and a spherical left ventricular model was used. Myocardial stiffness in terms of stiffness-stress relations out of diastolic pressure-volume relations of the entire left ventricles [20] corresponded well to myocardial stiffness in terms of stress-strain relations or stiffness-stress relations of isolated left ventricular papillary muscles.

Regarding left ventricular diastolic properties, filling characteristics of the entire left ventricular chamber (corresponding to chamber stiffness) as well as distensibility characteristics of the myocardial material itself (corresponding to myocardial stiffness) have to be distinguished [9, 25, 26].

Chamber stiffness depends on many factors, including the material properties of the heart wall, wall thickness to radius ratio, pericardial properties, completeness of ventricular relaxation, and residual volume from the preceding systolic effort [7, 13, 14, 19, 35]. Myocardial stiffness [25, 26] — or synonymous muscle [9, 20] or wall stiffness [10, 12] — depends on the material properties of the ventricular wall.

Left ventricular chamber stiffness was increased in SHR even in the younger age groups, thus resulting in altered filling characteristics of the hypertrophied ventricles in comparison to normal ventricles. Increase in chamber stiffness may be the consequence of left ventricular hypertrophy with increase in wall thickness to radius ratio or of left ventricular hypertrophy plus increase in myocardial stiffness.

In order to exclude alterations of distensibility characteristics of the myocardial material itself even at early stages of hypertrophy, myocardial stiffness was determined (1) from diastolic pressure volume relations of the entire left ventricles, taking into account geometric factors [20], as well as (2) from stress-strain and stiffness-stress relations of isolated left ventricular myocardium. If myocardial stiffness would be increased in the hypertrophied hearts — either due to ultrastructural or functional alterations of the myofibrils, architectural distortion and mal-alignment of myofibres [25, 26], or due to fibrosis — irreversible damage of the left ventricular wall might be expected and regression of hypertrophy would not, or at least not necessarily, result in a normal left ventricle. On the contrary, if myocardial stiffness is normal in the early stages of hypertrophy in spontaneous essential hypertension, regression of hypertrophy after relief of pressure load might lead to normal chamber stiffness and — since normal myocardial contractility per mass unit was found in the younger SHR — in normal systolic and diastolic left ventricular properties.

As could be shown by our results, myocardial stiffness was normal in the younger SHR in spite of marked left ventricular hypertrophy, indicating normal distensibility properties of the material of the ventricular wall and thus — since myocardial contractility was normal as well — pointing to normal material properties of the myocardium. Accordingly, the increase in chamber stiffness in the younger SHR was mainly due to an increase in the wall thickness to radius ratio, while intrinsic stiffness of the ventricular wall was normal. As shown by our results, pressure hypertrophy does not necessarily include increased myocardial stiffness, as was reported in pressure hypertrophy due to outflow tract banding [20]. Myocardial stiffness was increased only in 60—80-week-old SHR as in the stage of increased systolic wall stress and decreased left ventricular function (see Session A, Bürger and Strauer, I).

When relating left ventricular systolic and diastolic properties, close coincidence was found between increase in myocardial stiffness and decrease in ejection fraction or between increase in myocardial stiffness and increase in systolic wall stress, with the exception of one 10-week-old SHR with excessive high systolic pressure at the time of the experiment, high systolic wall stress, and subnormal ejection fraction, but normal slope of the isovolumic stress-volume relation (see Session A, Bürger and Strauer, I). Since increase in systolic wall stress was closely related to decrease in ejection fraction (see Session A, Bürger and Strauer, I), inverse correlation between myocardial stiffness and ejection fraction implies correlation between myocardial stiffness and systolic wall stress and vice versa. To decide whether the relations between myocardial stiffness and ejection fraction or between myocardial stiffness and systolic wall stress represent only a coincidence or a causal connection, further experiments, especially concerning basal molecular mechanisms are needed.

Summary

Mechanics of isolated left ventricular papillary muscles in isotonic, isometric, and isotonic afterloaded contractions showed normal contractility and normal relaxation parameters in the younger age groups of SHR in comparison to age-matched NR. Left ventricular hypertrophy in SHR thus differs from other types of pressure hypertrophy, where reduced myocardial contractility has been reported even at early stages of hypertrophy. At about 40 weeks of age, first isotonic shortening velocity tended to decrease while maximum isometric tension development was even increased. In 60—80-week-old SHR, isotonic shortening velocity was significantly reduced in comparison to age-matched NR. Likewise, other contraction and relaxation parameters tended to be diminished. In SHR as well as in NR there was an age dependent decrease in myocardial contraction velocity.

Left ventricular diastolic pressure volume relations showed a steeper course in SHR even at the younger age groups in comparison to NR, with increased slope of a tangent to the pressure-volume curve at each filling pressure. Accordingly, chamber stiffness was elevated in SHR, resulting in altered filling properties of the entire left ventricular chamber as a result of left ventricular hypertrophy. In contrast, myocardial stiffness (determined from stiffness-stress relations of the entire left ventricles as well as from stress-strain relations of isolated left ventricular papillary muscles) was normal in the younger age groups of SHR in spite of marked left ventricular hypertrophy, indicating normal distensibility properties of the material of the left ventricular wall itself. In 60—80-week-old SHR myocardial stiffness increased with a close correspondence between increase in myocardial stiffness and decrease in ejection fraction or between increase in myocardial stiffness and increase in systolic wall stress.

As shown by our results, in the early stages of hypertrophy in SHR systolic as well as diastolic left ventricular properties were normal. It has been discussed that relief of pressure load and regression of hypertrophy in the early stages of hypertrophy due to spontaneous essential hypertension might result in a normal left ventricle, while in the latest stage of hypertrophy irreversible damage of the left ventricular wall ought to be expected.

References

1. Averill DB, Ferrario CM, Tarazi RC, Sen S, Bajbus R (1976) Cardiac performance in rats with renal hypertension. Circ Res 38 : 280
2. Barry WH, Brooker JZ, Alderman EL, Harrison DC (1972) Analysis of ventricular compliance curves following pacing induced angina. Circulation [Suppl II] 45 : II—483
3. BertrandME, Rousseau MF, Lefebvre JM, Lablanche JM, Asseman PH, Carre AG, Lekieffre JP (1878) Left ventricular compliance in acute transmural myocardial infarction in man. Eur J Cardiol [Suppl] 7 : 179

4. Bing OHL, Matsushita S, Fanburg BL, Levine HJ (1971) Mechanical properties of rat ciardiac muscle during experimental hypertrophy. Circ Res 28 : 234
5. Bürger SB, Strauer BE (1978) Left ventricular geometry and wall stress in various stages of hypertrophy due to spontaneous essential hypertension. Circulation [Suppl II] 57/58 : II–158
6. Covell JW, Ross J Jr (1973) Nature and significance of alterations in myocardial compliance. Am J Cardiol 32 : 449
7. Dwyer CM (1970) Left ventricular pressure-volume alterations and regional disorders of contraction during myocardial ischemia induced by atrial pacing. Circulation 42 : 1111
8. Gaasch WH, Battle WE, Oboler AA, Banas JS, Levine HJ (1972) Left ventricular stress and compliance in man with special reference to normalized ventricular function curves. Circulation 45 : 746
9. Gaasch WH, Levine HL, Quinones MA, Alexander JK (1976) Left ventricular compliance: Mechnisms and clinical implications. Am J Cardiol 38 : 645
10. Gaasch WH, Bing OHL, Franklin A, Rhodes D, Bernard SA, Weintraub RM (1978) The influence of acute alterations in coronary blood flow on left ventricular diastolic compliance and wall thickness. Eur J Cardiol [Suppl] 7 : 147
11. Glantz SA, Kernoff RS (1975) Muscle stiffness determined from canine left ventricular pressure-volume curves. Circ Res 37 : 787
12. Glantz SA, Parmley WW (1978) Factors which affect the diastolic pressure-volume curve. Circ Res 42 : 171
13. Grossman W, McLaurin LP, Moos SP, Stefadouros M, Young DT (1974) Wall thickness and diastolic properties of the left ventricle. Circulation 49 : 129
14. Grossman W, McLaurin LP, Stefadouros MA (1974) Left ventricular stiffness associated with chronic pressure and volume overloads in man. Circ Res 35 : 793
15. Hamrell BB, Alpert NR (1977) The mechanical characteristics of hypertrophied rabbit cardiac muscle in the absence of congestive heart failure. The contractile and series elastic element. Circ Res 40 : 20
16. Heller LJ (1978) Cardiac muscle mechanics from Doca- and aging spontaneously hypertensive rats. Am J Physiol 235 : H 82
17. Jacob R, Ebrecht G, Kämmereit A, Medugorac I, Wendt-Gallitelli MF (1977) Myocardial function in different models of cardial hypertrophy. An attempt at correlating mechanical, biochemical and morphological parameters. Basis Res Cardiol 72 : 160
18. Kitabatake A, Suga H (1978) Diastolic stress-strain relation of nonexcised blood-perfused canine papillary muscle. Am J Physiol 234 : H 416
19. McLaurin LP, Rolett EL, Grossman W (1973) Incomplete ventricular relaxation and diastolic compliance. Am J Cardiol 31 : 146
20. Mirsky I (1976) Assessment of passive elastic stiffness of cardiac muscle: Mathematical concepts, physiologic and clinical considerations, directions to future research. Progr Cardiovasc Dis 18 : 277

21. Mirsky I, Parmley WW (1973) Assessment of passive elastic stiffness for isolated heart muscle and the intact heart. Circ Res 33 : 233
22. Moskowitz SE, Lewis BS, Halon DA, Amar R, Gotsman MS (1978) Computer prediction of left ventricular compliance throughout diastole in normal patients. Eur J Cardiol [Suppl] 7 : 121
23. Nayler WG, Williams A (1978) Relaxation in heart muscle: Some morphological and biochemical considerations. Eur J Cardiol [Suppl] 7 : 35
24. Okamoto K, Aoki K (1963) Development of a strain of spontaneously hypertensive rats. Japn Circ J 27 : 282
25. Peterson KL, Ricci D, Tsuji J, Sasayama S, Ross J Jr (1972) Evaluation of chamber and myocardial compliance in pressure overload hypertrophy. Eur J Cardiol [Suppl] 7 : 195
26. Peterson KL, Tsuji J, Johnson A, DiDonna J, Lewinter M (1978) Diastolic left ventricular pressure-volume and stress-strain relations in patients with valvular aortic stenosis and left ventricular hypertrophy. Circulation 58 : 77
27. Pfeffer MA, Pfeffer JM, Frohlich ED (1976) Pumping ability of the hypertrophying left ventricle of the spontaneously hypertensive rat. Circ Res 38 : 423
28. Rankin JS, Arentzen CE, McHale PA, Ling D, Anderson RW (1977) Viscoelastic properties of the diastolic left ventricle in the concious dog. Circ Res 41 : 37
29. Ritman EL, Heethaar RM, Robb RA, Pao YC (1978) Finite element analysis of myocardial diastolic stress and strain relationships in the intact heart. Eur J Cardiol [Suppl] 7 : 105
30. Schierek P, Boom HBK (1978) Left ventricular active stiffness: Dependency on time and inotropic state. Pfluegers Arch 373 : 135
31. Spann JF, Buccino RA, Sonnenblick EH, Braunwald E (1967) Contractile state of cardiac muscle obtained from cats with experimentally produced ventricular hypertrophy and heart failure. Circ Res 21 : 341
32. Strauer BE (1979) Das Hochdruckherz. Springer, Berlin Heidelberg New York
33. Strauer BE, Scherpe A (1975) Experimental hyperthyroidism II. Mechanics of contraction and relaxation of isolated ventricular myocardium. Basic Res Cardiol 70 : 130
34. Tomoda H (1978) Clinical evaluation of left ventricular myocardial stiffness. Japn Heart J 19 : 74
35. Tyberg JV, Misbach GA, Glantz SA, Moores WY, Parmley WW (1978) A mechanism for shifts in the diastolic, left ventricular, pressure-volume curve: The role of the pericardium. Eur J Cardiol [Suppl] 7 : 163
36. Vignola PA, Walker HJ, Gold HK, Leinbach RC (1977) Alteration of the left ventricular pressure-volume relationship in man and its effect on the mitral echocardiographic early diastolic closure slope. Circulation 56 : 586

Systemic Hemodynamics and Cardiac Function in the Spontaneously Hypertensive Rat: Similarities with Essential Hypertension

E.D. FROHLICH, M.A. PFEFFER AND J.M. PFEFFER

Introduction

In recent years attention has been refocused on the hemodynamic aspects of the hypertensive diseases [1, 2]. From this re-examination a major concept has evolved: hypertension should no longer be considered a single homogeneous pathophysiological problem; it must be considered according to clinical and experimental types, etiology, and implicated pressor mechanisms [3, 4]. The concept is of value not only scientifically but clinically with respect to diagnostic and therapeutic concepts.

This conceptual evolution of hemodynamic mechanisms also conveys a clearer understanding of the pathophysiologic changes associated with the natural history of the development of hypertensive heart disease [5–7]. Until recently much of our thinking about the function of the hypertrophied heart in hypertension has been extrapolated from knowledge about acquired valvular heart disease, myocardiopathies, and other cardiac diseases that may complicate systemic arterial hypertension [8]. Even in experimentally induced hypertensive heart disease, myocardial hypertrophy frequently was produced rapidly by surgical or pharmalogic interventions, and the natural development of a slowly progressing hypertrophic process was not involved. With the introduction of the spontaneously hypertensive rat (SHR) by Okamoto and his co-workers in Kyoto, Japan, it finally became possible to study naturally occurring and slower process systematically [9].

Considerations

This discussion is concerned with the employment of a laboratory model of experimental hypertension that is genetic in origin, that does not require surgical or pharmacologic means of laboratory intervention, and that develops slowly and progressively – the SHR of Okamoto and Aoki. This experimental model is generally acknowledged to be the best presently available laboratory counterpart for essential hypertension in man [10]. To be sure, two drawbacks to the thesis developed are obvious: (1) until we know more precisely the nature and inborn mechanism(s) underlying genetic essential hypertension in man, we shall never be certain that a true experimental laboratory counterpart exists, and (2) because this review is necessarily from the experience of one laboratory and research team, the discussion is, by design, biased. Nevertheless, with the admitted drawbacks the validity, pitfalls, and inconsistencies of the SHR are presented.

Methodological Approaches. Studies in small animals have required the adaptation of a variety of experimental techniques for hemodynamic evaluation. Thus, over a period of several years we have reported from our laboratory means for: indirectly recording rat tail pressures simultaneously with a calibrated reference pressure channel [11]; quantitative measurement of cardiac output in the rat using electromagnetic flowmetry [12]; assessing myocardial contractility by determining the acceleration of ascending aortic blood flow [13] as initially suggested by Noble [14]; confirmation of the reported hemodynamic findings in unanesthetized and unrestrained rats using the direct-Fick method [15] and the "reference sample" method of microsphere injection into the left ventricle [16]; adaptation of the microsphere methods for the quantitative determination of organ blood flows and derived vascular resistances in anesthetized or unanesthetized rats [17, 18]; and evaluation of the performance and structure of the hypertrophied myocardium of hypertensive rats at different stages in the progression of hypertensive heart disease [19—21].

Naturally Developing Hypertension. As indicated above, until recently the only means for assessing the pathophysiological problems posed by the slowly developing and progressive vascular disease of systemic arterial hypertension in a controlled fashion in the experimental laboratory animal was by artificially induced alterations. Thus, experimental models had been developed: by banding the outflow tract of either ventricle; by constricting renal arteries with and without nephrectomy, by salt-loading the animal with and without additional treatment with exogenous steroids; by denervation of baroreceptors; by extirpation of adrenal tissue, and so forth [2, 8]. Indeed, some of these maneuvers were performed in combination in an effort to develop hypertension rapidly and to observe the consequent pathophysiologic alterations. Each of these procedures, to be sure, had great value, but all suffered from the same major drawback — none provided the natural development of hypertension in a fashion that was analogous to essential hypertension in man, and none involved those mechanisms that seem to be operative so subtly in man [3, 4].

Further, if we are to learn how the myocardium adapts to a slowly progressing left ventricular afterload, the work imposed upon ventricular outflow should not be brought about acutely by dramatic change; this cardiac example is applicable to other functioning organ systems. As a result of the myriad of experimental approaches, conflicting concepts have evolved concerning the capability and performance of the hypertrophied ventricle in systemic arterial hypertension: some have suggested the heart performs normally; others report a subnormal capability; and still others demonstrated a supranormal ability.

Spontaneously Hypertensive Rat. It therefore was necessary for the investigator to be provided with an experimental model of naturally developing hypertension, preferably of genetic origin. In recent years at least five such models have been developed. One, involving horses, is totally impractical. The others, involving the rat, are highly practical for the following reasons: firstly, the rat life span normally is 3 years and the study of the natural history of the disease is feasible for prospective laboratory investigation; secondly, the costs for conducting these long-term studies are real but manageable (more so than with larger animals or the primate); and thirdly, techniques used with larger animals seem to be adaptable for this animal model and have the further advantage of permitting measurements of entire organs, if this be necessary. The studies which we report herein relate only to the Okamoto-Aoki strain of SHR.

It is true that there are many questions that can be raised about the model and its appropriate controls, but the direct (especially hemodynamic) mechanisms at this point may be sufficiently analogous with the clinical problem to permit certain insights and inferences. As indicated, we believe this model is appropriate for hemodynamic studies since: it is one of genetic, natural development; the afterload imposed upon the left ventricle progressively increases without the need for surgical or pharmacological intervention; the elevated arterial pressure can also be approached similarly by therapeutic modalities; and the natural history of both disorders (SHR and man with essential hypertension) seems to be of the same duration and with similar cardiovascular complications. Each of the other genetic rat models, except perhaps the Smirk (or New Zealand) strain [22], are somewhat different. Dahl's strain of rats depends on excessive salt intake [23] and Bianchi's Milan strain probably reflects an inborn renal defect [24]. While these models may well be more pertinent to man with essential hypertension, they have not been studied as extensively because of their limited availability to investigators. Thus, this presentation will be concerned primarily with studies performed in our laboratories involving the SHR and some correlations of the results derived with other studies in essential hypertensive man.

This discussion will also underscore certain of the limitations of the SHR model, especially those concerning its breeding, its "appropriate" controls, and the role of aging, weight, and sex as they relate to interpretation of cardiovascular and hemodynamic data. These data will also provide some insight into the validity of the frequently used term "prehypertensive state"; review the hemodynamic changes associated with the development of the SHR hypertensive disease; explore whether an increased cardiac output is truly necessary early in the developmental stages for the maintenance of sustained SHR hypertension; explore the performance of the hypertrophied myocardium; and refer to studies concerned with measurement of body fluid volumes, mean circulatory filling pressure, and the role of salt excess in the SHR.

SHR Breeding and Control Strains

Breeding. The SHR model of experimental hypertension is genetically produced and, as has been outlined by Okamoto and Aoki, must be maintained by strict brother-to-sister inbreeding [9]. We have followed these methods, and in our studies to date involving well over 2500 rats, we have encountered no SHR which has had a normal arterial pressure. This has not been the general experience of investigators who have purchased the SHR commercially or who have not followed rigid brother-to-sister inbreeding. For the most part, our studies have been conducted primarily in rats whose ages range from 3 to 4 weeks to over 95 weeks. However, in one recent study we demonstrated that intra-arterial pressure measured in rats under 10 days of age was not significantly different from normotensive control rats, but by 14 days of age the arterial pressure had become significantly elevated [25]. Finally, we underscore that since this is a hereditary form of hypertension, genetic record-keeping is essential.

Control Strains. With respect to the appropriate normotensive control strains, this subject requires some discussion. As stated, the SHR was developed by selective brother-to-sister inbreeding from a normotensive strain of rats, some of whom presumably had outlying members that had demonstrated abnormally elevated arterial pressures. Thus, a normotensive strain of rats, the Wistar-Kyoto (WKY) was the immediate progenitor of the SHR; this WKY strain was developed, in turn, from the American Wistar rat (NR).

In earlier studies in our laboratory we have found that approximately 20% of our normotensive Wistars had at least one weekly average systolic pressure in excess of 150 mm Hg (taken by the rat-tail plethysmographic method) [26]. Subsequently, we were able to breed these so-called labile hypertensive Wistars so that with each successive generation to the F_6 arterial pressure increased. By the F_6 generation over 90% of these Wistars had a lifetime average systolic pressure in excess of 160 mm Hg [27].

Therefore, there are two normotensive strains of Wistar rats from which the SHR was derived: the WKY and NR. Both can be used as controls for the SHR; the more valid one is the WKY, but both are better. There is still one more problem inherent with the control strains for the SHR. Recently, we have found that 15% to 20% of the normotensive WKY control rats may have biventricular hypertrophy that seems to be related to small circulatory shunts, probably in the pulmonary circulation [28]. This finding is extremely important, especially in studies concerned with development and regression of ventricular hypertrophy and in comparisons of systemic hemodynamics and organ blood flow distribution. Therefore, all investigators must be aware of these findings, since significant differences between the WKY and the SHR may reflect not only heretofore unexplained abnormalities in the SHR but also unrecognized biventricular hypertrophy and associated arteriovenous fistulas in the WKY.

Body and Cardiac Weights. Some very real differences may be observed in body weights between the three rat strains: SHR, WKY, and NR. Although the female rats of all three strains are lighter than the male, with both sexes the NR were always the heaviest and the SHR (except for the very young male rats) were the lightest. The WKY rats fall in an intermediate position but are closer to the body weight of the SHR, expecially at the younger ages (under 12–14 weeks).

The remainder of this discussion, however, will be concerned primarily with male rats of the three rat strains since the observations of the former were essentially similar to those of the female rats.

From the earliest ages, left ventricular mass is greater in the SHR than in both normotensive strains. Thus, since the SHR consistently demonstrates lesser body weight and increased cardiac mass, a ratio presenting cardiac to total body weight is necessary (Fig. 1). From this relationship it may be appreciated that even though left ventricular weight increases with body growth of both normotensive strains of rats, the proportion of (left or right) ventricular mass to total body weight is always increased in the SHR.

A most interesting finding was the increased right ventricular weight in the SHR with respect to both normotensive strains. (There was no difference in left or right ventricular mass between the two normotensive strains). Whether this increased right ventricular mass in the SHR is the result of an increased load imposed upon the right ventricle by a failing left ventricle, whether this biventricular enlargement is the result of a generalized SHR myocardiopathy independent of the hypertensive disease, whether the right ventricle enlarges because the entire myocardium is a single syncytium that eventually reflects

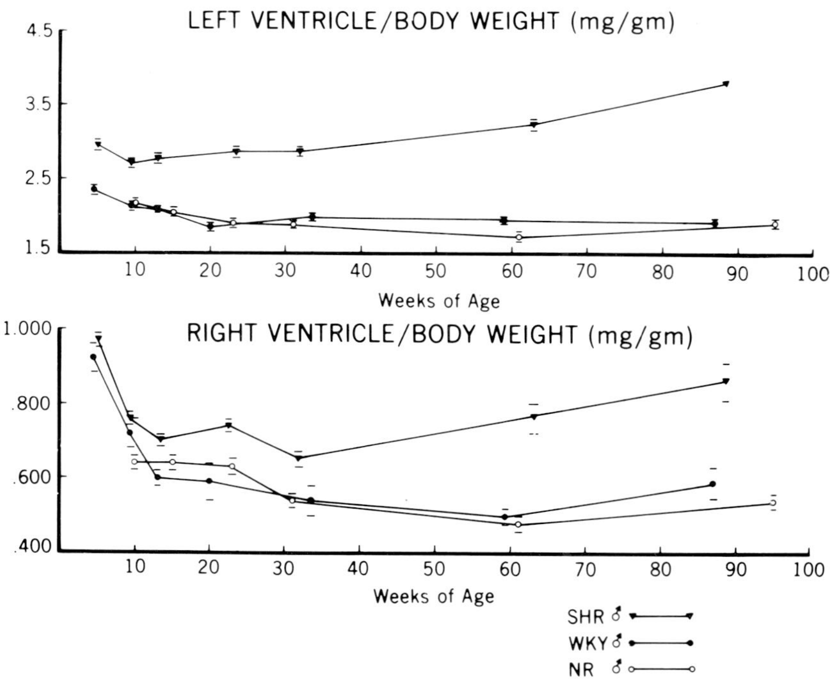

Fig. 1. Left ventricular to body weight ratios (*upper panel*) and right ventricular to body weight ratios (*lower panel*) of male SHR, WKY, and NR rats over a broad age range. Each point represents the mean (± 1 standard error of the mean). Curves represent the average data from approximately 2000 rats

left-sided changes upon the right ventricle [29], or whether still other factors are responsible for the right ventricular hypertrophy remains unknown at this time. Studies in many laboratories throughout the world are presently exploring these problems. Because of the differences in body and cardiac weights throughout the lifetime, it is not only important to express values in terms of ventricular to body weight ratios but, also rats of the same body weight should not be compared, since they may not be of the same age. Moreover, it follows then that since hemodynamic functions relate to age (infra) and not body weight (supra), the precise age of the rats must be known.

Arterial Pressure. Systolic and diastolic arterial pressure seems to achieve its maximum and remain at a plateau leven in both normotensive strains at about 6—10 weeks of age; it then remains stable throughout the rest of the life of the rat. In contrast, the arterial pressure of the SHR at 6 weeks of age is significantly higher (approximately 160/110 mm Hg) than both normotensive strains. This pressure continues to increase, so that by 28 weeks it is over 200/140 mm Hg. Arterial pressure thereafter seems to achieve a plateau for the remainder of the SHR lifetime (Fig. 2a). These systolic and diastolic pressures do not seem to be significantly different between the male and female rats of all threee rat strains. After 28 weeks mean arterial pressure is approximately 175 mm Hg as compared to approximately 115 mm Hg in both groups of normotensive rats (Fig. 2b). These pressures are significantly reduced when the animals are subjected to hemodynamic studies involving thoracotomy and placement of an electromagnetic flow probe. Under these circumstances, the mean arterial pressures of the SHR and normotensive strains are approximately 125 and 90 mm Hg, respectively.

Thus, at least from 14 days of age and older arterial pressure is significantly higher in the SHR than in either normotensive strain (WKY or NR). Whether the highter arterial pressures of the myocardial tension at 14 days of age are of sufficient magnitude to explain the increased cardiac mass observed at that time remains to be demonstrated. The tension developed by the left ventricle may indeed be sufficiently increased to warrant the increased mass. In contrast, it may also be argued that even at this early age there is a generalized myocardiopathy that seems to be associated with the increased arterial pressure associated with the hypertensive vascular disease.

Heart Rate. The heart rate of the unanesthetized and anesthetized SHR seems to be faster in all ages than in both normotensive control strains (Fig. 3). Although heart rate declines slightly with aging, the decline is proportional in all strains; even at the oldest ages, heart rate remains faster in the SHR.

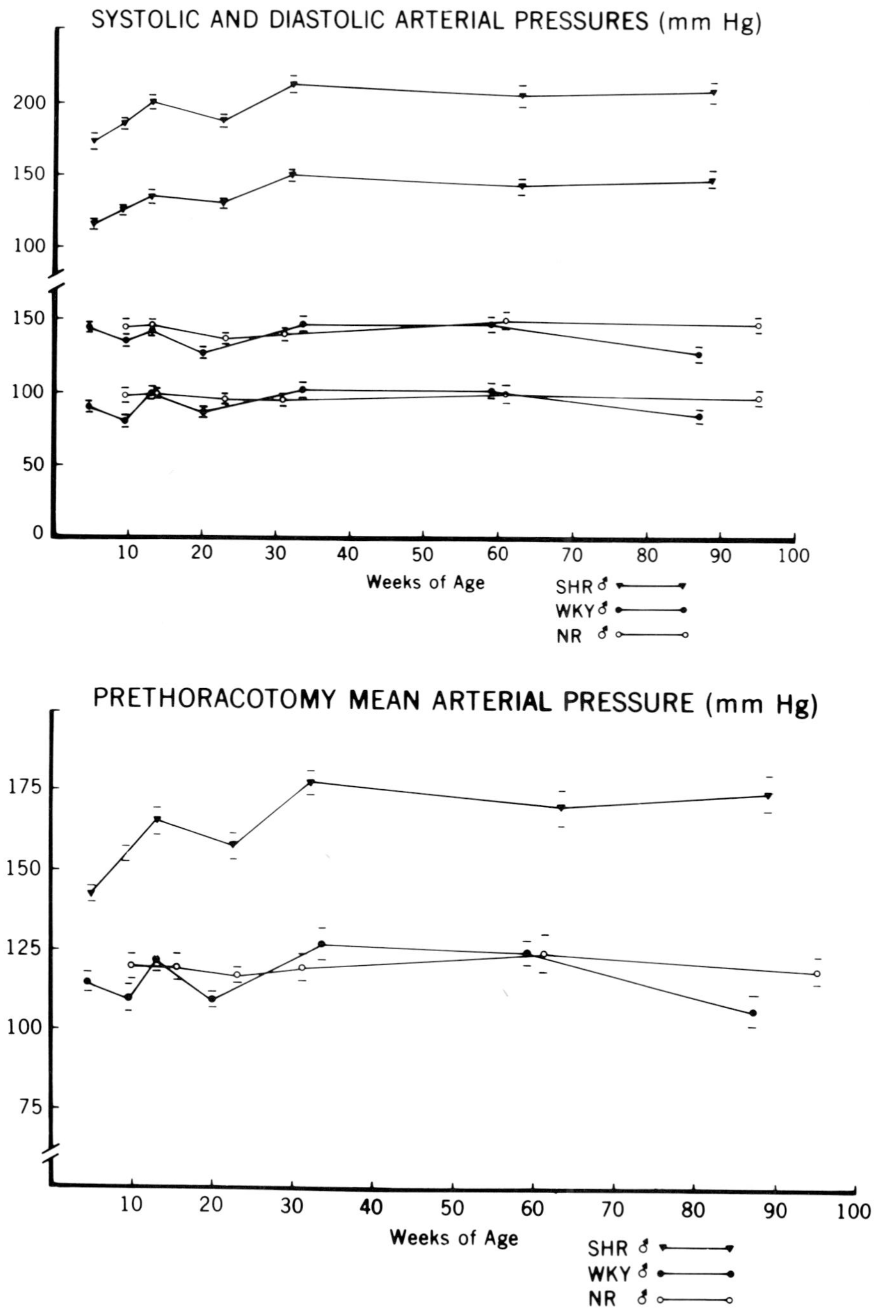

Fig. 2a, b. Systolic and diastolic arterial pressures (a) and mean arterial pressures (b) from approximately 2000 male SHR, WKY, and NR rats. These pressures were obtained during light ether anesthesia before thoracotomy was performed for other hemodynamic studies. Each *point* represents the mean (± 1 standard error of the mean)

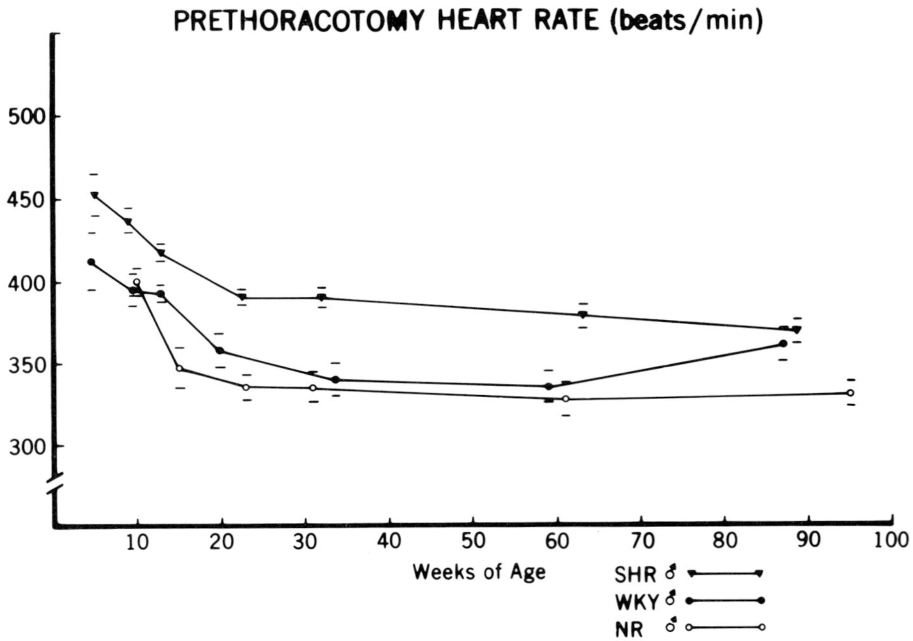

Fig. 3. Prethoracotomy heart rates obtained during light ether anesthesia in approximately 2000 SHR, WKY, and NR male rats. Each point represents the mean (± 1 standard error of the mean)

Hemodynamic Studies

Essential Hypertension. Before discussing the hemodynamic characteristics of the SHR and comparing these findings to essential hypertensive man, it may be useful to review briefly the hemodynamic characteristics in man. In earlier studies we compared the hemodynamic measurements in patients with essential hypertension with normotensive volunteer subjects [30]. These studies demonstrated that as arterial pressure increased progressively in groups of patients with borderline, to mild, to moderate, and then to severe hypertensive vascular disease, it did so in parallel with the total peripheral resistance. The heart rate of all groups of patients with essential hypertension remained faster than in the normotensive subjects, and there were no interhypertensive group differences.

In contrast, cardiac output and left ventricular ejection rate were increased in patients with labile (or borderline) hypertension and this was associated with a normal total peripheral resistance. However, if the cardiac output were increased to the same level in the normotensive individuals as was observed in the patients with borderline hypertension, total peripheral resistance would actually be reduced. Therefore, we suggested that the patients with borderline hypertension had an inappropriately normal or increased total peripheral resistance [7, 30, 31]. When autonomic influences upon the myocardium were blocked pharmacologically (with propranolol and atropine), cardiac output and heart rate became the same as in normotensive control subjects who were treated similarly [32]. This pharmacologic maneuver, which produced intrinsic cardiac function, unmasked the increased vascular resistance in borderline hypertension. In addition, patients with borderline hypertension had a somewhat higher level of plasma renin activity than the normal subjects or patients with essential hypertension of mild or moderate severity [30].

We have also classified patients with essential hypertension according to cardiac involvement: no cardiac involvement whatsoever, only electrocardiographic evidence of left atrial enlargement, and those with obvious left ventricular hypertrophy (chest X-ray and electrocardiographic criteria) [5]. Thus, as the heart becomes more involved, arterial pressure and total peripheral resistance increase pari passu, presumably the result of the progressively increasing afterload which the left ventricle must overcome. Even before obvious left ventricular hypertrophy is recognized clinically, the vigor with which the left ventricle ejects blood becomes impaired with evidence of left atrial abnormalities or enlargement. And all patients with left ventricular hypertrophy demonstrated left atrial abnormality. These findings demonstrate that left ventricular hypertrophy becomes manifest clinically very early as arterial pressure and total peripheral resistance progressively rise.

Spontaneously Hypertensive Rat. How do these findings in man relate to the laboratory model of SHR? First, with respect to the role of renin, early in the SHR life span renal renin content and plasma renin activity are increased [33]. These findings are consistent with observations in man with borderline hypertension [30, 34]. With respect to hemodynamic changes, Table 1 compares selected characteristics in the three groups of rats (SHR, WKY, and NR) at different ages; Fig. 4 and 5 summarize the hemodynamics over the life span. Certainly by 4 to 5 weeks arterial pressure is significantly higher and heart rate is faster..After thoracotomy is performed for electromagnetic flowmeter placement, arterial pressure is reduced in both groups, but this pressure continues to remain higher in the SHR. This is explained on the basis of a significantly increased total peripheral resistance and a slightly higher cardiac output; cardiac work is also increased. By 8 to 12 weeks body weight has increased, but this increase in mass is greater in the normotensive rats than in the SHR. By this age, SHR arterial pressure and heart rate are significantly greater and the mean arterial pressure following flowmeter placement is greater than both normotensive strains. The elevated arterial pressure is also explained by the significantly increased total peripheral resistance.

It is important to recognize that at this age there are also some very important hemodynamic differences between the two normotensive strains [19, 35, 36]. Arterial pressure and total peripheral resistance are higher in the NR than the WKY, and cardiac output and aortic blood flow acceleration are less in the NR. Aortic flow acceleration is used as an index of left ventricular contractility, since at this time in the cardiac cycle the left ventricle is acting as an impulse generator [14]. When the SHR is compared with the NR, one may infer that

Table 1. Selected hemodynamic features of male normotensive Wistar-Kyoto (WKY) and American Wistar (NR) and spontaneously hypertensive (SHR) rats. Each value represents the mean at the respective ages[a]

	4–5 Weeks		10 Weeks			24 Weeks		
	WKY	SHR	NR	WKY	SHR	NR	WKY	SHR
Prethoracotomy:								
Body weight (g)	95	97	225	228	210	378	284[c]	265[b, d]
Systolic/Diastolic (mm Hg)	145/90	172/114[b]	144/97	134/80[c]	185/126[b, d]	144/99	143/99	200/134[b, d]
Mean arterial pressure (mm Hg)	108	133[b]	113	98[c]	146[b, d]	114	114	156[b, d]
Heart rate (bpm)	412	455[b]	399	396	438[b, d]	348	393[c]	418[b, d]
Post-thoracotomy:								
Mean arterial pressure (mm Hg)	70	96[b]	82	69[c]	111[b, d]	90	86	129[b, d]
CI (ml/min/kg)	314	332	262	281	286[d]	199	260[c]	249[d]
TPRI (mm Hg/ml/min/kg)	0.218	0.298[b]	0.309	0.249[c]	0.388[b, d]	0.469	0.326[c]	0.516[b, d]
Acceleration (g)	—	—	6.56	7.47	8.29[d]	8.10	12.44[c]	13.93[d]
Min. work (g — meters)	27.6	41.3[b]	63.4	57.2	88.6[b, d]	89.6	81.5	113.5[b, d]

[a] CI = cardiac index; TPRI = total peripheral resistance index

[b] Significantly different from WKY

[c] Significantly different from NR

[d] Significantly different from NR

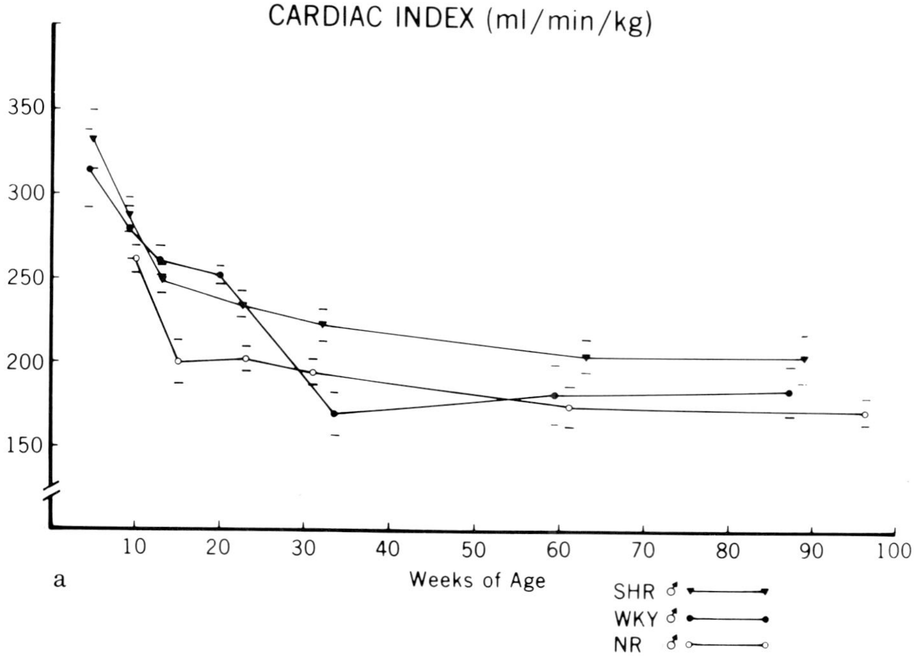

a

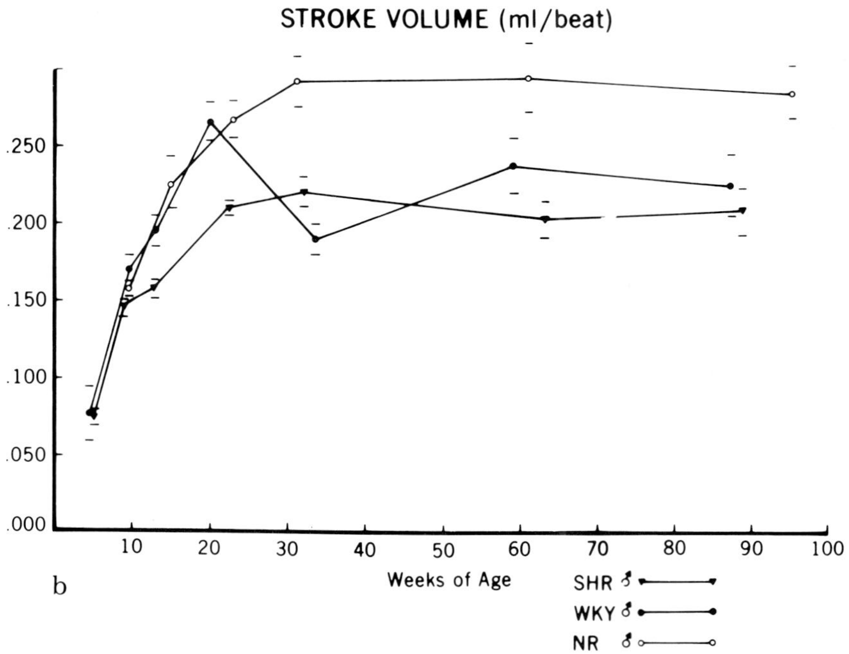

b

Fig. 4. (a) Cardiac indexes, (b) stroke volume, and (c) peak flow velocity (*upper panel*) and maximum ascending aortic flow acceleration (*lower panel*) of approximately 2000 SHR, WKY, and NR male rats. The values were obtained during ether anesthesia through thoracotomy, using a Statham electromagnetic flow probe. Each point represents the mean (± 1 standard error of the mean)

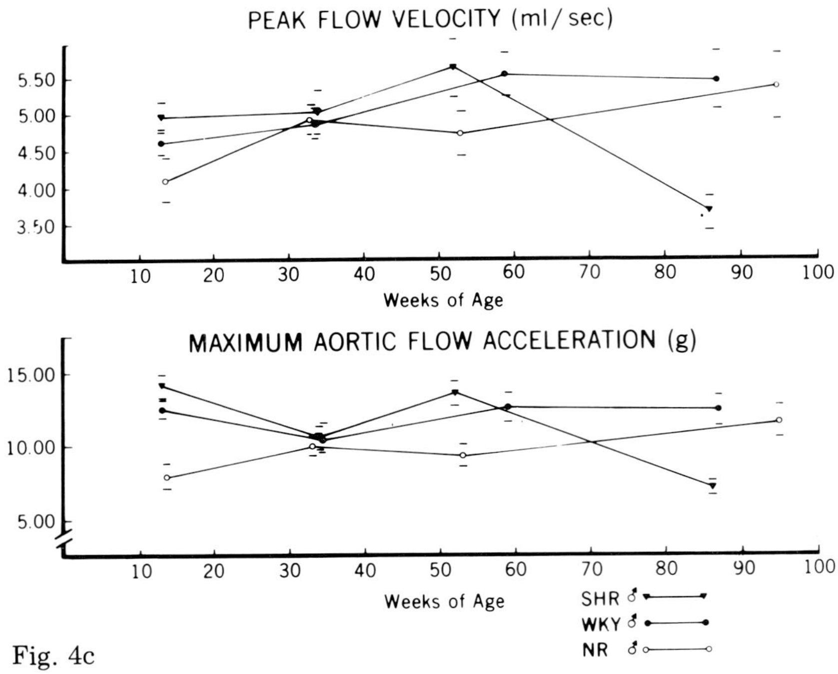

Fig. 4c

the hypertensive rat demonstrates a hyperkinetic circulation in comparison with the NR: cardiac output, heart rate, and aortic flow acceleration are increased, and the left ventricle is also performing increased work [35]. However, this is not confirmed when the SHR is compared with the WKY, underscoring the value of using two normotensive control strains [36]. By 6 months of age when the animals are fully mature and the hypertension is well-established, arterial pressure is magnificently elevated (to an average level of 200/134 mm Hg) and heart rate is still faster (Table 1). At this age the SHR is significantly lighter in weight in comparison with both normotensive strains, but the WKY also weighs less than the NR. The greater arterial pressure is also elevated during thoracotomy and is related to the increased vascular resistance. Even at this age the SHR cardiac output, heart rate, and left ventricular contractility remain greater than in the NR; this is explainable by the persistent significant hemodynamic differences between the two strains of normotensive rats.

Thus, we may summarize these concepts as follows: (1) the importance of utilizing two normotensive strains is clear; (2) early in hypertension there may be some evidence of a hyperkinetic circulation, at least when one compares the SHR with the NR; (3) the hemodynamic alterations observed in the SHR are very similar to those in man with essential hypertension; and (4) from the very earliest age that we have studied the SHR (14 days with only pressure measurements and from 4 weeks on with the other hemodynamic measurements), arterial pressure and total peripheral resistance remain elevated, and these are associated with an increased left ventricular mass.

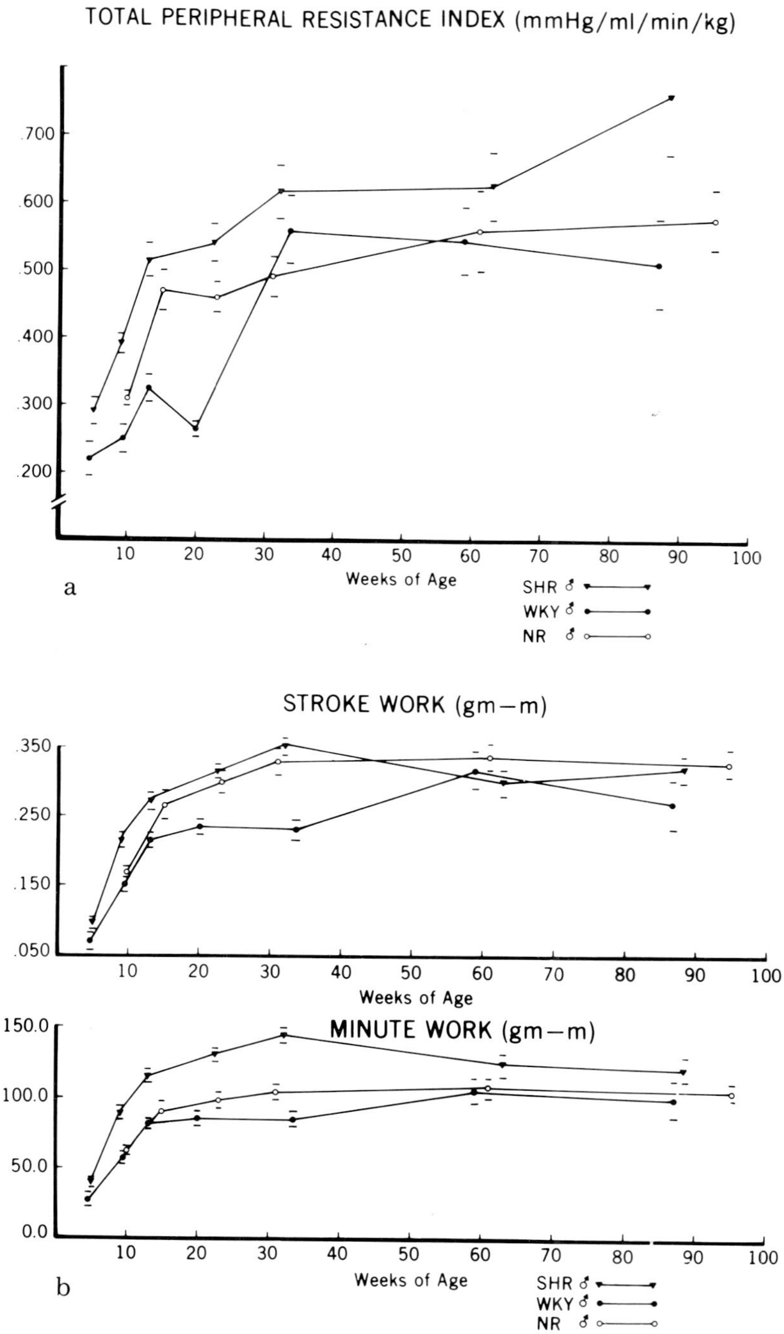

Fig. 5. (a) Total peripheral resistance index (*upper panel*), (b) left ventricular stroke work (*middle panel*) and minute work (*lower panel*) obtained by electromagnetic flowmetry in approximately 2000 SHR, WKY, and NR male rats during ether anesthesia. Each point represents the mean (± 1 standard error of the mean)

Regional Hemodynamics. Knowledge of the hemodynamic changes that we have discussed above has been extended with regional blood flow studies using radioactively labeled carbonized microspheres [16–18]. By coincidentally measuring cardiac output (by using either electromagnetic flowmetry during anesthesia or by using the direct-Fick method or the reference sample method in conscious rats) it is possible to quantify actual blood flows to each organ. Thus, the distribution of microspheres to each organ (as compared with the total amount injected) can be related to the actually measured cardiac output, thereby providing a numerical expression of organ flow and the means to determine the resistance to blood flow in each organ. From these studies we have determined that the blood flow in each organ. From these studies we have determined that the blood flow to each organ is normal in the SHR except for the heart. An increased myocardial flow may be explained on the basis of myocardial oxygen demand created by the greater minute work of the hypertrophied left ventricle. However, if we express this flow per gram of tissue, then the myocardial blood flow is normal. We may therefore conclude that the increased total peripheral resistance observed in the SHR from the earliest age seems to be evenly distributed throughout all the organs' vasculatures.

Special Cardiac and Hemodynamic Studies

Role of Increased Cardiac Output in Development of SHR Hypertension. In recent years there has been great interest in the role of an increased cardiac output in the pathogenesis of most forms of clinical and experimental hypertension [37]. An increased cardiac output has been attributed by Guyton and his colleagues to be the result of an expanded intravascular volume brought about by an inappropriately set pressure level in the kidneys to normally excrete extracellular fluid volume [38]. As a result, intravascular volume expands at normal pressure levels, and in hypertension, a higher arterial pressure in the kidney is necessary to maintain a normal extracellular fluid volume. Once that pressure is achieved, Guyton suggests that the intravascular volume will then contract and a reduced cardiac output (to normal level) will ensue. This adaptive phenomenon has been termed total body autoregulation and explains the conversion from a high cardiac output-normal total peripheral resistance systemic hemodynamic profile to one of a normal cardiac output and high total peripheral resistance.

To test the necessity of a high cardiac output to produce a sustained state of hypertension in the SHR, we treated WKY, NR and SHR rats from conception with either of two beta-adrenergic receptor-blocking drugs: timolol or propranolol [7, 36, 39]. These compounds reduced cardiac output from conception of the rats when given to the breeding parents, to the pregnant mother, and then to the offspring, who had remained treated first through the placental circulation and later, until weaning, through the mother's milk. After weaning the drugs were fed directly to the rats in their drinking water until hemodynamic studies were performed at 12 weeks of age. These animals demonstrated a normal growth and development (both normotensive and hypertensive rats), whether they received the beta-receptor blocking drugs or not. That the rats receiving these drugs were adequately blocked was shown by the significantly reduced heart rate and fluid consumption in both normotensive and SHR rats from the time of birth until hemodynamic studies were performed at 12 weeks of age. At that time, despite the reduced cardiac participation (manifested by a lesser heart rate, cardiac output, and aortic flow acceleration), arterial pressure followed the same course, whether or not beta-adrenergic receptor blocking therapy was used. These studies provide very strong evidence that hypertension could develop in the SHR without an elevated cardiac output-indeed, even with a reduced systemic flow. An additional finding was the persistence of left ventricular hypertrophy in the male SHR rats despite no change in arterial pressure. It was of further interest to observe that the female-treated SHR demonstrated a significant reduction in left ventricular mass, although arterial pressure was not reduced [39].

Exercise Studies. To determine whether left ventricular mass was maximal at any age induced by increased total peripheral resistance and arterial pressure, the SHR, WKY, and NR rats were exercised (continuous swimming) for 2 h each day for several weeks [20]. Body growth was similar in all three strains to those controls rats who were not exercised. Nevertheless, left ventricular and right ventricular to body weight indexes increased further in all three rat strains, demonstrating potential for augmented myocardial hypertrophy. Moreover, the kidney to body weight and adrenal to body weight ratios also increased as a result of exercise. These studies may also suggest that another factor, in addition to a hemodynamic stress, may participate in the phenomenon of increased organ mass as a result of exercise.

Ventricular Pumping Ability. There is need to know whether the slowly developing hypertrophy in the SHR is associated with normal pumping ability of the left ventricle. Some suggest myocardial performance is normal in hypertrophy, others suggest it may be enhanced, and still others suggest a diminished function exists. In order to assess this in SHR, we developed a technique, used originally in dogs by Bishop et al. [40], in which Tyrode's solution is rapidly infused intravenously over a 1-min period to permit a progressive rise in central venous pressure and enhanced ventricular performance [19]. Approximately 30 s after the infusion was begun, a plateau in the maximum cardiac output was achieved despite further increase in venous pressure. At this point, peak cardiac output and pumping ability of the left ventricle had been achieved. When we compared this pumping performance of the left ventricle in the NR, WKY, and SHR rats of 11–24, and 83-week age groups, the SHR demonstrated a normal pumping ability at 4 and 6 months of age. However, the oldest group of SHR (83 weeks of age) failed to demonstrate the same performance as either normotensive group of rats [19]. There was a dramatic diminution in the peak cardiac output, whether expressed in absolute terms or per gram of left ventricular myocardial tissue.

These studies demonstrated that the left ventricular hypertrophied heart was able to pump normally until later in life when maximum myocardial adaptability had been achieved. These findings, once again, are in accord with the clinical observation that persistently sustained hypertension is ultimately associated with a failing left ventricle when the myocardium no longer can adapt.

Other Studies. Time does not permit an elaboration of other studies conducted in our laboratory. These involve the measurement of fluid volume compartments in the SHR [25] and measurement of mean circulatory filling pressure, which seem to be increased in the SHR [41]. Since intravascular volume was not expanded and interstitial fluid pressure and volume were normal, it may be concluded from these studies that an increased venomotor tone exists in the SHR [42].

We have also demonstrated that the SHR is sensitive to sodium loads, and that when fed a sodium excess diet, the SHR will respond by an increased arterial pressure and total peripheral resistance [43]. In contrast, the WKY responds by a maintained arterial pressure associated with an increase in cardiac output. Thus, in response to sodium excess, the SHR increases its vascular resistance, whereas the WKY decreases its vascular resistance.

Conclusions

Therefore, we conclude that the systemic hemodynamics and cardiac function of the SHR provide some striking similarities with essential hypertensive man. Both have their hypertension based in a genetic origin. Both demonstrate similar progressive hemodynamic alterations in response to pregressive vascular disease. Early in hypertension there may be a hyperkinetic circulation, but this participation of increased cardiac output does not seem to be a pathogenetic factor in that it is not essential for the later development of increased total peripheral resistance in both man and SHR. Rather, the increased cardiac participation may reflect the participation of a generalized cardiovascular excitation. Both forms of hypertension, man and rat, respond similarly to long-term pharmacologic reduction of arterial pressure with improved morbidity and mortality. With respect to the pathophysiologic alterations, both forms of hypertension demonstrate some participation of the renopressor system early in the development of hypertension; neither however, demonstrates any apparent hormonal, volume-dependent, or humoral features (although altered kallikrein excretion seems to be present in both forms). Finally, both forms of hypertension seem to have important neural mechanisms participating in the development and maintenance of hypertension, and this thesis has been supported by studies from a variety of investigative centers, including ours.

References

1. Frohlich ED, Tarazi RC, Dustan HP (1969) Re-examination of the hemodynamics of hypertension. Am J Med Sci 257 : 9
2. Frohlich ED (1977) Haemodynamics of hypertension. In: Genest J, Koiw E, Kuchel O (eds) Hypertension: Physiopathology and treatment. McGraw-Hill, New York, p 15
3. Dustan HP, Tarazi RC, Hinshaw LB (1976) Mechanisms controlling arterial pressure. In: Frohlich ED (ed) Pathophysiology: Altered regulatory mechanisms in disease, 2nd edn. Lippincott, Philadelphia, p 49
4. Frohlich ED (1977) Pathophysiology of hypertension. In: Kurtzman NA, Martinez-Maldonado M (eds) Renal Pathophysiology. Thomas, Springfield Ill, p 881
5. Frohlich ED, Tarazi RC, Dustan HP (1971) Clinical-physiological correlations in the development of hypertensive heart disease. Circulation 44 : 446
6. Frohlich ED (1977) Cardiac participation in hypertension. Cardiovasc Med 2 : 109
7. Frohlich ED, Pfeffer MA (1975) Adrenergic mechanisms in human and SHR hypertension. Clin Sci Mol Med 48 : 225s–238s
8. Report of the Hypertension Task Force (1979) vol 3: Current research and recommendations from the task force subgroups on local and systemic hemodynamics. U.S. Department of Health, Education, and Welfare, National Institutes of Health. DHEW Publication No. (NIH) 76–1625
9. Okamoto K, Aoki K (1963) Development of a strain of spontaneously hypertensive rats. Jpn Circ J 27 : 282
10. Udenfriend S, Spector S (1972) Spontaneously hypertensive rats. Science 176 : 1155
11. Pfeffer JM, Pfeffer MA, Frohlich ED (1971) Validity of an indirect tail-cuff method for determining systolic arterial pressure in unaesthetized normotensive and spontaneously hypertensive rats. J Lab Clin Med 78 : 957
12. Pfeffer MA, Frohlich ED (1972) Electromagnetic flowmetry in anesthetized rats. J Appl Physiol 33 : 137
13. Pfeffer MA, Frohlich ED (1973) Hemodynamics of spontaneously hypertensive rats. I. Effects of pressure elevation. Am J Physiol 224 : 1066
14. Noble MIM (1968) The contribution of blood momentum to left ventricular ejection in the dog. Circ Res 23 : 663
15. Walsh GM, Tsuchiya M, Frohlich ED (1976) Direct Fick application for measurement of cardiac output in rat. J Appl Physiol 40 : 849
16. Nishiyama K, Nishiyama A, Frohlich ED (1976) Regional blood flow in normotensive and spontaneously hypertensive rats. Am J Physiol 230 : 691
17. Tsuchiya M, Ferrone RA, Walsh GM, Frohlich ED (1978) Regional blood flows measured in conscious rats by the combined Fick and microsphere methods. Am J Physiol 235 : H357
18. Ferrone RA, Walsh GM, Tsuchiya M, Frohlich ED (1979) Comparison of systemic and regional hemodynamics in conscious spontaneous and renovascular hypertensive rats. Am J Physiol 236 : H403

19. Pfeffer MA, Pfeffer JM, Frohlich ED (1976) Pumping ability of the hypertrophying left ventricle of the spontaneously hypertensive rat. Circ Res 38 : 423
20. Pfeffer MA, Ferrell BA, Pfeffer JM, Weiss AK, Fishbein MD, Frohlich ED (1978) Ventricular morphology and pumping ability of exercised spontaneously hypertensive rats. Am J Physiol 235 : H193
21. Pfeffer JM, Pfeffer MA, Fishbein MC, Frohlich ED (1979) Cardiac function and morphology with aging in the spontaneously hypertensive rat. Am J Physiol 237 : H461
22. Smirk FH, Hall WH (1958) Inherited hypertension in rats. Nature 182 : 290
23. Dahl LK, Heine M, Tassinari L (1962) Role of genetic factors in susceptibility to experimental hypertension due to chronic excess salt ingestion. Nature 194
24. Bianchi G, Fox U, DiFrancesco F, Bardi U, Radice M (1973) Hypertensive role of the kidney in spontaneously hypertensive rats. Clin Sci Mol Med 45 : 135s
25. Trippodo NC, Walsh GM, Frohlich ED (1978) Fluid volumes during onset of spontaneous hypertension in rats. Am J Physiol 235 : H52
26. Frohlich ED, Pfeffer MA, Weiss AK, Brecher GA (1972) Variability of arterial pressure in normotensive and spontaneously hypertensive rats. Proc Soc Biol Med 140 : 145
27. Peterson AL, Pfeffer MA, Weiss AK, Frohlich ED (1977) Development of a hypertensive strain of Wistar rats from previously normotensive but borderline normals. J Lab Clin Med 89 : 1163
28. Pfeffer MA, Pfeffer JM, Dunn FG, Nishiyama K, Tsuchiya M, Frohlich ED (1979) Natural biventricular hypertrophy in normotensive rats. I. Physical and hemodynamic characteristics. Am J Physiol 236 : H640
29. Grant RP (1953) Architectonics of the heart. Am Heart J 46 : 405
30. Frohlich ED, Kozul VJ, Tarazi RC, Dustan HP (1970) Physiological comparison of labile and essential hypertension. Circ Res [Suppl I] 27 : 55
31. Frohlich ED (1971) Beta-adrenergic blockade in the circulatory regulation of hyperkinetic states. Am J Cardiol 27 : 195
32. Julius S, Pascual AV, London R (1971) Role of parasympathetic inhibition in the hyperkinetic type of borderline hypertension. Circulation 44 : 413
33. Sen S, Smeby RR, Bumpus FM (1972) Renin in rats with spontaneous hypertension. Circ Res 31 : 876
34. Hamet P, Kuchel O, Genest J (1973) Effect of upright posture and isoproterenol infusion on cyclic adenosine monophosphate excretion in control subjects and patients with labile hypertension. J Clin Endocrinol Metab 36 : 218
35. Pfeffer MA, Frohlich ED (1973) Hemodynamic and myocardial function in young and old normotensive and spontaneously hypertensive rats. Circ Res [Suppl I] 32 : 28—38
36. Pfeffer MA, Frohlich ED, Pfeffer JM, Weiss AK (1974) Pathophysiological implications of the increased cardiac output of young spontaneously hypertensive rats. Circ Res [Suppl I] 34 : 235

37. Ferrario CM, Page IH (1978) Current views concerning cardiac output in the genesis of experimental hypertension. Circ Res 43 : 821
38. Coleman TG, Granger HJ, Guyton AC (1971) Whole-body circulatory autoregulation and hypertension Circ Res [Suppl I] 28 : 76
39. Pfeffer MA, Pfeffer JM, Weiss SK, Frohlich ED (1977) Development of SHR hypertension and cardiac hypertrophy during prolonged beta-blocking therapy. Am J Physiol 232 : H639
40. Bishop VS, Stone HL, Guyton AC (1964) Cardiac function curves in conscious dogs. Am J Physiol 207 : 677
41. Yamamoto J, Trippodo NC, Ishise S, Frohlich ED (1980) Total vascular pressure-volume relationship in the conscious rat. Am J Physiol 238 : H823
42. Yamamoto J, Trippodo NC, Frohlich ED (1981) Whole body venous capacity and effective total tissue compliance in SHR. Hypertension 3 : 104
43. Chrysant SG, Walsh GM, Kem DC, Frohlich ED (1979) Hemodynamic and metabolic evidence of salt sensitivity in spontaneously hypertensive rats. Kidney Int 15 : 33

Part II: Myocardial, Adrenergic and Noncontractile Responses

Reversal of Cardiac Hypertrophy by Antihypertensive Therapy

R.C. Tarazi and S. Sen

Introduction

Until recently the study of regression of cardiac hypertrophy was restricted to experimental animals, and even in those conditions studies were largely limited to the effect of surgical interventions or of digitalis therapy (for review, see [1]). Clinical studies were hampered by problems in the quantification of changes in ventricular mass. The development of ventriculography led to some studies in man following surgical correction of aortic valve lesions [2, 3], but the results were, to say the least, uncertain. Investigations remained, however, limited by the invasiveness of the procedure and, therefore, by the inability to evaluate by repeated studies the multiple factors involved, the time frame needed for reversal, and the effects of medical therapy.

Three practically contemporaneous developments have drastically altered the outlook in this problem and have led to a marked renewal of interest in the reversal of myocardial hypertrophy—particularly as regards hypertensive heart disease. The first was the demonstration that medical therapy could reverse hypertrophy in spontaneously hypertensive rats (SHR) [4, 5]. The second was the simultaneous and partly unexpected finding that control of hypertension alone was not sufficient for reversal of hypertrophy, and that all antihypertensive drugs were therefore not equivalent in that respect [1, 4, 6]. The third was the development of noninvasive techniques allowing more precise quantitative estimate of left ventricular mass in man [7, 8].

Growing experience with reversal of cardiac hypertrophy has led to important questions being asked [1]. The first question relates to the impact on cardiac performance of a reduction in myocardial mass; the second concerns the nature and importance of factors (other than blood pressure) that could modulate structural responses of the heart to antihypertensive measures. Frohlich and Tarazi [9] have recently summarized the evidence for a dissociation between arterial pressure levels and degree of ventricular hypertrophy. Nowhere is this dissociation better evident than in the response of the heart to different antihypertensive drugs.

Experimental Studies

Experimental models allow a direct determination of cardiac weight and thus appear to avoid the many uncertainties inherent in clinical studies of cardiac hypertrophy (vide infra). However, they also have their difficulties [1], not the least of which is the definition of a proper index of reference. Body weight is the more commonly used index, but the body weight of most hypertensive animals is smaller than that of their normotensive counterparts, and it could be influenced by the drugs used to control hypertension. The results of various studies must therefore be carefully examined to avoid unwarranted extrapolations.

Effects of Different Drugs

The early observations of Patton et al. [10] regarding regression of hypertrophy following nephrectomy in renovascular hypertensive rats were confirmed and extended by Hall et al. [11]. More directly relevant to most clinical problems was the reversal of ventricular hypertrophy by medical control of spontaneous hypertension in rats [4—6]. The essential results of these studies were confirmed by different centers [12—14], namely, that ventricular weight could be returned to normal with adequate antihypertensive drugs, both in SHR and in renovascular hypertensive rats. The important fracture, however, that stood out in these results was the divergent effect on cardiac weight of otherwise equipotent antihypertensive drugs [15].

Three effective antihypertensives were used in SHR by Sen et al. [4—6] in SHR, viz. methyldopa, hydralazine, and minoxidil. The three controlled arterial pressure equally but only methyldopa reduced ventricular weight. Cardiac hypertrophy was left unchanged by hydralazine and was even accentuated by minoxidil (Table 1). These results pointed out more forcefully than other models the importance of factors other than increased resistance to ejection in the modulation of cardiac hypertrophy [1, 4, 9, 15]. Observations to date suggest that

Table 1. Antihypertensive therapy and cardiac hypertrophy in SHR. (Data reproduced with permission, Sen et al 1977)

Group	BP (mm Hg)	Ventricular weight (mg/g)
Normal	120	2.6
SHR	188	3.4
Methyldopa	149	2.7
Hydralazine	123	3.4
Minoxidil	130	3.8

Results of antihypertensive therapy indicate that reversal of cardiac hypertrophy is not dependent on blood pressure control alone adrenergic stimulation is particularly potent in retarding the reversal of cardiac [16] or of vascular [17] hypertrophy in response to blood pressure control (vide infra).

More recently, our studies were extended to the use of a converting enzyme inhibitor (captopril) in both SHR [17] and rats with renovascular hypertension (unpublished observations). The results in SHR were of particular significance in that this model of hypertension was not regarded as "renindependent" [19]. Blood pressure was reduced moderately (151 ± 3 vs. 193 ± 5 mm Hg, $P < 0.001$) by increasing doses of captopril, while ventricular weight was practically normalized. Ventricular weight in untreated SHR averaged 962 ± 20 mg (3.3 ± 0.06 mg/g body weight); it was reduced to 814 ± 20 mg ($P < 0.001$) by 6 weeks of treatment. The ventricular weight in treated SHR was not significantly different from that of normotensive WKY controls (2.8 ± 0.05 vs. 2.95 ± 0.04 mg/g, P:N.S.) [18]. Control of blood pressure and reversal of hypertrophy were achieved by much smaller doses of captopril in rats with Goldblatt one-clip-2-kidney hypertension.

The aspect of that study that deserves singling out was the alteration in myocardial composition with reversal of hypertrophy by captopril. Previous experience with either methyldopa in SHR [4, 5] or nephrectomy in renovascular hypertension (Table 2) had demonstrated an increase in myocardial hydroxyproline concentration in hearts whose weights were reduced by treatment. The interstitial and supporting fibrous tissue that had increased pari passu with ventricular hypertrophy remained unchanged when the mass of contractile proteins was reduced [4]. In contrast, following 6 weeks of therapy with captopril, total myocardial hydroxyproline was reduced from 0.58 to 0.48 mg ($P < 0.05$) [18]. Similar results were obtained by combined treatment with captopril and hydrochlorothiazide, but not by diuretic therapy alone (Table 3). The reasons for the difference among different treatment schedules (methyldopa, nephrectomy, and captopril) as regards their effect on myocardial composition are not clear. Better understanding may lead to more effective interference for reversal of the structural lesions of hypertension.

In contrast with the relatively homogeneous results obtained with other forms of antihypertensive therapy are the controversies surrounding the effects of beta-adrenergic blockers. Initial reports by Vaughn-Williams and Raine [20] in normotensive rabbits and by Fernandez at al. [21] in renovascular hypertensive rats described marked reductions in ventricular weight by beta-blockers. This was not confirmed by subsequent studies either in normotensive or in hypertensive animals [22—24]; propranolol treatment for up to 3 months did not in our experience reduce ventricular weight in normotensive rabbits (Tarazi, Sen, and Erlandson, unpublished results). In SHR alterations in cardiac weight, although statistically significant, were minimal in magnitude [6]. In view of the proposed role of adrenergic influences on cardiac hypertrophy [16], these negative results deserve a more detailed discussion. The effect of beta-adrenergic blockade on cardiac hypertrophy appears to depend on a number of factors, which include among others the level of adrenergic drive in the model investi-

Table 2. Differences in the biochemical correlates of cardiac hypertrophy in Wistar rats. Averill et al. 1976

	Myocardial DNA		Myocardial RNA		Myocardial hydroxyproline	
	Content (mg)	Concentration (mg/g)	Content (mg)	Concentration (mg/g)	Content (mg)	Concentration (mg/g)
Normotensives (n=11)	1.97 ± 0.07	2.21 ± 0.10	2.73 ± 0.10	3.05 ± 0.09	0.65 ± 0.04	0.72 ± 0.03
Hypertensives (n=14)	2.47 ± 0.11	1.86 ± 0.05	4.36 ± 0.23	3.27 ± 0.12	1.30 ± 0.20	0.93 ± 0.09
P	< 0.005	< 0.005	< 0.005	(n. s.)	< 0.01	< 0.05

Table 3. Effect of converting enzyme inhibitor (CEI) on ventricular biochemical composition (reversal therapy). Sen et al. 1980

Treatment groups	RNA		DNA		Hydroxyproline	
	mg/g	mg (total)	mg/g	mg (total)	mg/g	mg (total)
SHR (untreated)	3.2	3.1	1.76 ± 0.06	1.67	0.50	0.53
	P = n. s.	*P* < 0.05	*P* = n. s.	*P* < 0.2	*P* < 0.1	*P* < 0.05
SHR and CEI	3.1	2.58	1.75	1.46	0.59	0.45
SHR and hydrochlorothiazide	3.4	3.04	1.65	1.45	0.566	0.52
	N	*P* < 0.05	*P* < 0.05	*P* < 0.4	*P* = n. s.	*P* < 0.05
SHR and hydrochlorothiazide + CEI	3.23	2.56	1.80	1.42	0.60	0.48

gated and the effect of the drug on arterial pressure. In recent experiments we found that a particular ratio of hydralazine to propranolol did reverse ventricular hypertrophy with moderate control of arterial pressure in SHR, whereas a smaller ratio of propranolol to hydralazine did not alter ventricular weight despite achieving better blood pressure control.

Factors Influencing Reversal of Hypertrophy

The experience detailed in the previous section confirmed in a strictly controlled experimental situation the many discrepancies reported clinically between blood pressure level and cardiac enlargement [25, 26]. These discrepancies had been repeatedly pointed out, but the difficulties and uncertainties of diagnosis in man reduced their impact. The data base is now stronger in favor of the suggestion that many factors, hemodynamic and adrenergic as well as humoral, play a significant role in myocardial hypertrophy. Raab [27] has stressed the importance of catecholamines in hypertensive heart disease. Our experience with reversal of hypertrophy by medical treatment in SHR is in agreement with his concept; adrenergic stimulation was a potent factor in preventing reversal of hypertrophy despite adequate blood pressure control [16] (Fig. 1). This was suggested in our early studies and further demonstrated by the results of various types of combined antihypertensive therapy [4—6].

Sen et al. [6] showed that methyldopa effectively prevented the increase in cardiac weight induced by minoxidil and, in fact, reduced it toward normal in SHR. More recent and as yet unpublished results indicate that propranolol could produce similar effects when added in adequate ratio to hydralazine treatment in SHR (Sen and Tarazi [48]). The finding that higher doses of propranolol must be given, helped explain our initial negative results [6]. This observation may also help explain part of the discrepancy among different investigators regarding the effect of beta-blockers on structural cardiovascular changes [20—24]. Taken altogether, results to date suggest that the degree of interference with adrenergic drive and the site of action of the drug used as well as the type and stage of evolution of hypertension may all influence the response of ventricular hypertrophy to the reduction of arterial pressure.

Catecholamines are certainly *not* the only factor that can modulate hypertrophic response to antihypertensive drugs; other factors include hemodynamic variables other than pressure and myocardial effects of angiotensin [1]. Furthermore, studies of SHR need to be repeated in other models of hypertension; early results from echocardiography in man appear, however, to confirm the initial conclusion of our experimental studies [28].

Alterations in Myocardial Composition with Regression of Hypertrophy

Following removal of the causative lesion or when arterial pressure is controlled, cardiac weight begins to decrease at different rates, depending on the circumstances; regression of hypertrophy can begin within 3 days of removal of outflow obstruction [29] and be almost complete in 1 week. In other instances, ventricular weight is back to normal only after 4–6 weeks of continued therapy [5]. Changes in cardiac weight during development and regression of hypertrophy are not due to fluctuations in water content; the ratio of wet to dry weight was not altered in these conditions in almost all models investigated[4, 5, 29, 30]. The most direct biochemical correlate of development and reversal of ventricular hypertrophy is the concentration of RNA per unit myocardial tissue (for review, see Rabinowitz and Zak [31]). A positive correlation exists between degree of hypertrophy and elevation of RNA, and contrariwise, both concentration and total myocardial RNA are significantly reduced to normal with reversal of hypertrophy which is induced either medically [5] or surgically [29].

In contrast with these rather homogeneous results is the variable response of myocardial collagen. The thick ventricles secondary to pressure overload contain more collagen [4, 32]; regression of hypertrophy could leave behind an increasing concentration of myocardial hydroxyproline. This was observed following methyldopa or surgical treatment of hypertension [5, 29]; however, blood pressure control by captopril led to actual reduction of total ventricular hydroxyproline [18]. In order to explain the lack of ready regression of collagen in earlier studies, Cutiletta et al. [29] had suggested that collagen fibers, once formed and extruded into the interstitial space, are not as accessible to removal as are intracellular components. Results with captopril (in the heart) as well as Hollander's results with penicillamine (in the aorta) indicate that particular drug effects on collagen metabolism must also be taken into account [18, 33].

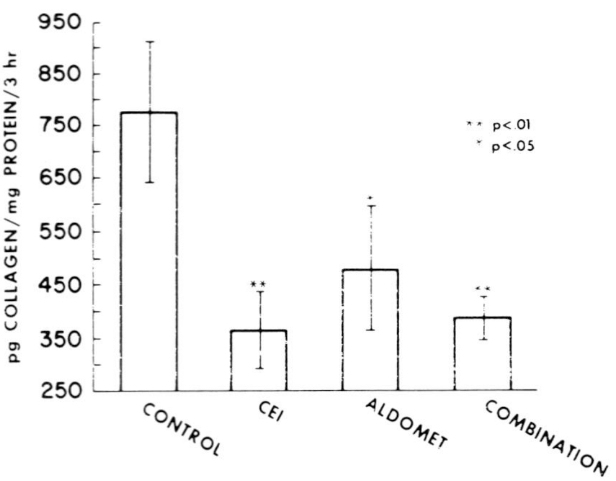

Fig 1. Effect of long-term antihypertensive therapy with three treatment regimens on the rate of myocardial collagen synthesis after prevention of hypertension in spontaneously hypertensive rats. *CEI*, converting enzyme inhibitor; *p*, probability. (Sen et al. 1979)

Furthermore, it would seem that the development of collagen is not uniform throughout the evolution of hypertension. Sen and Bumpus [34] described two stages in SHR with particularly increased collagen content of the myocardium, namely in very young rats and in older animals with well-established hypertension. The latter was related to development of arterial pressure, since it could be effectively prevented by antihypertensive therapy (Fig. 1). It is of interest to contrast the results of *prevention* with those of *treatment* of hypertension; methyldopa prevented the increase of collagen but could not reverse it in 6 weeks of therapy. Further studies will have also to consider the relative participation of different types of collagen in hypertensive conditions and their response to therapy. These changes in myocardial composition could carry potentially important implications for cardiac performance [15], just as structural vascular alterations can influence peripheral resistance and hemodynamic characteristics [35].

Clinical Studies

A review of available reports in 1978 did not allow definite conclusions because published studies were too few and results were difficult to interpret, due in large part to methodological problems [1]. In the short period since that review, the impact of echocardiography on the study of ventricular hypertrophy has been felt strongly [28, 36, 37].

In contrast with the inferential conclusions that could be drawn from electrocardiographic studies, echocardiography offers a direct approach to determination of ventricular wall thickness [7], calculation of left ventricular mass [38], and distribution of hypertrophy [8, 39, 40]. Reduction of left ventricular wall thickness and mass have been reported with successful treatment of hypertension [28, 41]. In our experience a reduction of left ventricular mass by 8%–25% was noted as early as 10–15 weeks after initiation of treatment with methyldopa in nine essential hypertensive patients. Alcocer and Aspe [28] have reported a reduction of left ventricular mass in hypertensive subjects by treatment with methyldopa, but not following beta-blockade therapy. Bibra and Richardson [41] reported early septal hypertrophy in man in response to hypertension, which returned to normal on antihypertensive therapy with either diuretics, beta-blockers, or methyldopa.

Attractive as these results are, it is important to stress the serious limitations to the indiscriminate use of M-mode echocardiography [7, 8]. This technique offers only a limited view of the left ventricle; calculations of left ventricular mass are based on the same assumptions as, and subject to the same limitations of, calculations of left ventricular volume. In our experience, based on autopsy-controlled studies of dogs, correlation of left ventricular weight with the mass calculated from M-mode tracings gave an index of determination of only 50% [8]. Although significant ($P < 0.001$), this level of correlation should caution against undue extrapolations. Measurement of wall thickness appeared much more reliable than calculations of "mass". On the other hand, two-dimensional echocardiography gave a very reliable estimate of left ventricular weight because it allowed direct determination of the left ventricular long-axis and also an overview of possible regional or segmental hypertrophy [8]. Prospective studies with two-dimensional echocardiography, presently underway, will be needed to answer in man the many questions raised by animal experiments.

Hemodynamic Sequelae of Reversal of Hypertrophy

Growing experience with reversal of hypertrophy has led to important questions, some of which could have been anticipated. Of particular importance is the implication for cardiac performance of a loss of muscle mass with relative increase in collagen concentration [4, 15]. Cardiac hypertrophy, especially in cases induced by pressure overload, is often associated with diminished performance. Would then a reversal of hypertrophy be hemodynamically beneficial or harmful?

Cardiac hypertrophy in hyperthyroid animals regresses after correction of the metabolic disorder, but contractility remains depressed [42, 43]. On the other hand, contractility was reportedly normalized after relief of a right ventricular pressure overload [44]. In our experience with SHR, treatment with methyldopa and reversal of hypertrophy were associated with marked improvement of cardiac performance, but this was related to reduction of afterload [45]. Although the rats' ventricles were smaller, this did not impair the heart's ability to sustain increased volume loads as compared to hypertrophied controls. In that respect the recent report by Limas [14] is potentially of considerable interest; the hypertrophied ventricles of SHR were shown to have a reduced calcium uptake and enhanced Ca^{++}ATPase activity, resulting in a lower stoichiometric ratio between calcium uptake and ATP hydrolysis. Following treatment with either methyldopa or hydralazine, blood pressure was controlled but the abnormality in calcium transport was improved only with the former drug (methyldopa) which also led to regression of cardiac hypertrophy. Hydralazine left cardiac weight and the lower calcium uptake unchanged [14].

Reversal of hypertrophy did not completely normalize the SHR heart — its performance at high volume overload was somewhat less than matched normotensive controls — but this reversal did not appear to injure it either. There was some question, however, regarding the regressed heart's ability to sustain a sudden increase of pressure [45]. Pfeffer et al. [46] came also to similar conclusion with antihypertensive therapy in old (1 year) SHR; reduction in cardiac mass was associated with restoration of cardiac performance toward normal as peak pumping ability was improved but pressure generating capacity was reduced. Much remains to be determined in this area, particularly as regards the influence of myocardial collagen on cardiac performance. Experiments during the development of hypertrophy suggest that collagen influences passive length-tension curves but not the contractility of papillary muscles [47]. Analogous studies following reversal of hypertrophy have not yet been reported.

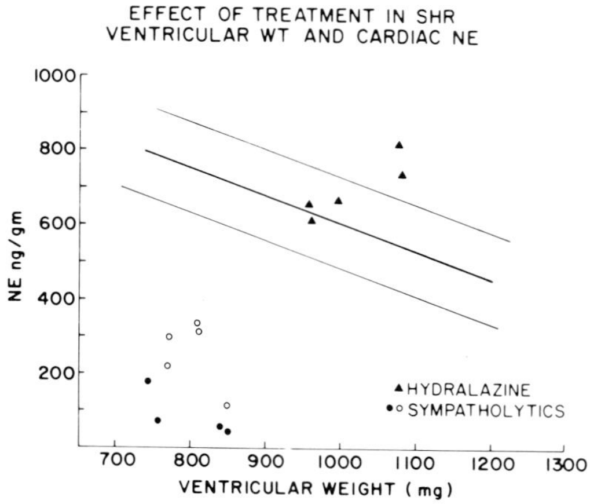

Fig. 2. Concentration of norepinephrine (*NE*) in myocardium was found to be inversely related to ventricular weight in both normal and weight-matched spontaneously hypertensive rats (*SHR*) (regression line and confidence limits of equation are shown in the graph. Against this background are plotted the results of treatment of SHR by reserpine or methyldopa (sympatholytics) and by hydralazine; all three drugs lowered arterial pressure, but reversal of cardiac hypertrophy was associated with concomitant reduction of ventricular NE. (Tarazi et al. 1979)

The effect in man of a reduction in left ventricular mass has not yet been determined with any real precision. Early indications from M-mode echocardiography did not suggest any obvious impairment at rest. Alcocer et al. [28] reported that the ejection fraction was unchanged in the smaller hearts following methyldopa treatment; our initial results are in agreement with theirs. Neither left ventricular end-diastolic volume nor its percent shortening (29% vs. 30%, P:N.S.) showed any significant change following reduction of ventricular mass in our patients. However, a larger number of observations are needed, particularly with two-dimensional echocardiography, as well as studies of ventricular response to stress and the use of more precise indexes of performance before any definite conclusions are possible.

Conclusion

In summary, reversal of cardiac hypertrophy has been proven to occur in experimental animals following some types of antihypertensive therapy. Evidence from man is highly suggestive but more studies are needed. Adrenergic factors seem to play an important role in modulating structural cardiac response to variations in arterial pressure. However, the effect of changes in muscle mass and composition still needs further evaluation. Of particular significance for the evolution and vascular complications of hypertension is the close correlation reported by Yamori et al. [17] between alterations in cardiac weight and protein synthesis in the mesenteric arteries in response to antihypertensive therapy. As facts become better known and conclusions become closer, the potential for adequate therapy is markedly increased, not only would we be able to prevent lesions by adequate blood pressure control but it might be possible to envision the possibility of reversing cardiovascular structural lesions.

References

1. Tarazi RC (1979) Reversal of cardiac hypertrophy; possibility and clinical implications. In: Robertson JIS, Caldwell ADS (eds) Left ventricular hypertrophy in hypertension. Academic Press, London, Royal Society of Medicine, London Royal Society of Medicine International Congress and Symposium Series, No. 9, pp 55—65
2. Kennedy JW, Twiss RD, Blackman JR, Merendino KA (1968) Hemodynamic studies one year after homograft aortic valve replacement. Circulation [Suppl II] 37/38 : 110—118
3. Baxley WA, Dodge HT (1971) Relationship of left ventricular performance and hypertrophy in humans. In: Alpert NR (ed) Cardiac hypertrophy. Academic Press, New York, pp 425—431
4. Sen S, Tarazi RC, Khairallah PA, Bumpus FM (1974) Cardiac hypertrophy in spontaneously hypertensive rats. Circ Res 35 : 775—781
5. Sen S, Tarazi RC, Bumpus FM (1976) Biochemical changes associated with development and reversal of cardiac hypertrophy in spontaneously hypertensive rats. Cardiovasc Res 10 : 254—261
6. Sen S, Tarazi RC, Bumpus FM (1977) Cardiac hypertrophy and antihypertensive therapy. Cardiovasc Res 11 : 427—433
7. Feigenbaum H (1976) Echocardiography, 2nd edn, Lea & Febiger, Philadelphia
8. Salcedo EE, Gockowski K, Tarazi RC (1979) Left ventricular mass and wall thickness in hypertension. Am J Cardiol 44 : 936—940
9. Frohlich ED, Tarazi RC (1979) Is arterial pressure the sole factor responsible for hypertensive cardiac hypertrophy? Am J Cardiol 44 : 959—963
10. Patton HS, Page EW, Ogden E (1943) The results of nephrectomy on experimental renal hypertension. Surg Gynecol Obstet 76 : 494—497
11. Hall O, Hall CE, Ogden E (1953) Cardiac hypertrophy in experimental hypertension and its regression following reestablishment of normal blood pressure. Am J Physiol 174 : 175—178
12. Tomanek RJ, Davis JR, Anderson SC (1979) The effects of alpha-methyldopa on cardiac hypertrophy in spontaneously hypertensive rats: Ultrastructural, sterological and morphometric analysis. Cardiovasc Res 13 : 172—182
13. Columbo M, Paddock J, Nagraj S, Hollander W (1979) Effects of hydralazine and propranolol on hypertensive cardiovascular disease in the SHR. Circulation [Part II] 60 : II—10

14. Limas CJ (1980) Effect of antihypertensive therapy on calcium transport by cardiac sarcoplasmic reticulum of spontaneously hypertensive rats (SHRs). Am J Cardiol 45 : 490
15. Tarazi RC, Ferrario CM, Dustan HP (1977) The heart in hypertension. In: Genest J, Koiw E, Kuchel O (eds) Hypertension physiopathology and treatment. McGraw-Hill, New York, pp 738–754
16. Tarazi RC, Sen S (1979) Catecholamines and cardiac hypertrophy. In: Mezey KC, Caldwell ADS (eds) Catecholamines and the heart. Academic Press, London, Royal Society of Medicine, London Royal Society of Medicine International Congress and Symposium Series, No 8, pp 47–57
17. Yamori Y, Nakada T, Lovenberg W (1976) Effect of antihypertensive therapy on lysine incorporation into vascular protein of the spontaneously hypertensive rat. Eur J Pharmacol 38 : 349–355
18. Sen S, Tarazi RC, Bumpus FM (1980) Effect of converting enzyme inhibitor (SQ 14,225) on myocardial hypertrophy in spontaneously hypertensive rats. Hypertension 2 : 169–176
19. Muirhead EE, Prewitt RL Jr, Brooks B, Brosius WL Jr (1978) Antihypertensive action of the orally active converting enzyme inhibitor in spontaneously hypertensive rats. Circ Res 43 : 1–53
20. Vaughan-Williams EM, Raine AEG (1974) Effect of prolonged beta-receptor blockade on the weight and electrophysiological responses of rabbit hearts. Lancet II : 1048–1049
21. Fernandes M, Onesti G, Fiorentini R, Kim K, Swartz C (1976) Effect of chronic administration of propranolol on the blood pressure and heart weight in experimental renal hypertension. Life Sci 18 : 967–970
22. Caspari PG, Gibson K, Harris P (1975) Changes in myocardial collagen in normal development and after beta-blockade. Recent Adv Stud Cardiac Struct Metab 7 : 99–104
23. Pfeffer MA, Pfeffer MJ, Weiss AK, Frohlich ED (1977) Development of SHR hypertension and cardiac hypertrophy during prolonged beta blockade. Am J Physiol 232 : H639–H644
24. Weiss L, Lundgren Y (1978) Left ventricular hypertrophy and its reversibility in young spontaneously hypertensive rats. Cardiovasc Res 12 : 635–638
25. Ehrstrom R (1946) Enlargement of the heart in hypertension. Acta Med Scand [Suppl] 206 : 86–93
26. Grant RP (1953) Aspects of cardiac hypertrophy. Am Heart J 46 : 154–158
27. Raab W, Lepeschkin E (1950) Biochemical versus haemodynamic factors in the origin of hypertensive heart disease. Acta Med Scand 138 : 81–93
28. Alcocer L, Aspe J (1979) The effect of antihypertensive treatment with methyldopa on left ventricular mass. In: Robertson JIS, Caldwell ADS (eds) Left ventricular hypertrophy in hypertension. Academic Press, London; Grune & Stratton, New York; Royal Society of Medicine, London (Royal Society of Medicine International Congress and Symposium Serie No. 9, pp 93–97)
29. Cutiletta AF, Dowell RT, Rudnik M, Arcilla RA, Zak R (1975) Regression of myocardial hypertrophy. I. Experimental model, changes in heart weight, nucleic acids and collagen. J Mol Cell Cardiol 7 : 767–781

30. Beznak M, Korecky B, Thomas G (1969) Regression of cardiac hypertrophies of various origin. Can J Physiol Pharmacol 47 : 579—586
31. Rabinowitz M, Zak R (1972) Biochemical and cellular changes in cardiac hypertrophy. Annu Rev Med 23 : 245—262
32. Fanburg BL (1970) Experimental cardiac hypertrophy. N Engl J Med 282 : 723—732
33. Hollander W (1973) Hypertension, antihypertensive drugs and atherosclerosis. Circulation 48 : 1112—1127
34. Sen S, Bumpus FM (1979) Collagen synthesis in development and reversal of cardiac hypertrophy in spontaneously hypertensive rats. Am J Cardiol 44 : 954—958
35. Folkow B (1978) Cardiovascular structural adaptation; its role in the initiation and maintenance of primary hypertension. Clin Sci Mol Med 55 : 3s 22s
36. Schlant RC, Feiner JM, Heymsfield SB, Gilbert CA, Shulman NB, Tuttle EP Jr, Blumenstein BA (1977) Echocardiographic studies of left ventricular anatomy and function in essential hypertension. Cardiovasc Med 2 : 477—491
37. Savage DD, Drayer JIM, Henry WL, Mathews EC Jr, Ware JH, Gardin JM, Cohen ER, Epstein SE, Laragh JH (1979) Echocardiographic assessment of cardiac anatomy and function in hypertensive subjects. Circulation 59 : 623—632
38. Troy BL, Pombo J, Rackley CE (1972) Measurement of left ventricular wall thickness and mass by echocardiography. Circulation 45 : 602—611
39. Safar ME, Lehner JP, Vincent MI, Plainfosse MT, Simon AC (1979) Echocardiographic dimensions in borderline and sustained hypertension. Am J Cardiol 44 : 930—935
40. Guazzi M, Fiorentini C, Olivari MT, Polese A (1979) Cardiac load and function in hypertension. Am J Cardiol 44 : 1007—1012
41. Bibra H von, Richardson PJ (1979) Left ventricular hypertrophy in patients with moderate essential hypertension: An echocardiographic study. In: Robertson JIS, Caldwell ADS (eds) Left ventricular hypertrophy in hypertension. Academic Press, London, Grune & Stratton, New York, Royal Society of Medicine, London (Royal Society of Medicine International Congrss and Symposium Series, No 9, pp 47—54
42. Van Liere EJ, Sizemore DA (1971) Regression of cardiac hypertrophy following experimental hyperthyroidism in rats. Proc Soc Exp Biol Med 136 : 645—648
43. Skelton CL, Sonnenblick EH (1974) Heterogeneity of contractile function in cardiac hypertrophy. Circ Res [Suppl II] 34/35 : 83—96
44. Cooper G, Satava RM, Harrison CE, Colemen HN (1974) Normal myocardial function and energetics after reversing pressure-overload hypertrophy. Am J Physiol 226 : 1158—1165
45. Spech M, Ferrario CM, Tarazi RC (1980) Cardiac pumping ability following reversal of hypertrophy and hypertension in spontaneously hypertensive rats. Hypertension 2/1 : 75—82

46. Pfeffer J, Pfeffer M, Flecther P, Braunwald E (1980) Improved cardiac performance with long term reduction of blood pressure in old spontaneously hypertensive rats. Am J Cardiol 45 : 490
47. Bing OHL, Fanburg BL, Brooks WW, Matsushita S (1978) The effect of the lathyrogen β-amino proprionitrile (BAPN) on the mechanical properties of experimentally hypertrophied rat cardiac muscle. Circ Res 43 : 632—637
48. Sen S, Tarazi RC, Bumpus FM (1980) Reveral of myocardial hypertrophy and influence of adrenergic system. (Abstract). Circulations 62 (Suppl. III): III—121

Left Ventricular Dynamics and Myocardial Function in Goldblatt Hypertension of the Rat
Biochemical, Morphological and Electrophysiological Correlates[1]

R. JACOB AND G. KISSLING

Introduction

The pathogenesis of hypertension in man as well as the nature and speed of development of secondary alterations in various organs, particularly those involving the heart, are not uniform. Thus, one cannot expect a given experimental model in animals to simulate all pathophysiological aspects of the heart in hypertension.

Despite a few peculiarities, the hypertrophied left ventricle of the rat following unilateral renal artery coarctation reveals structural and functional alterations which are unquestionably common to those found in certain forms of human hypertension. The goal of the present study was to characterize the changes in left ventricular dynamics and myocardial mechanics in the stage of pre-insufficiency and to interpret these alterations in terms of biochemical, morphological and electrophysiological findings insofar as the current state of knowledge permits. Special attention is given to the question of the significance of early manifested alterations as a cause of later impaired contractile performance. The study is based on investigations of our group in recent years [3, 6, 11, 13, 15, 17, 18, 20, 22—24, 29—32, 35, 40, 41] as well as some newer unpublished results.

Methods

In young male Wistar rats (body weight 140–170 g) arterial hypertension leading to left ventricular hypertrophy was induced by constricting one renal artery while the contralateral kidney was left intact (Goldblatt II). The animals were provided with a standard dry meal (ssniff, Intermast GmbH, Soest) and tap water ad libitum. Details of operation technique and plethysmographic measurement of arterial blood pressure are published elsewhere [20, 24, 32, 41]. The experiments were performed 4, 8, 12 and 24 weeks after operation. Sham operated rats of the same age served as controls.

---

1 Supported by the Deutsche Forschungsgemeinschaft

Measurement of Left Ventricular Dynamics in Situ. After opening the chest under urethane anaesthesia (1.2 g/kg body weight) an electromagnetic flow-probe was placed around the aortic trunk. Central systemic pressure was measured using a canula in the left carotid artery, and the left ventricle was pierced at the apex with a double-barreled canula for pressure and volume measurements. One bore was connected to a syringe, the piston of which was coupled with a linear potentiometer. This arrangement permitted direct measurement of changes in syringe, and thereby ventricular, volume as differences in electrical potential.

Two methods were used for determination of end-diastolic volume. The first procedure involved recording end-diastolic pressure-volume relations (as "relaxation curves") of the beating heart with carefully clamped artrioventricular border immediately after completion of an entire series of measurements. The individual end-diastolic volumes occurring at different times during an experiment were read from these curve using end-diastolic pressure values. In the alternative procedure the atrioventricular border was clamped several times during an experiment and the inner ventricular volume was reduced to zero by suction within 6 to 8 s. This method had the advantage that the absolute amount of end-diastolic volume could be measured several times during a single experiment.

Furthermore, this method makes direct allowance for the fact that the end-diastolic pressure-volume relations are variable to a certain extent due to stress relaxation and to changes in right ventricular filling. Volume measurements on chronically altered ventricles, however, yielded basically the same results with both procedures. In both methods incomplete relaxation was prevented by setting heart rate at approximately 160/min by vagal stimulation. Compared to measurements on the arrested heart, these procedures have the advantage that contracture during the measuring period was definetely excluded.

During an experiment isovolumetric contractions were obtained by brief occlusions of the ascending aorta. The end-diastolic volume of the left ventricle was varied by gradual obstruction of the inferior vena cava. The average wall stress [36] and the tangent elastic modulus in the middle of the ventricular wall [9, 34] were calculated assuming a thick-walled sphere.

Measurement of Myocardial Mechanics in the Isolated Strip Preparation. These experiments were carried out on trabecular preparations from the rear wall of the left ventricle. The muscle strips were fixed in a measuring apparatus described by Gülch [4]. A temperature controlled tyrode solution was used for perfusion (concentration in mM/l: glucose 25, NaCl 130.5, KCl 4,9, $CaCl_2$ 2.2, NaH_2PO_4 0.8, $NaHCO_3$ 20.0). The solution was constantly bubbled with 95% O_2 und 5% CO_2 (pH = 7.4). The temperature was set at 25 °C or 32 °C depending on the subject of the experiment. Under steady state conditions the isometric length-tension relations were recorded and the force-velocity relations were determined from afterloaded contractions as well as from isometric and isotonic quick release experiments [17, 20, 21].

Furthermore, trabecular preparations were glycerinated for at least 30 min. Quick-release experiments were performed after activation using solutions with defined Ca^{++} concentrations. The shortening velocity was plotted as a function of sarcomere length, which was measured using a light microscope [1, 2, 3].

Electrophysiological Investigations. The membrane potential was measured in trabecular preparations of the free wall of the left ventricle with conventional glass microelectrodes. Ca^{++} mediated action potentials were measured after depression of the fast inward current either by TTX or by partial depolarization under high extracellular K^{+} concentrations [6].

Morphological Studies. Thin isolated muscle strips from the rear wall of the left ventricle were investigated. The quantitative analysis of cell components was made by taking electronmicroscopic pictures at 10,000 magnifications, projecting them onto a dot rule glass screen and then evaluating them using a stereological point counting method [40, 41].

Biochemical Investigations. Tissue weight and content of basic constituents were determined, and proteins were fractionated [29]. The hydroxyproline concentration was measured in samples of 25 or 50 mg dry weight according to Stegemann [37]. The actomyosin solution was extracted from single left ventricles and purified by the dilution technique [27, 32]. Myofibrillar ATPase activity and Ca^{++} ATPase activity of myosin were determined by measuring the liberation of inorganic phosphate [30—32].

Results and Discussion

Development of blood pressure, body weight and heart weight. Within 2—4 weeks after operation systolic arterial pressure, measured by the tail cuff method, rose from a control level of 100 mmHg to 200 mmHg on the average, remained then substantially constant for 3—4 months and showed a tendency towards a slight decrease near the end of the 6-month observation period in most samples 20, 24, 41].

The average body weight of both control and Goldblatt animals was not significantly different after 4 weeks. At this time there was a 30%—50% increase in left ventricular weight as compared to the sham operated controls of the same age which were likewise still growing. Post-operative growth of Goldblatt rats was inhibited in the following weeks and further augmentation of ventricular mass was small. As a result of general inhibition in growth, the absolute left ventricular weight in some samples of Goldblatt rats was nearly equal to that of controls after 8 weeks. However, the weight of the left ventricle in relation to body weight was also still significantly increased in these animals.

Thus, the absolute extent of left ventricular hypertrophy depends not only on the level of blood pressure but also on the general development of the entire organism, which seems to be greatly influenced by hypertensive vasculopathy. An increase in left ventricular mass of more than 70% in comparison to controls is thus rarely obtainable.

Left Ventricular Pressure Volume Relations

As could be expected from the increase in muscular mass, the hypertrophied left ventricle of Goldblatt rats developed a higher isovolumetric pressure at a given end-diastolic pressure in comparison to controls, although the difference was no longer substantial by the 24-week stage. Thus, in the 4- and 8-week stage the curve of total pressure was shifted significantly upwards in the pressure-volume diagram (Fig. 1a, b). The distance between the curve of isovolumetric total pressure and the end-diastolic pressure-volume curve was increased as an indication of enhanced ventricular work capacity [22—24].

However, the typical features of concentric hypertrophy were not present in the 4-week stage. Instead, an augmentation of the diastolic ventricular size was

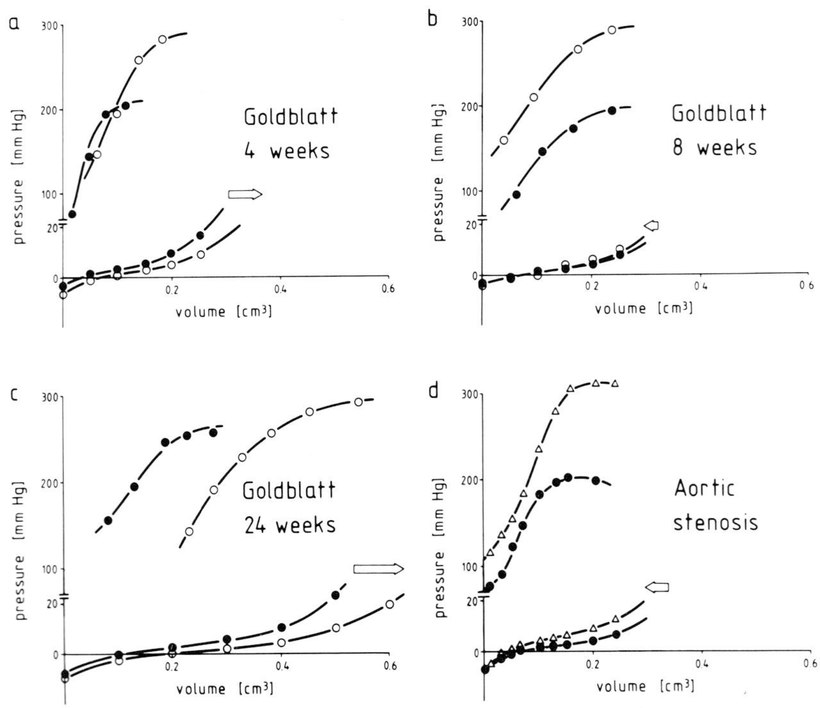

Fig. 1. Isovolumetric pressure-volume relations of the hypertrophied left ventricle of the rat in different stages of Goldblatt hypertension (a—c) and in the 7-week stage of experimental aortic stenosis (d). ○, Goldblatt hypertension 4 (a), 8 (b) and 24 weeks (c); Δ, aortic stenosis (d); ●, control animals of the same age

observed. This is certainly due to a significant (approximately 30%) increase in the circulating blood volume with simultaneously increased hematocrit values as we found in this stage (Goldblatt rats: plasma volume 38.6±1.1 ml/kg body wt., arterial hematocrit 54.9±0.1 vol%; controls: plasma volume 32±0.2 ml/kg body wt., arterial hematocrit 48.3±0.6 vol%). For comparison the pressure-volume relations under experimental aortic stenosis, 7 weeks after supravalvular constriction of the aorta ascendens, are shown as an example of concentric hypertrophy (Fig. 1d) [12].

In the 8-week stage the end-diastolic pressure-volume relations of Goldblatt rats and controls were not substantially different (Fig. 1b). We interpret this as a result of a relatively more intensive body and ventricular growth of the controls and a decreasing trend in the circulating blood volume of the Goldblatt rats [8] in this stage.

After 6 months, however, 7 of 21 specimens investigated to date revealed a significant rightward shift of the isovolumic pressure-volume relations both in diastole and systole (Fig. 1c). The other animals showed alterations similar to the 8-week stage. Although no signs of congestive failure were present and end-

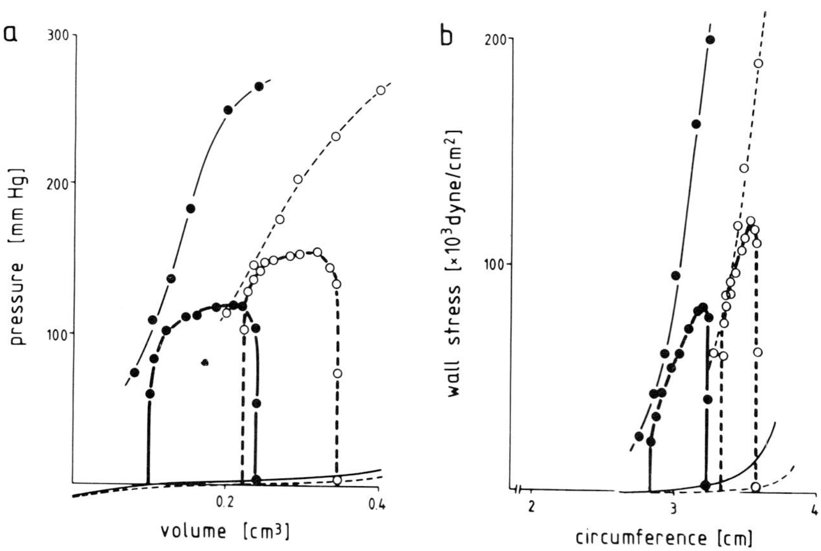

Fig. 2. (a) Representative left ventricular isovolumetric pressure-volume relations and pressure-volume loops of a Goldblatt heart in the 24-week stage and an age-matched control. (b) The mean wall stress, which was calculated under the assumption of a thick-walled spherical shell from the data of Fig. 2(a), is plotted as a function of the circumference at the middle of the ventricular wall. ●, control animal (body weight 450 g, left ventricular weight 0.872 g); ○, Goldblatt rat (body weight 400 g, left ventricular weight 1.119 g)

diastolic pressure was in a normal range, we have indications that structural dilatation was developing in a portion of the animals.

The altered performance of the dilated ventricles in 6-month stage can be deduced from Fig. 2a. This figure shows both the isovolumetric pressure-volume relations and the pressure-volume loop for an individual contraction cycle constructed by means of electromagnetic flow measurements. End-diastolic and end-systolic volumes are substantially increased, the ejection fraction being decreased as a result of altered geometrical conditions and partially also a moderate decrease in myocardial contractile capability (see below). In the 8-week stage, however, the end-diastolic and end-systolic volumes were fairly identical in controls and hypertensive animals, and thus the pressure-volume loop of the hypertensive rats merely deviated from the controls by showing higher pressures in the upper part of the loop (not depicted).

The relation between the isovolumic pressure-volume curve, on the one hand, and the end-systolic pressure-volume loop under normal afterloaded conditions, on the other hand, is of interest when considering a conceivable increase in frictional and deformational resistance due to increased myocardial mass. If a significant increase in intramyocardial resistances occurs during the ejection period at this approximately 40% hypertrophy, one should expect an impairment of fibre shortening such that the end-systolic pressure volume values would be shifted more to the right in relation to the curves of isovolumetric total pressure. This was neither the case, however, in the 8-week stage nor after 24 weeks.

Wall Stress and Length-Stress Relationship

Calculation of wall stress yields an indication of momentary wall loading in systole and diastole as well as of contractile capability [14]. Diastolic wall stress at the usual in situ end-diastolic pressure was only increased in the 4-week stage. Due to the augmentation in ventricular mass, systolic wall stress during normal afterloaded performance equalled the control values in the 8-week-stage despite systemic hypertension. In the 24-week stage, however, wall stress is substantially higher in the dilated ventricles than in controls throughout the entire ejection period, although the end-systolic value is still lower than the value at the end of the isovolumetric period (Fig. 2b). Whereas the absolute degree of fibre shortening is small, stroke volume is in a normal range as a result of the geometric conditions.

Thus, it is obvious that in the 6-month stage a dilatation as defined by Linzbach [25] is beginning in a portion of the animals. Wall growth is not sufficient to prevent an increase in systolic wall loading, i.e. the required wall stress development. As illustrated in Fig. 3, average systolic wall stress compared to controls remained constant in the initial weeks (when disregarding the immediately postoperative stage) and was accompanied by a decreasing ratio of inner radius to wall thickness, whereas in later stages wall loading increased markedly as a result of limited mass increase.

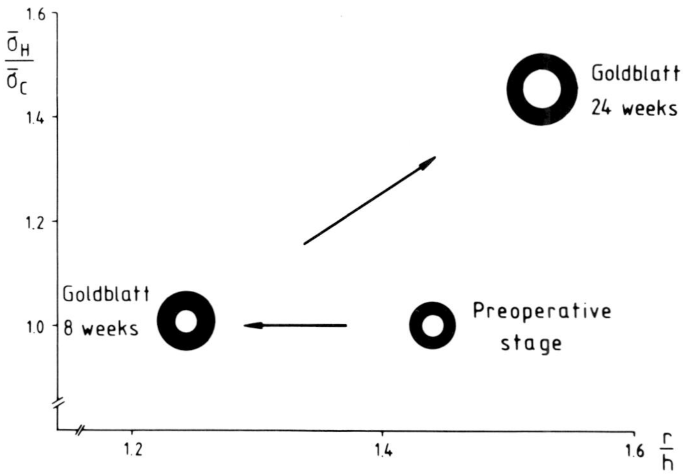

Fig. 3. According to the formula $\sigma = \frac{P \cdot r}{2 \cdot h}$, wall stress depends on ventricular pressure (P), (inner) ventricular radius (r) and ventricular wall thickness (h). The quotient of mean systolic wall stress of the hypertrophied ventricles to age-matched controls expressed as a function of the inner radius/wall thickness ratio is shown for the 8-week stage and the dilated ventricles in the 24-week stage of Goldblatt hypertension, starting from the preoperative stage

Correlation of Hemodynamic Values

Due to differences in heart size, the results varied depending on whether haemodynamic values were correlated with end-diastolic ventricular volume (V_d) or pressure (EDP). Thus, the advantage of plotting the results in the form of pressure-volume diagrams is obvious. Nevertheless, consideration of the time course of ventricular contraction yields additional indications of cardiac dynamics. The parameters (isovolumic pressure, maximum rate of pressure rise, stroke volume, maximum flow rate) of the ventricles dilated in the 24-week stage were still higher than, or in the range of, age-matched control values when plotted as a function of end-diastolic pressure. Thus, power capacity of the ventricle as a whole was still increased due to the augmentation of muscle mass. Yet, stroke volume, maximum flow rate and acceleration were reduced when related to end-diastolic volume, in agreement with Fig. 2.

A decrease in acceleration ($d^2 V/dt^2$) was observed early as the 8-week stage of Goldblatt hypertension, and was even noticeable after a few weeks of swimming training. Thus, such an alteration in cardiac dynamics is no viewed as an early sign of insufficiency, but rather as a characteristic of the hypertrophied heart.

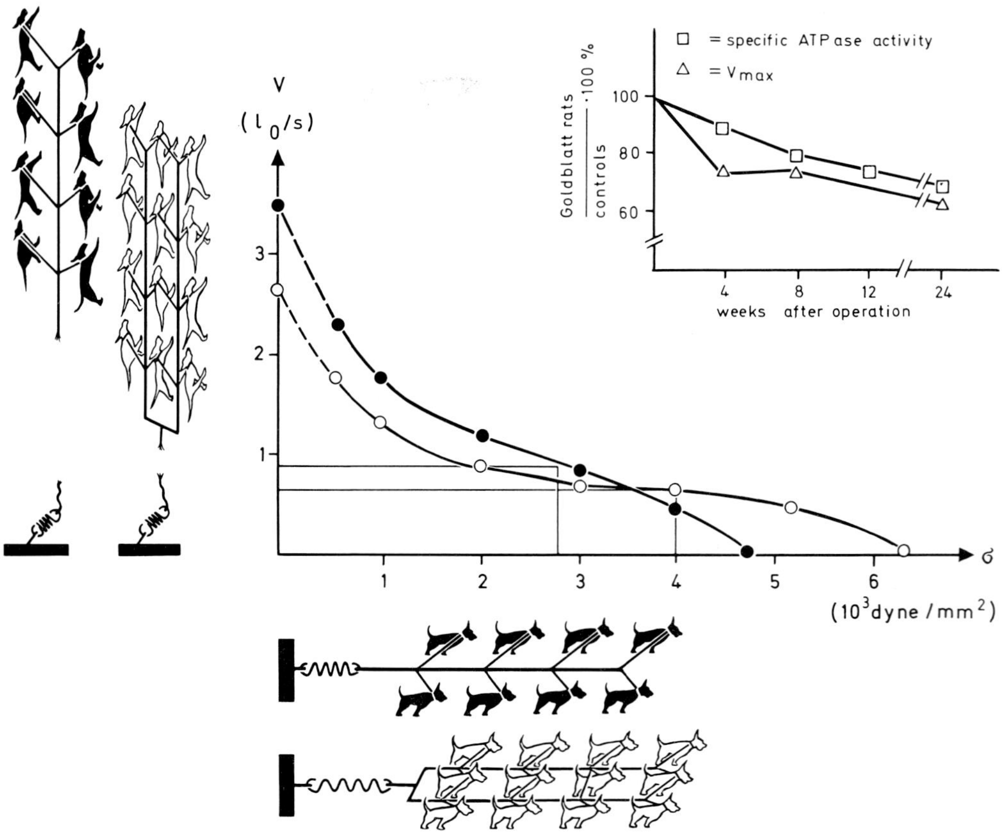

Fig. 4. Force-velocity relations measured from afterloaded contractions on isolated trabecular muscle strips of the left ventricle. The intersection of the curves is caused by a decrease in unloaded shortening velocity in the hypertrophied preparations (*ordinate*), while developed tension is increased (*abscissa*). The maximum momentary power (*maximum rectangle* under the force-velocity curve), however, is not reduced in early stages of hypertrophy. ○, Goldblatt hypertension, 8-week stage; ●, age-matched controls. The schematic presentation illustrates the density of interaction sites between actin and myosin and the load of the cross bridges. Inset, maximum shortening velocity (△) as well as specific Ca^{++}ATPase activity of myosin (□) decline continuously over the period of observation in Goldblatt myocardium. From (16)

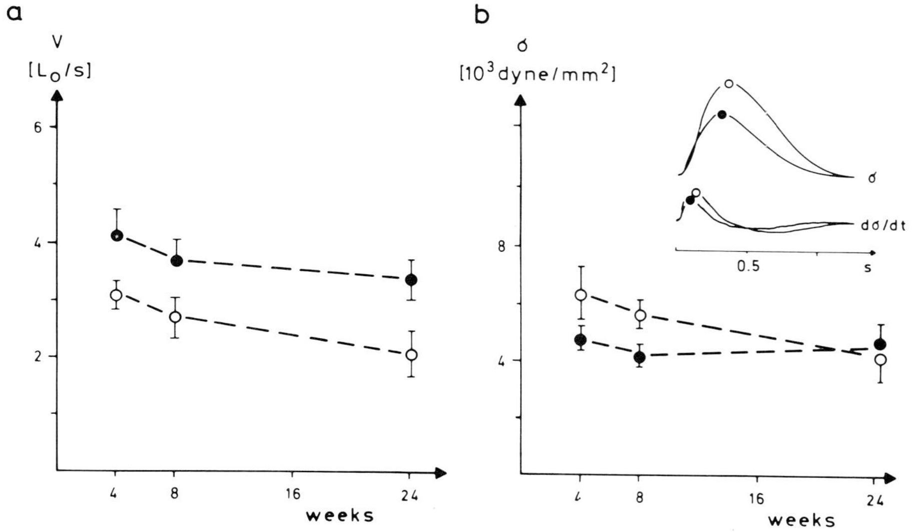

Fig. 5. Time-dependent changes of (a) V_{max} (V) and (b) developed tension (σ) during the period of observation. Measurements on isolated trabecular muscle strips of the left ventricle. *Inset:* Comparison of the isometric mechanograms in the early stage of Goldblatt hypertension. ○, Goldblatt hypertension in the 4-, 8- and 24-week stages; •, age-matched controls. From [20].

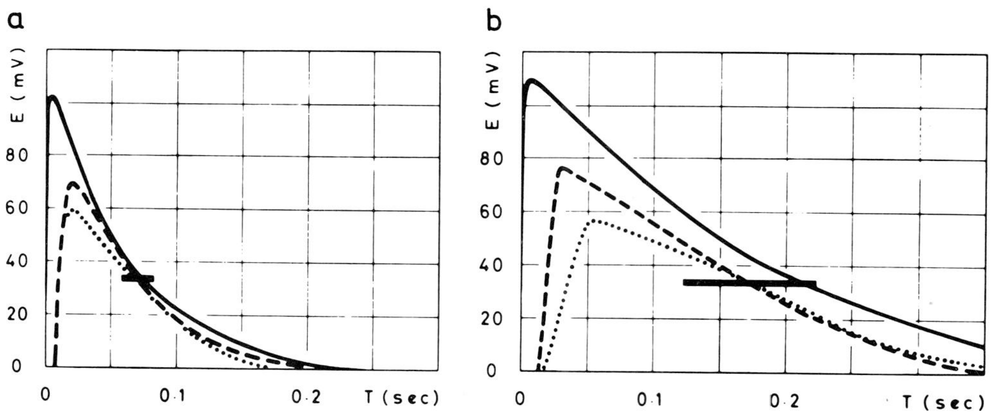

Fig. 6. Mean action potential constructed from measurements on Goldblatt rats in the 12 week stage (b) and on corresponding controls (a).
———, standard solution; - - - - - -, 13 m*M* K^+, 2.2 m*M* Ca^{++}; · · · · · ·, 13 m*M* K^+, 0.55 m*M* Ca^{++}. Note that all action potentials are superimposed starting from the same baseline. The standard deviation is indicated by the *horizontal bars*. From [6]

Myocardial Contractile Capability in Whole Heart and Isolated Strip Preparations in Different Stages of Goldblatt Hypertension

In the isolated hypertrophied myocardial preparations, the initial rate of tension development is markedly slower than in controls (Fig. 5 inset). Nevertheless, in the earlier stages of Goldblatt hypertension, the maximum rate of tension rise and peak isometric tension were increased, accompanied by a prolonged time to peak [6, 17, 20]. This is in agreement with the enhanced isovolumetric stress of the whole left ventricle in early stages [24], whereas isometric stress attains at best control values in most other models of pressure-induced hypertrophy.

In the course of the first 6 months the initially increased (isometric or isovolumic) stress returned to or below control levels both in the whole heart and in the isolated preparations (Fig. 5b). [Quantitative differences in the calculated stress values, on the one hand, and the measured results in the isolated myocardium, on the other hand, are certainly due to the fact that the usually employed concentration of free Ca^{++} ions (2.2 m*M*) and the temperature do not correspond to the actual physiological conditions.]

In contrast, maximum shortening velocity under external zero load was already reduced by about 25% in the early stage of hypertension, as determined on the basis of afterloaded contractions or by isotonic quick release experiments. This results in a crossing of the tension-velocity curves when the usual graphical presentation for afterloaded contractions is employed (Fig. 4). As Fig. 5a and Fig. 4 (inset) show, the apparent V_{max} continually decreased over the first 6-month period. A slight age-dependent reduction in V_{max} was also seen in the controls. Maximum instantaneous power, which was not substantially altered or even slightly increased in the early stage, showed a corresponding reduction below the control norm over the same period [20].

Interpretation of Hypertrophy-Induced Alterations in Myocardial Mechanics on the Basis of Biochemical, Morphological, and Electrophysiological Investigations

The described alterations in muscle mechanics and the time course thereof suggest several questions of principle significance:

1. How can the discrepancy between unloaded shortening velocity and developed tension be explained, particularly the initially increased isometric tension?
2. Is the reduction in V_{max} due to processes of excitation and electromechanical coupling or to alterations in contractile proteins, particularly altered specific ATPase activity of myosin?
3. Could a reduction in the latter parameters be a partial cause of conceivable later contractile failure?
4. What other alterations contribute to contractile impairment?

Additional methodological approaches were required for dealing with these questions.

Contractile Material Content

The ratio of the volume of myofibrils to total cell volume was significantly (by 7%—12%) increased in all stages of Goldblatt hypertension [17, 40, 41], the concentration of contractile protein being increased [15, 29, 32].

The relative augmentation in contractile material content should indicate an increase in the number of available interaction sites per unit cross section and thus an increase in developed tension as illustrated by a closer arrangement of the white dogs in the scheme of Fig. 4. This aspect, a variability of fibril content in chronic myocardial alterations, apparently receives too little attention in the pathophysiological literature. It is not possible, however, to attribute the reduction in developed tension between the 4- and 24-week stage to a decrease in actomyosin concentration. For actomyosin content was clearly increased after 6 months in comparison to controls (178±6 and 148±5 mg/g dry wt., respectively) despite the increase in hydroxyproline concentration (3.49±0.3 and 2.87±0.2 μg/mg dry wt., respectively).

In contrast, unloaded shortening velocity should be independent of the number of interaction sites — in the ideal case (Fig. 4, ordinate). The possible relationship between unloaded shortening velocity, on the one hand, and ATPase activity, on the other hand, will be discussed below. Both values showed a roughly parallel decrease during the period of observation [16, 17, 32] (Fig. 4, inset). It is difficult, however, to relate unloaded shortening velocity to a certain biochemical parameter (e.g. ATPase-activity) because the apparent value of V_{max} is also influenced by the Ca^{++} concentration [5]. In Goldblatt myocardium one finds electrophysiological and mechanical alterations which suggest changes in the rate, intensity and duration of Ca^{++} activation.

Action Potential

The most remarkable electrophysiological feature of the pressure-hypertrophied myocardium is a considerable prolongation of the plateau phase of the action potential (Fig. 6) [6]. The halfwidth of the action potential increased with increasing degree of hypertrophy. The so-called Ca^{++} action potentials obtained in partially depolarized myocardium under various Ca^{++} concentrations were also prolonged. These alterations are probably the result of a delayed inactivation of the slow transmembrane influx which prolongs the period of activation and should also increase the amount of Ca^{++} available for intracellular storage.

Thus, the prolonged duration of the action potential explains the increased time to peak tension and is also a partial cause of the increased isometric tension development in the early stage of Goldblatt hypertension.

In view of the Ca^{++} diffusion distance, the intracellular conduction system and Ca^{++} stores are of particular interest. As demonstrated by electron microscopic investigations, the internal membrane systems clearly show signs of hypertrophy and enlargement. As a result, the ratio of inner tubuli (T-system and sarcoplasmic reticulum) to total cell volume was not reduced in the investigated stages [40, 41].

Dysfunction of the Ca^{++}-sequestering system has been described in other models of hypertrophy [7, 33, 38]. Although our own investigations on the Goldblatt myocardium have not yet been completed, it can be assumed that there are comparable alterations in the later stages of this model as well. Incomplete relaxation seen at high stimulation frequency, however, is rather due to prolonged time to peak tension than to decreased relaxation rate [18]. On the other hand, the retarded force development in the earliest phase of tension rise as described above (Fig. 5, inset) could indicate an initially retarded Ca^{++} release.

In view of these different alterations which could be related to Ca^{++} activation, it was necessary to perform measurements on native preparations under more defined conditions of electromechanical coupling as well as on glycerinated preparations under given Ca^{++} concentrations [3, 18].

Experimental increase of external Ca^{++}concentration under simultaneous reduction of sodium in native preparations could not raise the apparent V_{max} to the same level attained by controls under identical conditions, and also had moderate influence on developed tension. This does not suggest that processes of electromechanical coupling are the decisive factor in the reduction of contractile capability in this model.

Investigations on glycerinated fibres also showed Ca^{++} independent alterations in V_{max} of Goldblatt myocardium. The *apparent* value of V_{max} under external zero load was clearly influenced by Ca^{++}. However, consideration of an internal load by extrapolation of the lenght-velocity relations to the starting length of the respective quick release yields serious indications for a Ca^{++} independent V_{max} as was shown in normal myocardium [2]. A reduced value of unloaded shortening velocity was obtained on the basis of this concept as well [0.91 ML/s in Goldblatt myocardium and 1.28 ML/s in controls (temperature 5 °C)]. In myocardium of the same ventricles the myofibrilar ATPase activity was reduced from 0.23 to 0.15 μM $P_i \cdot mg^{-1} \cdot min^{-1}$ [3].

Myofibrillar Proteins; Myofibrillar and Myosin ATPase Activity

The described Ca^{++} independent alterations suggest that changes in the contractile proteins themselves must be present which cause a reduction in shortening velocity. As already mentioned, unloaded shortening velocity and myofibrillar ATPase activity were reduced to a comparable degree (to 71.1% and 65.2%, respectively) in glycerinated fibres. Thus, our results are compatible with the assumption of an intrinsic relationship between both parameters. The Ca^{++} ATPase activity of myosin revealed alterations in the same direction (Fig. 4, inset) [16, 32].

Recently a reduction in the apparent V_{max} was shown in chemically skinned preparations from a model of hypertrophy which could be more suitable for clarification of this special problem [26], although fibrosis has been excluded in our preparations. However, the relation between ATPase activity and isometric force development in chronically altered myocardium seems to require further clarification.

The question of the extent to which alterations in stoichiometry of different myosin components play a role in reduced ATPase activity has not been definitively answered [28, 31]: the myosin light chains to heavy chains ratio (LC/HC) as well as the ratio of light $chain_1$ to light $chain_2$ (LC_1/LC_2) was slightly decreased in the 24-week stage of Goldblatt hypertension [31]. Furthermore, changes in the heavy chain of myosin might also be responsible for a change in the isoenzyme pattern.

Indications of an influence of the process of hypertrophy on the troponin-tropomyosin system were not found. Neither a change in cooperativity nor in Ca^{++} sensitivity of troponin occurs in Goldblatt myocardium [35].

The significance of structural alterations in the contractile proteins for the development of contractile impairment is disputable [16, 39] (see also Session B, Alpert et al.). In our opinion the decrease in ATPase activity is certainly not the primary cause of heart failure. Nevertheless, even if we assume that reduced ATPase activity improves efficiency of the individual contractions [see Session B, Alpert et al.], we must also consider the continuous decrease in myocardial power with decreasing V_{max}, which is represented by the area below the force-velocity curve. Thus, we should not exclude the possibility that these alterations could be an unfavourable factor in later stages.

Hypertensive Vasculopathy; Mitochondrial Alterations and Connective Tissue Content

In the 24-week stage vascular alterations with hyperplasia and hypertrophy of the media and frequent diffuse fibrosis became evident [40, 41]. Whereas a continuous decrease in mitochondrial volume and mitochondria-myofibril ratio was generally observed, marked qualitative mitochondrial alterations occured only in a portion of the specimens, probably due to O_2 deficiency caused by vascular alterations [41]. Occasionally scars could be seen macroscopically. In some specimens such alterations already occurred at an earlier stage. Obviously those preparations with the highest connective tissue content showed the worst mechanical performance [3, 18]. This must be considered when correlating V_{max} and ATPase activity in the later stages.

Thus, hypertensive vasculopathy appears to be an important factor contributing to morphological and functional alterations in later stages of Goldblatt hypertension with altered mitochondrial ultrastructure, myocardial cell necroses, fibrosis and structural dilatation. Catecholamine depletion due to chronic haemodynamic overloading could be intensified by the concurrent appearance of vasculopathy as well.

Myocardial Elasticity in Goldblatt Hypertension

A decrease in myocardial distensibility is always measured in preparations from the 24-week stage or calculated from the diastolic pressure-volume relationship

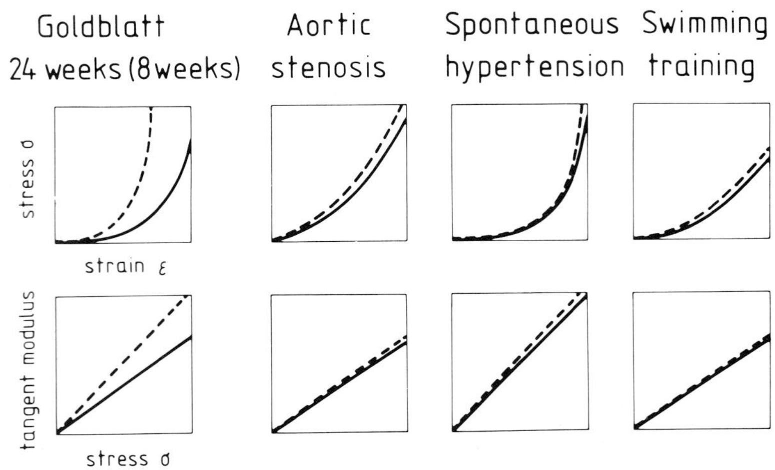

	Goldblatt	Aortic stenosis	Spontaneous hypertension	Swimming training	
Hypertrophy	3.49	3.36	4.17	2.90	µg hydroxyproline/mg dry wt
Control	2.87	3.02	3.36	2.91	
Degree of hypertrophy	51%	18%	50%	15%	

Fig. 7. Stress-strain relations, tangent modulus-stress relations and hydroxyproline concentrations in various models of cardiac hypertrophy. Goldblatt hypertension: In the early stages diastolic distensibility can be unchanged or already decreased. Aortic stenosis: 7 weeks after operation. Spontaneous hypertension: The animals were 40-week-old; controls were provided by normal Sprague-Dawley rats of the same age (SuT: SDT strain, Süddeutsche Versuchstierfarm, Tuttlingen). Swimming training: 2 hours daily for 10 weeks. From [10–12, 18, 20, 21, 29]

of the whole ventricle at this stage. The relation between tangent modulus and stress is substantially steeper, indicating a "fibrosis type" [10, 11, 19] of decreased distensibility (Fig. 7). However, a pronounced increase in stiffness can also appear in earlier stages, apparently due to the above mentioned vascular alterations.

This decrease in distensibility is not reversible by withdrawal of Ca^{++} or by administration of Ca^{++} antagonists [10] and must probably be directly attributed to the increase in collagen tissue. Discrepancies between elastic properties and collagen content, which we assumed to occur in early stages of Goldblatt hypertension [18, 20, 41], could have had methodological causes, because both parameters were not determined in the same individual strip preparations. The arrangement of connective tissue may also be involved. A significant increase in stiffness, however, is obviously not an intrinsic characteristic of hypertrophy process, as is shown by comparison with some other models in Fig. 7.

Conclusions

In Goldblatt rats defects due to hypertensive vasculopathy are increasingly superimposed on the alterations resulting from pressure-induced cardiac overloading. The complexity of the resulting changes make this model less suitable for clarification of specific questions concerning the process of fibre hypertrophy per se. However, the model presents some features common to heart disease in certain forms of human hypertension and — with the above restriction — appears well suited to the study of the interesting phase of pre-insufficiency.

Summary

Left ventricular dynamics and myocardial mechanics in the first 6 months following unilateral renal artery coarctation are analysed on the basis of biochemical, electrophysiological and morphological investigations. The early manifested alterations are interpreted in view of their potential significance for a later decrease in contractile capability. The signs of concentric hypertrophy are found in the first months of hypertension with augmented work capacity and ventricular mass increase — which seldom excedes 70% of the age-matched control value and is accompanied by a general inhibition of body growth. The diastolic pressure-volume relation in the 4-week stage is modified by an increased circulating blood volume. In the 24-week stage a portion of the animals reveal a significant left ventricular dilatation with increased rest volume and systolic wall stress under normal afterloaded performance, but without signs of congestive heart failure. The calculated value of active isovolumic tension as well as the measured isometric tension in the isolated preparation are significantly increased in the 4-week stage and then decrease continually to slightly below the control level by the 24-week stage. In contrast, the apparent value of unloaded shortening velocity is already reduced by about 25% in the 4-week stage and continues to decrease during the following weeks.

The discrepancy between active tension development and V_{max} can be partially explained by increased contractile material content and prolonged duration of the action potential (prolonged plateau phase of the action potential and prolonged "Ca^{++} action potential") under reduced myofibrillar ATPase activity. The relation between tension development and ATPase activity requires further clarification, however, in order to evaluate the significance of a change in cross-bridge kinetics. In glycerinated preparations from Goldblatt myocardium a Ca^{++}-independent reduction in maximum unloaded shortening velocity was demonstrated — by consideration of an internal load. This is compatible with the assumption of an intrinsic relation between V_{max} and myofibrillar ATPase activity. A peculiarity of the Goldblatt model is the early onset of hypertensive vasculopathy with qualitative mitochondrial alterations, myocardial cell necroses and increased connective tissue content, especially in the perivascular space. The decrease in myocardial distensibility can probably also be sufficienctly explained by the increasing collagen content.

The effects of vasculopathy are superimposed on the alterations induced by hemodynamic overloading, i.e. the process of myocardial hypertrophy itself, and appear to be an important factor contributing to functional alterations in later stages of Goldblatt hypertension.

References

1. Brenner B (1979) Indirekter Nachweis einer dehnungsinduzierten Ca^{++}-Freisetzung aus dem sarkoplasmatischen Retikulum glyzerinisierter Skelett- und Herzmuskelpräparate. Basis Res Cardiol 74 : 177—202
2. Brenner B, Jacob R (1978) A theoretical and experimental approach to determination of the true value of maximum unloaded shortening velocity (V_{max}) in muscle. Pfluegers Arch [Suppl] 377 : 1
3. Ebrecht G, Brenner B, Jacob R (1979) Ca^{++} independent reduction of the unloaded shortening velocity of hypertrophic left ventricular myocardium of Goldblatt rats. Biennial Meeting of the International Society for Heart Research European Section, Dijon
4. Gülch RW (1974) A critical analysis of myocardial force velocity relations obtained from damped quick-release experiments. Basic Res Cardiol 69 : 32—46
5. Gülch RW (1977) The effect of preload and Ca^{++}-ions on the timecourse of the isometric force and on the force-velocity relation: Is V_{max} dependent on the number of activated cross-bridges? Basic Res Cardiol 72 : 102—108
6. Gülch RW, Baumann R, Jacob R (1979) Analysis of myocardial action potential in left ventricular hypertrophy of Goldblatt rats. Basic Res Cardiol 74 : 69—82
7. Heilmann C, Lindl T, Müller W, Pette D (1980) Characterization of cardiac microsomes from spontaneously hypertonic rats. Basic Res Cardiol 75 : 92—96
8. Helmchen U (1973) Der relative Reninismus als ein pathogenetisches Prinzip der renalen Hypertonie. Habilitationsschrift, University of Tübingen

9. Hepp A, Hansis M, Gülch R, Jacob R (1974) Left ventricular isovolumetric pressure-volume relations, "diastolic tone" and contractility in the rat heart after physical training. Basic Res Cardiol 69 : 516–532
10. Holubarsch C, Holubarsch T (1979) Stress-strain relationships and tangent modulus in anoxic and hypertrophied myocardium. Pfluegers Arch [Suppl] 379 : 4
11. Holubarsch C, Jacob R (1979) Evaluation of elastic properties of myocardium. Experimental models of fibrosis and contracture in heart muscle strips. Z Kardiol 68 : 123–127
12. Horneff G, Holubarsch C, Jacob R (to be published) Left ventricular isovolumetric pressure-volume relations, wall stress and elastic modulus in rats with experimental aortic stenosis. Basic Res Cardiol
13. Jacob R (1976) Pathophysiologie der Herzmuskelinsuffizienz. In: Erkrankungen des Herzmuskels. Thieme, Stuttgart, pp 25–36
14. Jacob R, Gülch R, Holubarsch C, Kissling G (1975) Die Bewertung der myokardialen Leistungsfähigkeit. Muskelphysiologische Grundlagen und methodische Probleme. Med Klinik 70 : 1347–1365
15. Jacob R, Kämmereit A, Medugorac I (1975) Significance of actomyosin concentration for the contractile capability of the hypertrophied myocardium. Internat. Study Group for Res. Cardiol. Metabolism, European Section, Bruessel 80 (abstr.)
16. Jacob R, Kämmereit A, Medugorac I, Wendt-Gallitelli MF (1976) Maximalgeschwindigkeit der lastfreien Verkürzung (V_{max}), myokardiale Leistungsfähigkeit und „Kontraktilitätsindizes" beim hypertrophierten Myokard. Z Kardiol 65 : 392–400
17. Jacob R, Ebrecht G, Kämmereit A, Medugorac I, Wendt-Gallitelli MF (1977) Myocardial function in different models of cardiac hypertrophy. An attempt at correlating mechanical, biochemical and morphological parameters. Basic Res Cardiol 72 : 160–166
18. Jacob R, Brenner B, Ebrecht G, Holubarsch C, Medugorac J (1980) Elastic and contractile properties of the hypertrophied myocardium in Goldblatt hypertension and experimental aortic stenosis of the rat. Methodological and pathophysiological considerations. Basic Res Cardiol 75 : 253–261
19. Jacob R, Holubarsch C, Moser H, Brenner B (1980) Quantification of changes in myocardial elasticity under hypoxia. Model experiments on whole heart preparations and isolated muscle strips. In: International Symposium Advances Clinical Cardiol, Quantification of myocardial ischemia, Vol 1 : 211–228, Witzstrock New York
20. Kämmereit A, Jacob R (1979) Alterations in rat myocardial mechanics under Goldblatt hypertension and experimental aortic stenosis. Basic Res Cardiol 74 : 389–405
21. Kämmereit A, Medugorac I, Steil E, Jacob R (1975) Mechanics of the isolated ventricular myocardium of rats conditioned by physical training. Basic Res Cardiol 70 : 495–507
22. Kissling G, Wendt-Gallitelli MF (1977) Dynamics of the hypertrophied left ventricle in the rat. Effects of physical training and chronic pressure load. Basic Res Cardiol 72 : 178–183

23. Kissling G, Gassenmaier T, Gülch R, Jacob R (1974) Probleme der Kontraktilitätsbewertung am Beispiel des hypertrophierten Rattenherzens. Verh Dtsch Ges Kreislaufforsch 40 : 262—266
24. Kissling G, Gassenmaier T, Wendt-Gallitelli MF, Jacob R (1977) Pressure-volume relations, elastic modulus, and contractile behaviour of the hypertrophied left ventricle of rats with Goldblatt II hypertension. Pfluegers Arch 269 : 213—221
25. Linzbach AJ (1959) Morphologische Gesichtspunkte der Herzdynamik. Herzinsuffizienz und Digitaliswirkungen. Springer, Berlin Göttingen Heidelberg (Bad Oeynhausener Gespräche 3, 1958, p 20)
26. Maughan D, Low E, Litten R, Brayden J, Alpert NR (1979) Calcium-activated muscle from hypertrophied rabbit hearts. Circ Res 44 : 279—287
27. Medugorac I (1975) Bedeutung und Problematik der Reindarstellung von Myosin. Instrum Forsch 4 : 22—30
28. Medugorac I (1975) Subunits of myosin. Relations to ATPase activity and mechanical function of muscle. Basic Res Cardiol 70 : 467—479
29. Medugorac I (1976) Different fractions in the normal and hypertrophied rat ventricular myocardium: An analysis of two models of hypertrophy. Basic Res Cardiol 71 : 608—623
30. Medugorac I (1977) Characteristics of the hypertrophied left ventricular myocardium in Goldblatt rats. Basic Res Cardiol 72 : 261—267
31. Medugorac I (1980) The myofibrillar ATPase activity and the substructure of myosin in the hypertrophied left ventricle of the rat. Basic Res Cardiol 75 : 163—170
32. Medugorac I, Jacob R (1976) Concentration and adenosintriphosphatase activity of left ventricular actomyosin in Goldblatt rats during the compensatory stage of hypertrophy. Hoppe Seylers Z Physiol Chem 357 : 1495—1503
33. Meerson FZ (1976) Insufficiency of hypertrophied heart. Basic Res Cardiol 71 : 343—354
34. Mirsky I, Parmley WW (1973) Assessment of passive elastic stiffness for isolated heart muscle and the intact heart. Circ Res 33 : 233—243
35. Rupp H (1980) Cooperative effects of calcium on myofibrillar ATPase of normal and hyperthropied heart. Basic Res Cardiol 75 : 157—162
36. Sandler H, Dodge HT (1963) Left ventricular tension and stress in man. Circ Res 13 : 91—104
37. Stegemann H (1958) Mikrobestimmung von Hydroxyprolin mit Chloramin-T und p-Dimethylaminobenzaldehyd. Hoppe Seylers Z Physiol Chem 311 : 41
38. Suko J, Vogel HK, Chidsey CA (1970) Intracellular calcium and myocardial contractility. III. Reduced calcium uptake and ATPase of the sarcoplasmic reticular fraction prepared from chronically failing calf hearts. Circ Res 27 : 235
39. Swynghedauw B, Schwartz K, Leger JJ (1977) Cardiac myosin. Phylogenic and pathological changes. Basic Res Cardiol 72 : 254—260
40. Wendt-Gallitelli MF, Jacob R (1977) Time course of electron microscopic alterations in the hypertrophied myocardium of Goldblatt rats. Basic Res Cardiol 72 : 209—213

41. Wendt-Gallitelli MF, Ebrecht G, Jacob R (1979) Morphological alterations and their functional interpretation in the hypertrophied myocardium of Goldblatt hypertensive rats. J Mol Cell Cardiol 11 : 275–287

Catecholamines in Experimental and Essential Hypertension[1, 2]

H. GROBECKER, J.M. SAAVEDRA AND P. DOMINIAK

Summary

Catecholamines and catecholamine-synthesizing enzymes have been investigated in specific brain areas, plasma, and adrenal glands during the development of high blood pressure in spontaneously hypertensive rats (SHR) and rats made hypertensive by administration of deoxycorticosterone and sodium chloride (DOCA-salt hypertensive rats). Changes in catecholamine metabolism were localized to regions of the brain implicated in the regulation of blood pressure. In SHR noradrenaline (NA) levels and dopamine-β-hydroxylase (DBH) activities were decreased in specific nuclei of the hypothalamus and in the nucleus interstitialis striae terminalis ventralis, in both young and adult rats. The decrease in the formation of NA can result in a reduced activation of central α-adrenergic receptors in depressor areas, which may be related causally to the onset of hypertension. The activity of the adrenaline-forming enzyme, phenyl ethanoloamine-N-methyltransferase (PNMT) was increased in brain stem areas of young SHR (A_1, A_2, area postrema), but it was normal in adult hypertensive animals. Adrenaline (A) levels in these areas were decreased in young SHR. In DOCA-salt hypertensive rats, enhanced PNMT activity occurred in A_1, area postrema, and locus coeruleus and extended to A_2 area with prolonged treatment and higher blood pressure. Plasma NA and DBH activity were increased in young SHR. In addition plasma A was increased in young stroke-prone SHR. In DOCA-salt hypertensive rats plasma NA was increased.

In adrenal glands of young SHR activities of tyrosine hydroxylase (TH), DBH, and PNMT as well as A content were decreased. In adult SHR, only TH turned to an enhanced activity. Also in DOCA-salt hypertensive rats, TH activity and A content of adrenal glands were increased. Administration of PNMT inhibitors or depletion of adrenal catecholamines by an adrenergic neurone blocking drug result in a normalization of the blood pressure in both models studied.

The results suggest that central and peripheral catecholaminergic neurons may play a role during onset and maintenance of genetic and experimental hypertension.

---

1 Supported by a grant from the Deutsche Forschungsgemeinschaft (Gr 274/10)
2 Dedicated to Prof. F. Gross on the occasion of his 68th birthday

In patients with essential hypertension circulating NA levels were not significantly different from normotensive subjects. Also, no changes in resting plasma NA and A could be observed in patients with stabilized essential hypertension before or after acute or chronic administration of propranolol. However, during propranolol treatment exercise significantly increased circulating NA.[3]

Introduction

In recent years the involvement of the sympathetic nervous system and the adrenal glands during the development and maintenance of high blood pressure in models of experimental hypertension and essential hypertension has been studied intensively [3]. In SHR [23] and DOCA-salt hypertensive rats [7], peripheral noradrenergic nerves, the adrenal medulla, and central noradrenergic and adrenergic neurons may play a role in the course of development of high blood pressure. The introduction of sensitive and specific radiometric assays for catecholamines and their synthesizing enzymes in combination with the microdissection of specific brain nuclei has made it possible to study changes in specific brain areas of rats implicated in the regulation of blood pressure [32]. Moreover, these quantitative radiometric methods of assessing sympathetic function were applied to measure circulating catecholamines and DBH activity in hypertensive rats and patients with essential hypertension [10, 27]. In the present paper results of experiments in the two animal models and in patients with essential hypertension are reported.

Material and Methods

Experimental Models of Hypertension

Male SHR and normotensive rats of the Wistar-Kyoto substrain, from which SHR were derived, were obtained from Taconic Farms, Germantown, New York, and maintained under identical conditions for 1 week until killed. Unilaterally nephrectomized rats, obtained from Zivic-Miller Laboratories, Allison Park, Pennsylvania, were made hypertensive by injection of deoxycorticosterone pivalate (25 mg/kg subcutaneous injection weekly of Percorten, Ciba Geigy Corp.) and sodium chloride 1% as drinking fluid. Controls received tap water as drinking fluid.

Systolic blood pressure was measured by a tail cuff plethysmographic method using a pneumatic pulse transducer and a programmed electrosphygmomanometer (Narco Biosystems, Houston, Texas).

Brain dissection was performed as described elsewhere [16, 30, 33]. The rats were killed by decapitation of 9 a.m., the brains were quickly removed and

3 Note added in proof: In young hypertensive patients elevated plasma concentrations of NA and A could be observed. (Dominiak, P., Kunkel, G., Grobecker, H., 1980), Abstract No. 0506. 1. World Conference on Clinical Pharmacology and Therapeutics, London

immediately frozen on dry ice, and serial sections 300 μm thick were cut in a cryostat at -10^0 C. Specific areas and brain nuclei were located under a dissecting microscope and dissected by the use of a needle with an internal diameter of 0.5 mm.

Blood samples were collected from a chronic arterial catheter in the tail artery and prepared for assay of DBH activity and catecholamines as described previously [10].

Adrenal glands were rapidly removed after decapitation of the animals, homogenized in cold isotonic sucrose, and aliquoted for determination of catecholamines and catecholamine-forming enzyme activities.

Biochemical Methods. The catecholamines dopamine, NA and A were assayed simultaneously by a modification of recently described isotopic radioenzymatic assays [5, 26] or NA was measured by the method of Henry et al. [13]. In brain nuclei PNMT and DBH were assayed as previously described [30, 32]. In the adrenal A and NA were measured according to Anton and Sayre [1]. Tyrosine hydroxylase was determined by the method of Nagatsu et al. [21], and DBH according to Molinoff et al. [20]. PNMT activity was measured by the method of Axelrod [2].

Proteins were measured in aliquots of brain and adrenal homogenates by the method of Lowry et al. [19]. Drugs used were: 2-guanyl-1, 2, 3, 10, 12, hexahydro-1, 2, a-pyrazinoindole hydrochloride, EMD 21 192, E. Merck AG. Darmstadt, West Germany; 2, 3-dichloro-*a* methyl-benzylaminehydrochloride (DCMB), Lilly Research Lab., Indianapolis, Indiana, United States and 3-Methyl-1, 2, 3, 4-tetrahydro [1] benzothieno-[3, 2-c] pyridine hydrochloride (SKF 7698), Smith, Kline and French Laboratories, Philadelphia, Pennsylvania, United States.

Human Investigations

During a screening program for search of high blood pressure 76 volunteers, age, sex, and race matched, were selected. Blood pressure was measured and the subjects divided into a hypertensive group (blood pressure over 140/80 n=40) and a normotensive group (blood pressure 100/70 to 135/80, n=36). After a rest of 30 min in supine position, a blood sample was taken from an antecubital vein for resting circulating NA and another two samples after standing for 5 and 10 min. Plasma NA was assayed according to Henry et al. [13].

In 12 patients with essential hypertension (WHO stage II) plasma catecholamines were assayed before and after acute or chronic treatment with propranolol. Hypertensive patients were diagnosed as having essential hypertension if there was no sign of associated diseases or complications. Blood pressure was measured in the radial artery by means of a Statham pressure transducer. Physical exercise was performed with an electrically braked bicycle ergometer in a supine position. Noradrenaline and A were assayed according to Passon and Peuler [24].

Table 1. Noradrenaline concentrations (NA) dopamine-β-hydroxylase (DBH) activity in forebrain nuclei of SHR and Wistar-Kyoto rats (WKY).[a] (Modified from Saavedra and Grobecker 1979)

	NA at age of 4 weeks		14 weeks		DBH at age of 4 weeks		14 weeks	
	WKY	SHR	WKY	SHR	WKY	SHR	WKY	SHR
Nucleus interstitialis striae terminalis ventralis	54.9±6.1	35.1±4.7[b]	58.0±8.7	32.1±3.4[b]	3.2±0.3	1.5±0.4[b]	5.1±0.6	2.5±0.2[b]
Hypothalamus								
Nucleus anterior	25.0±2.9	14.4±1.2[b]	19.6±2.0	9.4±1.2[b]	1.7±0.3	2.0±0.3	2.0±0.1	1.4±0.2[b]
Nucleus periventricularis	38.1±3.1	25.1±2.3[b]	34.5±3.5	20.5±3.9[b]	3.7±0.2	2.9±0.1[b]	4.7±0.2	3.0±0.3[b]
Nucleus paraventricularis	16.0±2.2	8.8±1.2[b]	19.6±1.2	12.9±2.0[b]				
Nucleus ventromedialis	19.6±3.1	15.1±2.6	21.1±2.9	16.5±2.2	2.0±0.2	2.2±0.3	2.9±0.2	2.1±0.2[b]
Nucleus dorosomedialis	25.9±2.8	17.8±2.5[b]	21.1±2.5	13.7±1.1[b]	2.8±0.2	2.3±0.1	4.2±0.4	3.7±0.3[b]

[a] Results are expressed as ng/mg protein (NA), or nmol octopamine/mg/protein/h (DBH) from groups of 14 rats; (mean ± s.e.m.)

[b] $P < 0.05$

Results

Catecholamines in Spontaneously Hypertensive Rats (SHR)

Changes in Central Catecholaminergic Neurons

In certain forebrain areas of young (4-week-old) and also adult SHR a decrease of the NA content was observed. These changes were localized in specific nuclei of the hypothalamus and closely related areas (Table 1). Similar changes in the activity of the noradrenaline-forming enzyme, DBH, were detected in the same areas of both young and adult rats (Table 1).

In the brain stem, where A-containing neurons are localized, the activity of the A-forming enzyme, PNMT, was increased in the A_1 and A_2 areas and the area postrema, but it was normal in these areas in adult SHR. Adrenaline levels in these areas were decreased in young SHR. However, not all brain stem areas showed the same reversed changes in A levels and PNMT activities. In the A_2 area the A content was unchanged, whereas the PNMT activity was increased. In the locus coeruleus the A content was significantly decreased, without an increase in PNMT activity (Table 2).

Table 2. Adrenaline concentrations and PNMT activity in brain stem areas of SHR and WKY (Wistar-Kyoto).[a] (Saavedra and Grobecker 1979)

Age	Area	Adrenaline WKY	SHR	Percent change	PNMT Percent change
4 weeks					
	A_1	1.84±0.14	[b]0.79±0.10	−47	+26[b]
	A_2	2.18±0.37	2.03±0.39	− 7	+23[b]
	Area postrema	2.90±0.61	[b]1.00±0.20	−65	+40[b]
	Locus coeruleus	1.63±0.24	[b]0.86±0.22	−47	−16
14 weeks					
	A_1	0.40±0.10	0.40±0.06	0	+ 2
	A_2	0.60±0.05	0.56±0.09	− 7	+ 4
	Area postrema	1.76±0.36	1.11±0.10	−37	+23
	Locus coeruleus	0.30±0.07	0.28±0.03	− 7	+13

[a] Results are expressed as ng/mg protein (A), or pmol/mg protein/hr (PNMT) for groups of 15 rats; (mean ± s.e.m.)

[b] $P < 0.05$

Plasma Catecholamines and DBH Activity

Plasma NA and DBH activity were increased in young SHR. In addition plasma A was increased in young stroke-prone SHR. At this time (4 weeks of age) blood pressure was significantly higher in SHR than in the WKY controls (Table 3).

Biosynthetic Enzymes and Catecholamines in Adrenal Glands

In adrenal glands of young SHR (4 weeks of age) activities of TH, DBH, and PNMT as well as A content were decreased. In adult SHR, TH turned to an enhanced activity, whereas DBH and PNMT activities were not different from WKY controls (Table 4). Depletion of catecholamines in adrenal glands of adult SHR by an adrenergic neuron blocking drug (EMD 21 192) resulted in a decline of blood pressure (Table 5).

Catecholamines in DOCA-Salt Hypertensive Rats

Changes in Central Catecholaminergic Neurons

In the brain stem regions A_1, area postrema, and locus coeruleus early increases of PNMT activity were found. After prolonged treatment with DOCA and salt the A_2 area also showed a significant increase in PNMT activity (Table 6).

Table 3. Plasma catecholamines and dopamine-β-hydroxylase activity in 4-week-old spontaneously hypertensive rats (SHR) and Wistar-Kyoto rats[a]

	WKY	SHR	SHR SP[d]
Noradrenaline	360 ± 23	425 ± 25[b]	432 ± 21[b]
Adrenaline	294 ± 21	319 ± 34	445 ± 47[c]
DBH	5.46 ± 0.29	8.23 ± 0.34[d]	
BP (mmHg)	93 ± 1	114 ± 3[c]	108 ± 3[c]

[a] Results are expressed as pg/ml (NA and A) or nmol octopamine/h/ml plasma (DBH), for groups of 9—10 rats (mean ± s.e.m.)

[b] $P < 0.05$

[c] $P < 0.01$, when compared with Wistar-Kyoto rats

[d] $P < 0.001$, SHR SP = stroke-prone rats

Table 4. Catecholamine synthesizing enzymes in the adrenal gland of SHR and Wistar-Kyoto rats.[a] (Modified from Grobecker, Saavedra and Axelrod, submitted for publication)

Enzymes	4 Weeks WKY	SHR	14 Weeks WKY	SHR
Tyrosine hydroxylase	11.9 ± 0.4	8.6 ± 0.2	56.6 ± 3.4	67.6 ± 2.8[b]
Dopamine β-hydroxylase	25.6 ± 2.6	17.7 ± 0.9	134 ± 12	149 ± 11
Phenylethanolamine N-methyl transferase	8.4 ± 0.1	5.3 ± 1.1	14.7 ± 1.1	15.2 ± 1.2
Blood pressure	105 ± 5	122 ± 6[b]	125 ± 8	210 ± 10[b]

[a] Results are expressed as nmol product/hr/adrenal gland, (mean ± s.e.m.) for groups of 6—14 animals. Blood pressures are expressed in mmHg

[b] $P < 0.05$ compared with control animals

Table 5. Effect of EMD 21 192 on blood pressure and catecholamine content in adrenal glands of SHR[a]

		Controls (SHR 14 weeks old)	EMD 21 192 (21.5 mg/kg IP, 7 days)
Blood pressure (mmHg)		201 ± 5	152 ± 7[c]
Catecholamines in	A	450 ± 40	206 ± 24[c]
adrenal glands (μg/g)	NA	158 ± 28	80 ± 12[b]

[a] Groups of 8—10 rats, mean ± s.e.m.

[b] $P < 0.05$

[c] $P < 0.001$

Table 6. PNMT activity in brain stem areas of DOCA-salt hypertensive rats.[a] (From Saavedra and Grobecker 1979)

Length of treatment (weeks)	Percent changes in PNMT activity areas A_1	A_2	Area postrema	Locus ceruleus
2	+ 92	− 4	+ 25[b]	+ 45[b]
4	+ 119	0	—	+ 42[b]
10	+ 109	+ 56[b]	+ 33[b]	+ 31[b]

[a] Results represent mean ± s.e.m. for groups of 12 rats. Percent changes in PNMT activity (pmol/mg protein/hour)

[b] $P < 0.05$

Plasma Catecholamines and DBH Activity

In DOCA-salt hypertensive rats circulating NA was increased (controls 0.25 ± 0.03 ng/ml, DOCA-salt: 0.44 ± 0.02 ng/ml, mean ± s.e.m., $p < 0.01$). No consistent change of DBH activity was observed.

Biosynthetic Enzymes and Catecholamines in Adrenal Glands

After only 1 week of treatment with DOCA and saline, TH activity in adrenals was significantly higher than in controls. TH activity increased further after 2 weeks of treatment. At this time blood pressure was elevated when compared with controls. After 4 weeks of administration of DOCA and saline, TH activity was still increased, whereas DBH and PNMT activity showed only a small but insignificant increase in hypertensive animals. The increase in TH activity was accompanied by a significant increase in adrenaline content. Noradrenaline levels showed also a small increase, which was not statistically significant. Administration of SKF 7698, an inhibitor of PNMT, reduced the activity of PNMT and adrenaline content and blood pressure declined (Table 7).

Table 7. Catecholamine synthesizing enzymes and catecholamine levels in the adrenal gland of DOCA-saline hypertensive rats and effect of SKF 7698. (Modified from Grobecker, Saavedra and Axelrod, submitted for publication)[a]

	Control	DOCA-Saline (4 weeks of treatment)	DOCA-Saline +SKF 7698(4)
Enzymes (1)			
Tyrosine hydroxylase	29.2 ± 2.1	47.9 ± 4.5[b]	89.9 ± 8.4[c]
Dopamine β-hydroxylase	217 ± 15	232 ± 27	141 ± 29[c]
Phenylethanolamine N-methyl transferase	16.8 ± 1.3	19.3 ± 1.1	10.9 ± 1.5[c]
Catecholamines (2)			
Noradrenaline	2.4 ± 0.5	3.3 ± 0.6[b]	2.6 ± 0.2
Adrenaline	9.2 ± 0.6	11.7 ± 0.6[b]	1.9 ± 0.2[d]
Blood pressure (3)	120 ± 6	158 ± 5[b]	120 ± 3

[a] Enzyme activities are expressed as nmoles product/hr/adrenal gland. Catecholamine levels represent µg/gland. Blood pressure is expressed in mmHg. 4 × 200 mg/kg, p.o. Results represent mean values ± s.e.m. for groups of 6—14 animals

[b] $P < 0.05$

[c] $P < 0.01$

[d] $P < 0.001$ compared with control animals

Circulating Catecholamines in Patients with Essential Hypertension

Plasma levels of circulating noradrenaline in age matched hypertensive patients were not significantly different from normotensive subjects (normotensive patients 284 ± 23 pg/ml; n=36; hypertensive patients 339 ± 19 pg/ml; n=40). There was also no difference in the increase of circulating NA levels after standing for 5 to 10 min between the normotensive and hypertensive subjects. In addition no consistent changes of DBH activity could be detected (but c. f. p. 110 footnote).

Plasma Catecholamines in Patients with Stabilized Essential Hypertension During Physical Exercise and Treatment with Propranolol

In 12 hypertensive patients (WHO stage II) resting NA and adrenaline levels were in the range of concentrations reported for normotensive subjects. After exercise on a bicycle ergometer (150 Wa for 5 min) in a supine position, a significant increase in NA and A concentrations was seen. Acute treatment with propranolol (80 mg orally 100 min before exercise) reduced the increase in heart rate and blood pressure during exercise, but elevated the increase in NA concentration in plasma to significantly higher levels than obtained without blockade of β-adrenoceptors. Chronic administration of propranolol (240 mg/day for 60 days) decreased blood pressure and heart rate significantly. No change in resting NA or A levels was observed. Although a significant increase of circulating NA during exercise after the treatment with propranolol for 8 weeks could be seen, the exaggerated response of sympathethic nerves observed after a single dose of propranolol was somewhat diminished after chronic treatment of the patients.

Discussion

In the rat brain as possible neurotransmitters dopamine, NA and more recently A as well as the enzymes involved in their biosynthesis, i.e., TH, DBH and PNMT, were found in specific areas [4, 15]. Some of the catecholamine-rich areas in the brain that have been proposed to be involved in cardiovascular regulation are localized in the anterior and posterior hypothalamus of the brain stem [8, 9, 12, 14, 22]. The changes in catecholamine metabolism described in this paper are specifically localized in the forebrain (hypothalamus) and the brain stem. Although the changes are complex and they may represent causative and/or adaptive mechanisms during the development of high blood pressure in genetic or experimental hypertension, the selective defect of central NA neurons in young SHR might be a primary phenomenon, which is already present when the blood pressure in SHR is at the borderline to high values. The reduction in NA levels was accompanied by a decrease in DBH activity. These changes in DBH activity were restricted to the areas showing decreases in NA content. Therefore, it is likely that a diminished synthesis of the neurotransmitter could lead to a diminished stimulation of postsynaptic α-receptors in selective hypothalamic areas and could explain the central hypotensive effects of α-receptor stimulant drugs such as clonidine and α-methyldopa [34, 36].

Located in the anterior hypothalamus is a depressor area and in the posterior hypothalamus, a pressor area [12]. An imbalance between these two areas in SHR could result in an enhanced pressor impulse flow from the posterior hypothalamus, thereby leading to an activation of peripheral sympathetic nerves. The coincidence of the decreased levels of A in specific brain stem structures (areas A_1, A_2, area postrema and locus coeruleus) and the increased activity of the A-forming enzyme, PNMT, could represent an enhanced release or metabolism of this amine during the early phase of the development of genetic hypertension. These changes are no longer present in adult rats, when the hypertension is fully developed. Thus, the increased PNMT activity in these areas could be a compensatory mechanism to an early increased release of the transmitter.

In young SHR also sympathoneuronal activity is increased, whereas medullary activity is depressed. It is likely that this depressed adrenal medullary activity is a compensatory mechanism related to the increased peripheral sympathetic nerve activity and/or to changes in catecholamine neurons in the hypothalamus or brain stem [10]. The increase in circulating NA in young SHR could lead to a decrease in the numbers of β_2-adrenoceptors in blood vessels, thereby leading to an increased peripheral resistance [18]. In adult SHR the enhanced TH activity in the adrenals may reflect increased synthesis of catecholamines and an increased release of catecholamines into circulation, thereby maintaining enhanced blood pressure.

In DOCA-salt hypertensive rats the described increase in PNMT activity in brain stem areas could also be a compensatory mechanism related to an enhanced sympathoneuronal and sympathoadrenal activity. The increase in plasma NA concentrations and an increase in TH activity as well as in A content in adrenal glands of DOCA-salt hypertensive rats indicates a contribution of sympathetic nerves and adrenal medulla to elevated blood pressure in this form of hypertension. As in SHR, increased circulating NA could lead to an desensitization of β-adrenoceptors. In the heart of DOCA-saline hypertensive rats a decreased number of β-adrenoceptors has been reported recently [35].

Administration of a PNMT inhibitor diminished both the PNMT activity and the A content in the adrenal glands of hypertensive rats. Blood pressure fell to normal values. Hypotension in DOCA-saline rats was also observed after adrenalectomy [6]. However, the decrease in blood pressure elicited by SKF-7896 might also be due to its α-adrenergic receptor blocking potency, since administration of an α-receptor blocker could mimic the effect of an acute adrenalectomy [6]. On the other hand, it has been shown that systemic administration of the PNMT inhibitor, which is without α-receptor blocking activity, to adult SHR (DCMB 2, 3-dichloro-α-methyl-benzylamine), results in a normalization of the blood pressure after several days of treatment [29]. Another possiblity for the antihypertensive effect of a PNMT inhibitor could be through inhibition of brain PNMT [31]. If a central or peripheral inhibition of PNMT by specific enzyme inhibitors is shown to be causally related to their antihypertensive effects, these or similar drugs [11], which deplete adrenal catecholamine stores, could be of importance in the future treatment of hypertension.

In contrast to the increase in plasma catecholamines in the two animal models studied, there is no unequivocal evidence for an increase in the activity in sympathetic nerves in human essential hypertension [28]. The result that no difference in circulating NA levels between normotensive subjects and hypertensive patients could be observed is in agreement with other studies [17, 25, 28]. However, these results are in disagreement with other studies [cf. 2]. It may be concluded that differences in plasma noradrenaline or catecholamine levels found in these studies may have been due to the small numbers of patients not age matched, as well as to a lack of appropriate normotensive groups, and other differences, e.g., the use of different methods to assay circulating catecholamines. However, the reported negative results do not rule out abnormal NA or A function in localized brain areas nor possible abnormalities in sympathetic neuronal function in special forms of essential hypertension.

Since the measurement of plasma catecholamines both under basal and stimulated conditions and after acute or chronic administration of β-adrenoceptor blockers may give a reliable biochemical index of the sympathetic nervous activity, it would be worthwhile to investigate a subgroup of young patients with essential hypertension and the appropriate normotensive subjects in order to evaluate an altered sympathetic activity as an important factor in the development of their elevated blood pressure.

References

1. Anton AH, Sayre DF (1962) A study of the factors affecting the aluminium oxide-trihydroxyindole procedure for the analysis of catecholamines. J Pharmacol Exp Ther 138 : 360–375
2. Axelrod J (1962) Purification and properties of phenylethanolamine-N-methyltransferase. J Biol Chem 237 : 1657–1660
3. Axelrod J (1976) Catecholamines and hypertension. Clin Sci Mol Med 51 : 415–421
4. Dahlström A, Fuxe K (1964) Evidence for the existence of monoamine containing neurons in the central nervous system. I. Demonstration of monoamines in the cell bodies of brain stem neurons. Acta Physiol Scand [Suppl 232] 62 : 1–55
5. Da Prada M, Zürcher G (1976) Simultaneous radioenzymatic determination of plasma and tissue adrenaline, noradrenaline and dopamine within the fentomole range. Life Sci 19 : 1161–1174
6. De Champlain J, van Ameringen MR (1972) Regulation of blood pressure by sympathetic nerve fibers and adrenal medulla in normotensive and hypertensive rats. Circ Res 31 : 617–628

7. De Champlain J, Krakoff LR, Axelrod J (1967) Catecholamine metabolism in experimental hypertension in the rat. Circ Res 20 : 136—145
8. Eferakeya A, Buñag RD (1974) Adrenomedullary pressor responses curing posterior hypothalamic stimulation. Am J Physiol 227 : 114—118
9. Gebber GL, Snyder DW (1970) Hypothalamic control of baroreceptor reflexes. Am J Physiol 218 : 124—131
10. Grobecker H, Saavedra JM, McCarty R, Chiueh CC, Kopin IJ (1977) Dopamine-β-hydroxylase activity and catecholamine concentrations in plasma: Experimental and essential hypertension. Postgrad Med J 53 : 43—48
11. Grobecker H, Roizen FM, Jacobowitz DM, Kopin IJ (1977) Effect of prolonged treatment with adrenergic neuron blocking drugs on sympathoadrenal reactivity in rats. Eur J Pharmacol 46 : 125—133
12. Hayward JN (1977) Functional and morphological aspects of hypothalamic neurons. Physiol Rev 57 : 574—658
13. Henry DP, Starman BJ, Johnson DG, Williams RH (1975) A sensitive radioenzymatic assay for norepinephrine in tissues and plasma. Life Sci 16 : 374—384
14. Hilton SM, Spyer KM (1971) Participation of the anterior hypothalamus in the baroreceptor reflex. J Physiol (Lond) 218 : 271—293
15. Hökfelt T, Fuxe K, Goldstein M, Johannson O (1973) Evidence for adrenaline neurons in the rat brain. Acta Physiol Scand 89 : 286—289
16. König JFR, Klippel RA (1963) The rat brain, a stereotaxic atlas of the forebrain and lower parts of the brainstem. Williams & Wilkins, Baltimore
17. Lake CR, Ziegler MG, Coleman MD, Kopin IJ (1977) Age-adjusted plasma norepinephrine levels are similar in normotensive and hypertensive subjects. N Engl J Med 296 : 208—209
18. Limas CJ, Limas C (1979) Decreased number of beta-adrenergic receptors in hypertensive vessels. Biochim Biophys Acta 582 : 533—536
19. Lowry OH, Rosebrough NJ, Farr AL, Randall RJ (1951) Protein measurement with the folin phenol reagent. J Biol Chem 193 : 265—275
20. Molinoff PB, Weinshilboum R, Axelrod J (1971) A sensitive enzymatic assay for dopamine-β-hydroxylase. J Pharmacol Exp Ther 178 : 425—431
22. Nathan MA, Reis DJ (1975) Fulminating arterial hypertension with pulmonary edema from release of adrenomedullary catecholamines after lesions of the anterior hypothalamus in the rat. Circ Res 37 : 226—235
21. Nagatsu T, Levitt M, Udenfriend S (1964) Tyrosine hydroxylase: The initial step in norepinephrine biosynthesis. J Biol Chem 239 : 2910—2917
23. Okamoto K, Aoki K (1963) Development of a strain of spontaneously hypertensive rats. Jpn Circ J 27 : 282—293
24. Passon PG, Peuler JD (1973) A simplified radiometric assay for plasma norepinephrine and epinephrine. Anal Biochem. 51 : 618—631
25. Pedersen EB, Christensen NJ (1975) Catecholamines in plasma and urine in patients with essential hypertension determined by double isotope derivative techniques. Acta Med Scand 198 : 373—377
26. Peuler JD, Johnsson GA (1977) Simultaneous single isotope radioenzymatic assay of plasma norepinephrine, epinephrine and dopamine. Life Sci 21 : 625—636

27. Reid JL, Jones DH, Dargie HJ (1977) Plasma noradrenaline and hypertension. Postgrad Med J 53 : 40—42
28. Reid JL, Jones DH, Hamilton CA (1978) Adrenoceptors and essential hypertension. In: Szabadi E, Bradshaw CM, Bevan P (eds) Recent advances in the pharmacology of adrenoceptors. Biomedical Press, Elsevier/North Holland, pp 261—267
29. Saavedra JM, Grobecker H (1979) Central and peripheral catecholamines in experimental and genetic hypertension. In: Meyer P, Schmitt H (eds) Nervous system and hypertension. Wiley, Flammarion, Paris, pp 223—233
30. Saavedra JM, Palkovits M, Brownstein MJ, Axelrod J (1974) Localisation of phenylethanolamine-N-methyl transferase in the rat brain nuclei. Nature 248 : 695—696
31. Saavedra JM, Grobecker H, Axelrod J (1976) Adrenaline-forming enzyme in brainstem: Elevation in genetic and experimental hypertension. Science 191 : 483—484
32. Saavedra JM, Grobecker H, Axelrod J (1978) Changes in central catecholaminergic neurons in the spontaneously (genetic) hypertensive rat. Circ Res 42 : 529—534
33. Schlumpf M, Waser P, Lichtensteiger W, Langemann H, Schlup P (1974) Standardized excision of small areas of rat and mouse brain with topographical control. Biochem Pharmacol 23 : 2447—2449
34. Struyker-Boudier HAJ, Smeets GWM, Brouwer GM, van Rossum JM (1974) Hypothalamic alpha adrenergic receptors in cardiovascular regulation. Neuropharmacology 13 : 837—846
35. Woodcock EA, Funder JW, Johnston PJ (1978) Decreased cardiac β-adrenoceptors in hypertensive rats. Clin Exp Pharmacol Physiol 5 : 545—550
36. van Zwieten PA (1975) Antihypertensive drugs with a central action. Prog Pharmacol 1 : 1—63

Session B: Cardiac Mechanochemistry and Morphology in Various Forms of Hypertensive Heart Disease

Chairmen: R. Jacob/Tübingen (FRG), J. Linzbach/Göttingen (FRG)

Part I: Contractile Proteins and Contraction Energetics

Cardiac Myosin in Heart Overloading

B. SWYNGHEDAUW, K. SCHWARTZ, G. LACOMBE, J.J. LEGER, N.V. THIEM AND A.M. LOMPRE

The heart, like most types of tissues, can adapt to envirommental factors and, more specifically, to its load. Overloading a heart as well as changing its initial length may increase work by means of two successive adaptational processes: (1) immediately by bringing the muscle's own mechanical properties into play and (2) at a later stage by changing muscle mass and structure.

In skeletal muscle chronic overloading, cross-innervation can induce changes both in contractile activity and the isozymic pattern of myosin and glycolytic enzymes. Chronically overloading of the heart may also be connected with isozymic changes in lactate dehydrogenases, although it may be the result of increase in the number of fibroblasts, and in myosin.

The modifications of myosin were of special interest since it is now well established that the myosin ATPase correlates with the shortening speed in phylogeny as well as in physiology and in skeletal as well as in cardiac muscle [1, 2].

Myosin and Myosin Isozymes

No matter what tissue myosin is extracted from, it always possesses several fundamental characteristics. (1) It is a polymer (mol. wt. 500 000) composed of two heavy chains (HC), and four light chains (LC). (2) Every myosin molecule can be cut by a mild tryptic hydrolysis into a soluble globular head(the heavy meromyosin), where both the ATPase and actin-binding sites are located, and an insoluble helical tail. (3) The ATPase activity is activated by millimolar concentration of calcium in a low ionic strength medium, by potassium or sodium in the absence of any divalent cations, and by actin in the presence of magnesium. An increasing amount of data suggest that myosins from a variety of sources have related light chains of only two distinct types: the alkali type and the phosphorylated type. The presence of three light bands on the electrophoretic pattern of white skeletal muscle myosin is presumably due to the existence of two different populations of myosins, each one containing both LC types.

Several publications have demonstrated some clear-cut differences between the primary structures of cardiac, fast skeletal and smooth muscle myosins.

When compared to skeletal muscle myosin, rabbit cardiac myosin is characterized by: (1) a lower ATPase specific activity, less sensitive to the activating effects of actin and SH reagents and more easily denatured by a mild alkaline treatment; (2) a slow rate of tryptic hydrolysis; (3) the absence of 3-methyl histidine as a consequence of the lack of the cytoplasmic methylating enzyme; the 13 amino acid peptides surrounding the 3-methyl histidine in skeletal myosin or the corresponding histidine in cardiac myosin were isolated and several amino acid substitutions have been demonstrated; (4) four light chains (mol. wt. 27 000 and 18 000), the sequences of which are related to those of the skeletal myosin, although their sizes and their sensitivity to dithionitrobenzene vary substantially with the two muscles; and (5) a specific antiserum [3]. When compared to smooth muscle, cardiac muscle is characterized by: (1) a higher calcium activated ATPase; (2) a faster tryptic hydrolysis; (3) two light chains which differ by their molecular weight and amino acid composition; and (4) a specific antiserum [3]. In contrast several authors have emphasized the similarity which exists between the cardiac myosin and the slow (red) skeletal muscle myosin and between the smooth myosin and the myosin extracted from nonmuscular tissues.

Three different laboratories (referred to in [3]) have simultaneously found that the cardiac myosin ATPase activity of small mammals, such as a mouse or rat, is higher than that of larger animals, such as a dog or rabbit. The calcium ATPase activity of rat heart myosin is approximately twice that of guinea pig heart myosin. Comparative cardiac myosin ATPase activities in order of decreasing size were: mouse, rat, guinea pig, pig or dog, human, and rabbit. Several data are also suggestive of changes in the primary structure [5]. From a physiologic point of view these structural variations correlate with the speed of shortening in muscles. The pioneer in this field was Barany [1], who found a correlation between Ca^{2+} as well as actin-activated ATPase of myosin and the maximal speed of shortening in skeletal and smooth muscles. Similar data were observed in mammalian hearts in our laboratory [2].

Myosin molecules not only vary from one species to the other or from one type of muscle to the other but can also change in the same muscle after cross innervation, stimulation, overloading, or thyroxine treatment. Clear-cut evidence has been published on the transformation of a fast skeletal muscle myosin into a slow one by *cross innervation* with a slow muscle nerve [6]. A similar result was obtained by a continuous pacing at a slow rate of a fast muscle [7], which suggests that the changes were induced by the work itself and not by some neurofactor. When the skeletal muscle *work* was directly affected some authors have reported slight but reproducible changes of myosin or myofibrillar ATPase. For example, a decrease of 10% was noted in the soleus after a double tenotomy of the contro-lateral muscles. Physical training does not apparently modify rat skeletal myosin ATPase but an increase of this activity by 30% to 50% affecting the reactivity of SH groups was observed in the heart [8]. Among the hormonal effects on cardiac myosin, those of *thyroxine* are certainly the most documented. Thyroxine treatment is able to induce a significant heart hypertrophy, with an increase in the contractility of both fresh and glycerinated cardiac fibers and a significant activation of cardiac myosin ATPase (by 200%) [8].

Myosin ATPase in Heart Overloading

The increase of cardiac work induced by an experimental aortic stenosis or incompetence is not basically different from that observed with the skeletal muscle after tenotomy or during exercise. The only well-defined myosin abnormality which has been reported in this condition concerns the enzymatic activity of the molecule. Several authors have found a decrease of cardiac myofibrillar ATPase activity by 20% to 40% in chronic overloading. Similar depression of ATPase activity was reported in highly purified preparations of myofibrils or myosin, although these data were sometimes contradictory [9].

Most of the authors found the defect by measuring the Ca^{2+}ATPase of myosin or myofibrils in low ionic strength. Results concerning the Mg^{2+}ATPase and the K^{+}EDTA ATPase are known to be poorly reproducible, and this probably explains why they were less conclusive. It is obvious that Ca^{2+}ATPase does not represent the "physiological" ATPase as well as the Mg^{2+}ATPase of myofibrils, nevertheless they both are closely related when simultaneously measured in comparative biochemistry.

The defect correlates with the heart enlargement. It obviously occurs only when the hypertrophy reaches a sufficient magnitude, which very likely changes according to the type of overloading. This has been shown in the following experiments: (1) in rats, while the myofibrillar ATPase is unaffected even after a long period by an aortic stenosis (which slightly increases the heart weight by 30%), the ATPase falls sharply by 25% when a further increase in the protein synthesis is induced by addition of aortic incompetence[10]; (2) human heart myofibrillar ATPase measured on 70 autopsy samples correlates negatively with heart weight, but the relation is not linear and in fact the ATPase falls sharply when a threshold of heart weight of 500 g is reached [11]. It must be emphasized that the degree of cardiac hypertrophy in humans is usually very far away from that observed in experimental models. Most of our knowledge concerning the pathogenesis of heart failure was obtained with failure occurring on very mild hypertrophy (+50%), whereas in humans chronic failure usually occurs with hearts which have gained at least + 300% of their own weight.

From a methodological point of view the numerous contradictory data reported could mainly be due to two technical problems. (1) Most of the experiments were dealing with the hypertrophy induced by an abdominal aortic stenosis in the rat or a pulmonary stenosis in cat or dog. As mentioned previously, such an overloading does not enlarge the heart by more than 50%. This is very far away from man, where heart hypertrophy commonly reaches 200% to 300%. (2) The myosin ATPase is one of the most complex activities to measure: the purity of the preparations must be checked routinely by electrophoresis and other methods; the integrity of the molecule has to be preserved by preparing the myosin within

24 h from a well-frozen tissue in the presence of EDTA and checked, for example, by measuring the burst size as below.

Experimental Models of Cardiac Hypertrophy

The study of structural changes requires amplification of growth and doubling of heart weight because of the poor sensitivity of most of the analytical techniques.

A large hypertrophy comparable to that observed in man can be obtained in rats by aortic stenosis or aortic incompetence alone in one case out of ten. The most accurate method for stenosis uses a calibrated forceps and hemoclips. An aortic incompetence can be produced by forcing a stiff polyethylene catheter through the aortic value.

Swimming increases heart weight. We tried to combine swimming (from 5 min to 6 h per day until the age of 3 months) and abdominal stenosis: 3 months of swimming and aortic stenosis increased ventricular weight by 60% compared to 30% in the aortic stenosis alone. Unfortunately, swimming also scattered the results.

In fact the only routine technique which produces a bulky hypertrophy (by 100% or more) was a combination of two successive overloadings. Aortic stenosis followed two weeks later by incompetence usually increases heart weight in rats by a factor of 2. A similar result can be obtained when an aortic insufficiency was performed in spontaneous genetic hypertension (P. Y. Hatt, personal communication).

Myosin Structure in Heart Overloading

Data concerning the structure of the molecule in this condition were still rare and poor. Recent observers reported the existence of several *myosin isozymes* in the ventricles; as in skeletal muscle, their charges differ in a non-dissociating medium [12]. Such myosin isozymes cannot of course be distingished by their light subunits, since heart myosin has a paired number of light chains. We have shown in rats [13] that an increase in cardiac work induces preferential synthesis of a cardiac myosin isozyme. Cardiac overloading was obtained by two-step overloading or by one-time stenosis or insufficiency. The rats exhibited 60% to 120% hypertrophy. A change in the isozyme pattern was demonstrated by three processes: (1) steady-state myosin Ca ATPase dropped by 50% and this was not due to any artifactual denaturation, since each preparation has a normal phosphate burst size. Moreover the heavy chains on SDS gel electrophoresis were homogeneous. This is in full agreement with previous observations [14]; (2) Antibodies raised against native or SDS denatured heavy meromyosin were tested by microcomplement fixation. They showed a vertical shift in the maximum amount of C complement fixed when made to react with myosin from hypertrophied heart compared to the control [15]. Several papers have shown that in phylogeny such a change indicates amino acid sustitutions; and (3) Electrophoresis in a nondissociating medium has shown that there are differences between the respective charges of several skeletal myosins [12]. In normal rat ventricles, there are three isozymes with a relative ratio of 3 < 2 << 1. This pattern was reversed after overloading with a great predominance of 3 in the larger hearts and an intermediary pattern in the less affected hearts [13].

This isozyme change tending toward lower myosin ATPase activity is undoubtedly related to the diminished maximum speed of shortening, since in overloading this speed was inversely proportional to heart weight, as in phylogenic studies. Moreover, such an isozyme change may correct the initial diminution of efficiency induced by overloading. This could be the first myocardial adaptational step observed in overloading. As such, it would precede the functioning of the heterometric and peripheral compensatory mechanisms.

References

1. Barany M (1967) ATPase activity of myosin correlated with speed of muscle shortening. J Gen Physiol 50 : 197–216
2. Delcayre C, Swynghedauw B (1975) A comparative study of heart myosin ATPase and light subunits from different species. Pfluegers Arch, 355 : 39–47
3. Leger JJ, Berson G, Delcayre C, Schwartz K, Leger J, Stephens M, Swynghedauw B (1975) Heart contractile proteins. Biochimie 55 : 1249–1273
4. Klotz C, Aumont MC, Leger JJ, Swynghedauw B (1975) Human cardiac myosin ATPase and light subunits. A comparative study. Biochim Biophys Acta 386 : 461–469
5. Schwartz K, Bouveret P, Sebag C, Swynghedauw B (1977) Immunochemical evidence for the species-specificity of mammalian cardiac myosin and HMM. Biochim Biophys Acta 425 : 24–36
6. Buller AJ, Mommaerts WFHM, Seraydarian K (1969) Enzymatic properties of myosin in fast and slow twitch muscles of the cat following cross-innervation. J Physiol (London) 205 : 581–597
7. Sreter FA, Elzinga M, Mabuchi K (1975) The N-methylhistidine content of myosin in stimulated and cross re-innervated skeletal muscles of the rabbit. FEBS Lett. 57 : 107–111
8. Katagiri I, Stone Freedberg A, Morkin E (1975) The effect of N-ethylmaleimide on the ATPase activities of cardiac myosin from thyrotoxic rabbit. Life Sci 16 : 1079–1087
9. Swynghedauw B, Leger JJ, Schwartz K (1976) The myosin isozyme hypothesis in chronic heart overloading. J Mol Cell Cardiol 8 : 915–924
10. Stephens M, Leger JJ, Preteseille M, Swynghedauw B (1979) The relationship of a decline in myofibrillar ATPase activity to the development of severe left ventricular hypertrophy in the rat. Pathol Biol (Paris) 27 : 41–44
11. Leclercq JF, Swynghedauw B (1976) Myofibrillar ATPase and OHPro content of human hypertrophied heart. Eur J Clin Invest 6 : 27–33

12. D'Albis A, Gratzer WB (1973) Electrophoretic examination of native myosin. FEBS Lett 48 : 292—296
13. Lompre AM, Schwartz K, D'Albis A, Lacombe G, Thiem NV, Swynghedauw B (1979) Myosin isoenzyme redistribution in chronic heart overloading. Nature 282 : 105—107
14. Swynghedauw B, Klotz C, Leger JJ, Preteseille M (1973) Heart myosin ATPase and light subunits in experimental rabbit's chronic aortic insufficiency. J Mol Cell Cardiol 5 :501—514
15. Schwartz K, Bouveret P, Bercovici J, Swynghedauw B (1978) An immunochemical difference between myosins in normal and hypertrophied rat hearts. FEBS Lett 93 : 137—140

Properties of Myocardial Myosin in Left Ventricular Hypertrophy Due to Spontaneous Essential Hypertension in Rats[1]

G.W. Mayr, S. Bürger and B.E. Strauer

Introduction

Spontaneously hypertensive rats (SHR) represent a useful model of chronic pressure overload of the heart. This strain of rats, firstly separated by selectively inbreeding Wistar Kyoto rats by Okamoto and Aoki in 1962 [10] show significant elevation in blood pressure as early as 4 weeks after birth, reaching maximum degree of hypertension, according to blood pressure values of more than 200 mm Hg, between the 25th and 30th week of age [4, 11]. Normotensive, age-matched Wistar Kyoto rats of the same progenitor strain (NR) may serve as controls, since showing always less than 140 mm Hg of blood pressure even at an advanced age.

In our laboratory myocardial changes during development and progress of spontaneous hypertension in these rats in comparison to normotensive rats have been examined (see session A, Bürger and Strauer). Myocardial muscle mechanics, as recently evaluated from isolated left ventricular papillary muscles by my colleagues and reported in a previous session, showed some differences between SHR and NR as depicted in Fig. 1.

The maximum isometric tension developed (P_0) was higher in SHR up to the 40th week, but it was only at week 20 that the difference, as compared with NR was significant at 5% probability level. In contrast to this finding, velocity parameters, as indicated by the values of dl/dt_{max} and $dT/dt_{max}/P_0$, were lower in SHR than in NR, the difference increasing with age. The significance of this reduction in dl/dt_{max} at 40 and 70 weeks could be elicited.

Another finding to be pointed out is the age dependence of the contractile parameters determined. As shown, apart from the above-mentioned specific alterations in SHR as compared with NR, both groups showed an overall decline in tension and length-dependent parameters of contraction.

Since the elementary work of Barany [2], who in various types of muscles from same and different species demonstrated good correlation between speed of

---

1 Supported from the Deutsche Forschungsgemeinschaft

mechanical parameters of isolated papillary muscles (left ventricle)

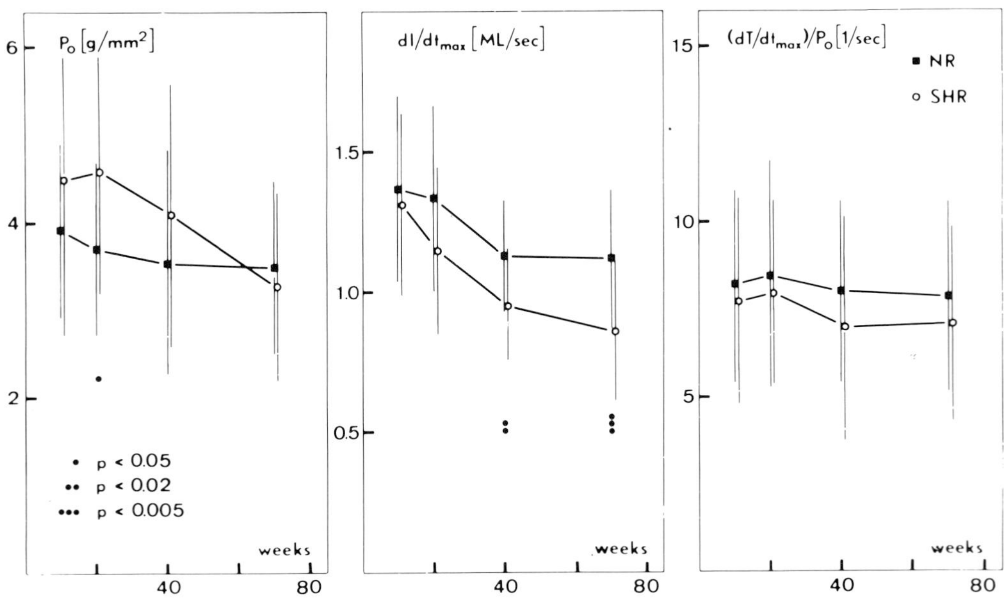

Fig. 1. The parameters as indicated on the panels (maximum tension (P_0), maximum isotonic shortening velocity (dl/dt_{max}), and normalized maximum rate of isometric force development [$(dT/dt_{max})/P_0$] were determined at mean ages as indicated on the *abscissa* from 76 (NR) and 71 (SHR) isolated left ventricular papillary muscles. Preload was chosen in such a way that maximum tension was developed isometrically. Parameter dl/dt_{max} was measured from isotonic twitches of muscles preloaded this way. *Vertical bars* indicate SD values

muscle shortening and myosin Ca^{++}-ATPase, some authors have also suggested the validity of this correlation for the ventricular muscle of a single species, differing only in contractile status [5, 7]. On the other hand, there seems to be no corresponding change (see [2]) in myosin ATPase, if maximum tension per unit cross section changes at constant velocity. For such an alteration, an increase in myofibrillar protein content can be responsible.

From these findings in muscle mechanics, one should therefore expect as changes in left ventricular myosin of SHR as compared with NR:

1. Corresponding to rise in maximum tension per unit cross section, an increase in actomyosin content per unit left ventricular mass, and

2. A fall in specific Ca^{++} activated myosin ATPase paralleling the fall of maximum shortening velocity.

Experimental methods

A total of 56 age-controlled male SHR (strain Okamoto-Aoki) and 83 age-matched NR (strain Wistar Kyoto), fed commercial stock chow diet and water ad libitum with blood pressure controlled by the water plethysmographic tail cuff method of Pfeffer [12] before killing, were used for the experiments.

In four age groups (10—11, 20—25, 40—45 and 75—80 weeks) three preparations of myosin were done from four to eight pooled left ventricles of freshly excised hearts, similar to the method described by Shiverick et al. [13]. To prevent sulfhydryl group oxidation, 0.5 m*M* dithiothreitol was included in all preparation steps.

Ventricular myosin content was estimated from protein content of the initial crude myosin extract. Although this crude myosin is not completely free of thin filament and other contaminant proteins and solubility at extraction conditions might be somewhat changed in SHR preparations, it might serve as a coarse estimate of myocardial myofibrillar protein content, assuming a rather constant contribution of myosin to total myofibrillar protein content of about 55% [8]. Although extraction was done over 60 min in a tissue homogenate, there will be an underestimation of the true myosin content by incomplete extraction, but this error was taken to be similar in both NR and SHR preparations.

In the final, highly purified fraction of myosin molecular integrity and preparation purity were routinely checked by SDS gel electrophoresis and UV absorption spectra. At any time by gel electrophoresis only the normal myosin chains (HC, LC1, LC2) could be detected. There were no proteolytic fragments as reported by others [14], although we did not use a protease inhibitor in our preparations. The ratio of A_{280mm}/A_{260mm} was never below. 1.57 (1.57 to 1.72), thus indicating absence of significant nucleotide contamination. In this final myosin fraction the assays were done as follows: In all assays reaction medium containing substrate was preincubated for 10 min at a temperature of 28 °C. Reaction was started by addition of myosin. After times as indicated below, the reaction was stopped by addition of the same volume of cold 10% TCA and stirring, and after removal of protein precipitate by centrifugation at 5000 g, the amount of phosphate liberated was determined by a modified Fiske Subbarow method, applied for small samples.

Special conditions: Ca^{++}-ATPase and EDTA-ATPase were measured over 10 min with 0.05 mg/ml myosin in medium containing 50 m*M* Tris buffer, CA^{++}-ATPase at 10 m*M* $CaCl_2$ and 2 m*M* ATP, and EDTA-ATPase at 2 m*M* EDTA and 5 m*M* ATP, with both ATPases at pH values and KCl concentrations as indicated in the figures. Mg^{++}-ATPase was measured over 30 min at a protein concentration of 0.1 to 0.2 mg/ml in 20 m*M* Tris-maleate, pH 7.5, which included 2 m*M* $MgCl_2$ and 1 m*M* ATP and KCl as indicated in figures.

Results and Discussions

As can be seen in Fig. 2 (left side), the mean heart weight of SHR, already at 10 weeks of age significantly higher than that of NR, clearly showed a faster rise until week 40, reaching a constant level thereafter. On the other hand the slower rise in NR heart weight further proceeded after the 40th week.

In the middle, changes of the heart to body weight ratio over the same period of age are plotted. At the earlies age determined, the 5th week, the ratios already showed a significant difference, the ratio in SHR being about 23% higher. With the rapid falling of NR ratio until the 40th week and a further increase of the SHR ratio, a difference of about 115% was reached at this age. After the 40th week the values remained almost constantly at about 2 for NR and 4.3 for SHR. These results clearly indicate pronounced ventricular hypertrophy in SHR due to beginning pressure overload at the 5th to 10th week as characterized by a heart to body weight ratio elevated by 50% until week 10 and a further increase of hypertrophy up to week 40.

On the right part of Fig. 2 the crude myoson yield, as calculated in mg/g of heart wet weight, is depicted. In SHR of 10 to 40 weeks of age a 10% to 15% higher yield was obtained, whereas a value similar to that in NR was found at 80 weeks of age.

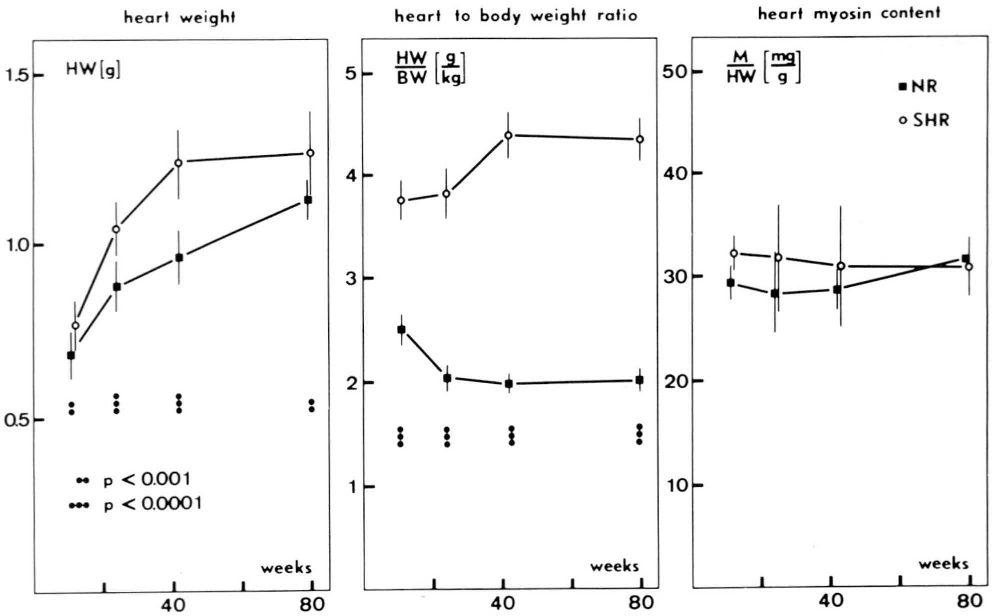

Fig. 2. Total heart (left + right ventricle) wet weights and body weights were measured at mean ages as indicated on the *abscissa* in 81 NR and 56 SHR. Crude myosin yield was determined, as indicated in the methods section, in each set of 12 preparations from NR and SHR. *Vertical bars* indicate SD values

This time course of crude myosin yield may express, as previously mentioned, a corresponding increase in myofibrillar protein content per unit mass of ventricle, privided solubility of myosin at extraction conditions and subunit composition of myofibrils was not significantly changed. The rise in maximum tension per unit cross section as expected could then be explained by a rise in myofibrillar protein content. Results of ultrastructural studies in SHR [6] clearly showed sarcomerogenesis and an increase in the fractional volume of myofibrils at the 15th and 21th week of age, thus corresponding well to what we found with the myofibriallar protein content. Fig. 3 + 4 show results of the ATPase

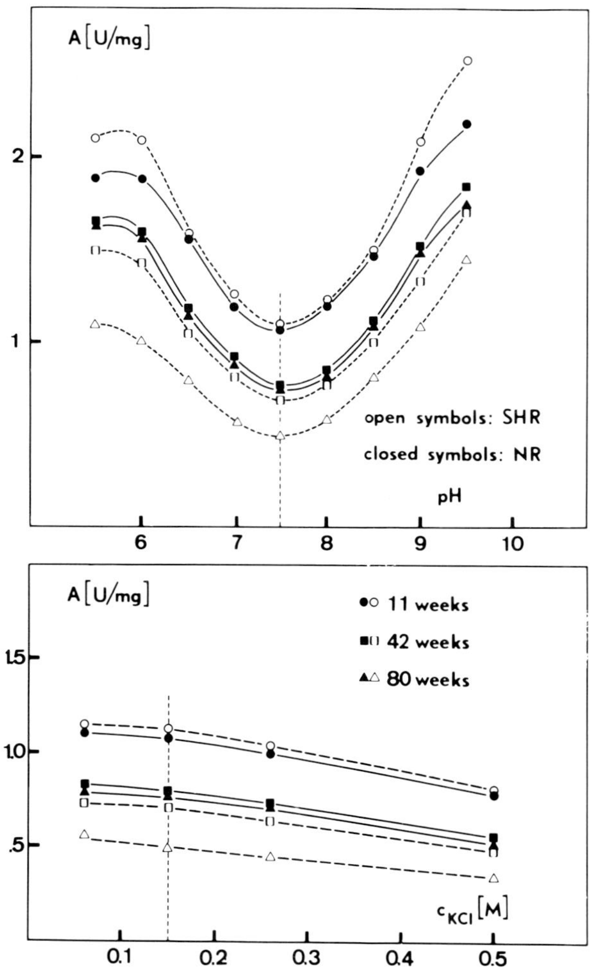

Fig. 3. Left ventricular myosin Ca^{++}-ATPase with pH (*above*) and KCl concentration (*below*) varied. *Dashed vertical lines* indicate same conditions in upper and lower graphs. Each curve represents the means of three assays done from different myosin preparations. Assaying conditions were as indicated in methods section

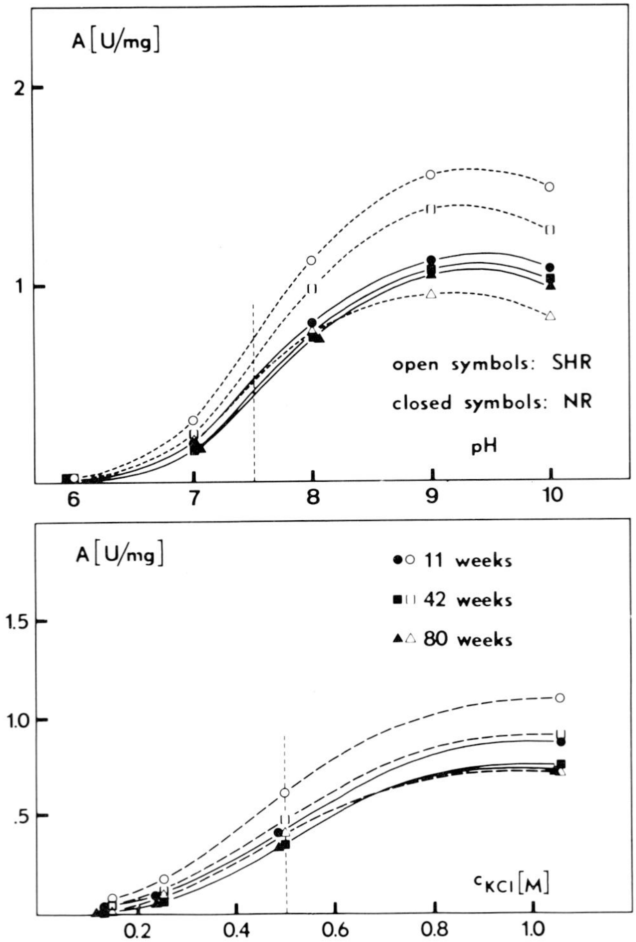

Fig. 4. Left ventricular myosin EDTA-ATPase with pH (*above*) and KCl concentration (*below*) varied. Each *curve* represents the means of three assays done from different myosin preparations. Assaying conditions as indicated in methods section. *Dashed vertical lines* indicate same conditions in upper and lower graphs

assays done. The pH profiles of Ca^{++}-ATPase in SHR and NR, determined for single groups of age (Fig. 3, upper graph), apart from the well established characteristic shape of each pH profile with maximums at pH 5.5 and 10 and a minimum at pH 7.5 [8], clearly showed some differences between the single groups of age and between SHR and NR.

In NR, with increase of age there was an activity fall by nearly the same absolute extent at each pH value, whereas in SHR activity at each pH value fell proportionally to the initial value. Moreover, the activity decline, levelling off with increasing age in NR, proceeded constantly and more pronounced in SHR.

As depicted in the lower part of Fig. 3, which shows Ca^{++}-ATPase activity at various concentrations of KCl, the same time-dependent behavior of ATPase was exhibited. The vertical dashed lines indicate same conditions in upper and lower graphs and shall be referred to later. The overall activity decrease from 10th to 80th week as 29% for NR and 57% for SHR in maximum.

Something unexpected was found in EDTA-ATPase (Fig. 4). Although pH profiles (above) for NR and SHR exhibited similar bell shape, activities in SHR at the age of 10 weeks already showed a large elevation of about 40% at each pH value. In the dependence on KCl concentration (below) a corresponding elevation was found and was yet relatively higher (up to 75%) at lower ionic strength. The second feature different in both groups was the time-dependent activity decline. Whereas in SHR preparations the decrease from 10th to 80th week was large (30% to 82%), the decrease in NR was very small (8% to 30%) at all conditions. Age dependence of EDTA-ATPase thus seemed to be similar to that of Ca^{++}-ATPase, in spite of the large difference in absolute activity levels.

Mg^{++}-ATPase, determined as defined in the methods section for the single groups of age at increasing concentrations of KCl (Fig. 5), in SHR at 10th week of age already showed significantly reduced activity (by 15%) as compared with NR. A subsequent fall in activities (by again 15%) took place in NR as well as in SHR, but whereas in NR the decline nearly stopped at 40th week, it still proceeded up to 80th week in SHR.

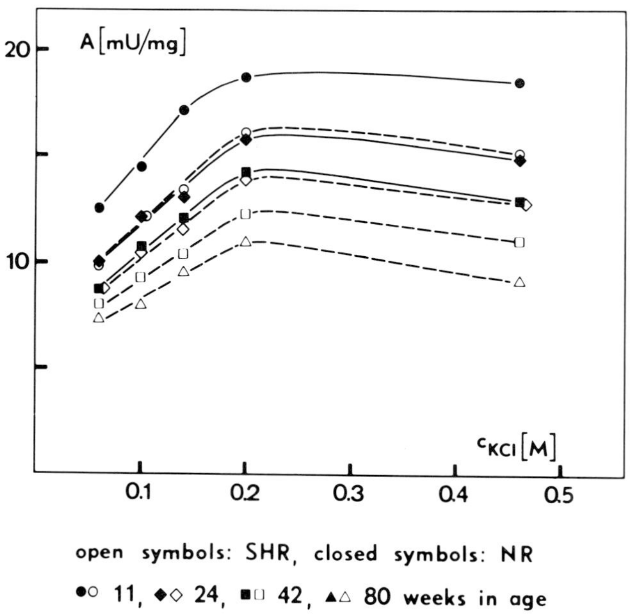

Fig. 5. Left ventricular myosin Mg^{++}-ATPase with KCl concentration varied. Each *curve* represents the means of threee assays done from different myosin preparations

In Fig. 6 the time-dependent changes of the three types of ATPase, measured at conditions for Ca^{++}- and EDTA-ATPase as were indicated by the dashed vertical lines on graphs of pH dependence just before and at conditions as indicated for Mg^{++}-ATPase, are lined out separately. A time course of Ca^{++}-ATPase as well as of Mg^{++}-ATPase activities can be seen, which corresponds well to the one we have found in the contraction parameter dl/dt_{max}, namely an early decrease in SHR which decreases faster with age than in NR. Only activities at 10 weeks deviate somewhat, since Mg^{++}-ATPase in SHR at this age already is significantly lowered.

In EDTA-ATPase, as shown in the middle at two pH values, a completely different behavior, as mentioned above, is exhibited. Whereas only a small decline of activity takes place in NR, the SHR acitvity, which is 40% above the value in NR at 10 weeks, rapidly falls with increasing age.

From these experiments the following conclusion can be drawn for left ventricular myosin ATPase:

1. In both groups of rats an approximately hyperbolic activity decline with increase of age takes place. Similar age-dependent behavior in rats has been reported by other authors [3]. In SHR this decline is more pronounced and seems to get steeper again after the 40th week, which is best seen in Ca^{++}- and EDTA-

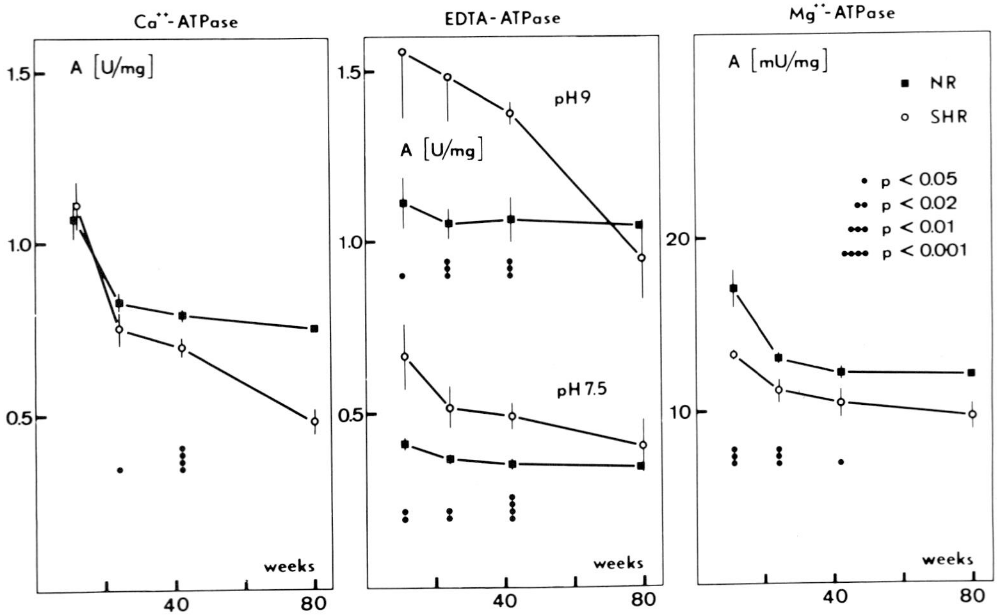

Fig. 6. Time courses of Ca^{++}-ATPase, EDTA-ATPase, and Mg^{++}-ATPase. KCl concentrations and pH values for calcium ATPase and EDTA-ATPase are the same as indicated by the *dashed vertical lines* in Figs 3 and 4, KCl concentrations for Mg^{++}-ATPase is 0.14 *M*. Further conditions as indicated in methods section. *Vertical bars* indicate SD values

ATPase. Concerning age, the latter observation coincides with beginning impairment of myocardial function as observed by other authors [9] and also by my colleagues (see session A, Bürger and Strauer).

2. Off from 20th week, Ca^{++}- and Mg^{++}-ATPase seem to correlate with maximum shortening velocity dl/dt_{max}.

3. EDTA-ATPase, already at the 10th week of age significantly higher in SHR, perhaps indicates a primary difference near the active center, at least in part of left ventricular myosin. Other observations suggesting this are the already strong reduction of Mg^{++}-ATPase at 10th week and, as pointed out in the pH profiles of Ca^{++}-ATPase, the differnt kinds of activity decrease in SHR myosin.

To confirm the above mentioned correlation between speed of muscle shortening and myosin ATPase, age-corresponding couples of activity and dl/dt_{max} values, taken from means of our experiments, were subjected to linear regression analysis. As depicted by the figures (see Fig. 7), a highly significant correlation between dl/dt_{max} and Ca^{++}-ATPase as well as Mg^{++}-ATPase was found.

This might be the largest set of contractile status in one species for which the validity of this correlation has been demonstrated, and it is the first time it has been shown for Mg^{++}-ATPase. On the other hand, no correlation was evaluated for EDTA-ATPase.

Provided good correspondence between changes in activities of myosin Ca^{++}- or Mg^{++}-ATPase and those of Ca^{++} activated actomyosin as well as myofibrillar

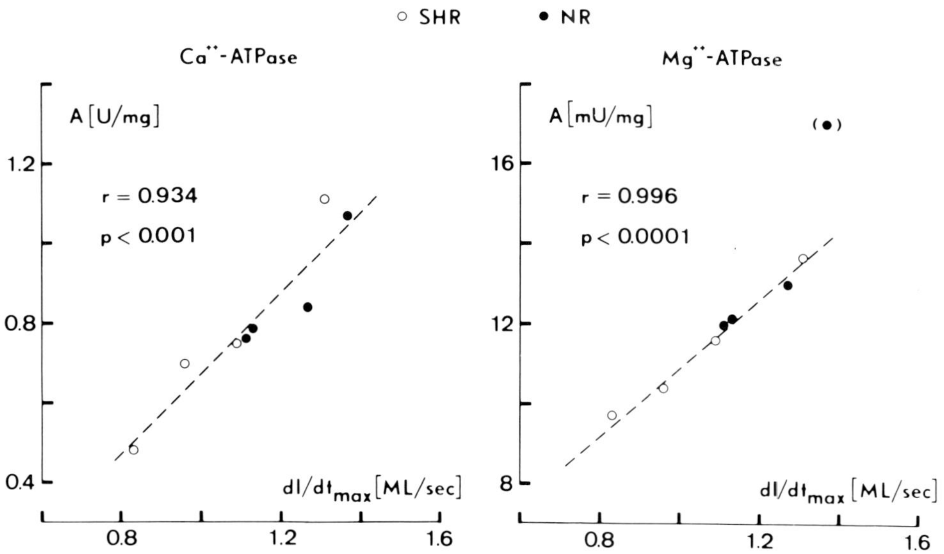

Fig. 7. Correlations of dl/dt_{max} with LV-myosin Ca^{++}-ATPase and Mg^{++}-ATPase activity. *Points* represent age corresponding couples of mean values. The outlying couple of values of Mg^{++}-ATPase and dl/dt_{max} in NR at 11 weeks of age was omitted in regression analysis

ATPase (in SHR, see [1]), the latter being more physiological systems, for an explanation of the above finding, a decrase of maximum rate of substrate hydrolysis, then also occurring in actomyosin during contraction, should cause a corresponding decrease in maximum rate of cross bridge turnover and thus in shortening velocity.

What kind of alteration takes place in the myosin molecule causing the ATPase activity changes observed could not be elucidated by our experiments, although in further experiments which shall do this. As possible alterations causing these functional differences in myosin one should take into account (1) changes in the primary structure of myosin or part of it, preferably in segments forming the active center (this means a change in myosin isozyme pattern) and (2) modifications of polypeptide chains of myosin after synthesis, as by phosphorylation, other modifications of amino acid residues, SH-group oxidation or by proteolytic cleavage in the way only a small fragment of the chain is lost. A cleavage of myosin into larger fragments can be excluded, since our gel electrophoretic runs of myosin never exhibited a gross change of the molecular weights in myosin chains (HC, LC1, LC2) from SHR left ventricles.

To summarize the conclusions:

1. The age-dependent decrease of velocity paramters of contraction, in particularly of maximal shortening velocity, to a significanctly greater extent in SHR is almost exactly paralleled by both Ca^{++}- and Mg^{++}ATPase, thus confirming linear correlations between velocities of shortening and of substrate hydrolysis.

2. A temporary increase in maximum tension seems to be due to a corresponding increase in contractile protein content of the myocardium and may indicate that heart hyperthrophy is in a functionally compensated status.

3. The acceleration of activity fall in SHR Ca^{++}-ATPase after the 40th week as well as the relatively steep decline of other ATPases and of dl/dt_{max} in this age period obviously indicate beginning impairment of myocardial contractile performance.

4. From results obtained with the EDTA-ATPase, a difference in at least part of the heart myosin seems to exist in SHR, either from birth, and then is perhaps of a genetic origin, or from the earliest state of hypertension or hypertrophy, which then is secondary. As indicated by the initially unchanged Ca^{++}-ATPase, it is not necessarily of physiological importance.

References

1. Aoki K, Ikeda N, Yamashita K, Hotta K (1974) ATPase activity and Ca^{++} interaction of myofibrils and sacroplasmic reticulum isolated from the hearts of spontaneously hypertensive rats. Jpn Heart J 15 : 475—484
2. Barany M (1967) ATPase activity of myosin correlated with speed of muscle shortening. J Gen Physiol 50 : 197—218

3. Chesky JA, Rockstein M (1977) Reduced myocardial actomyosin adenosine triphosphatase activity in the ageing male Fischer rat. Cardiovasc Res 11 : 242—246
4. Dietz R, Schömig A, Haebara H, Mann JFE, Rascher W, Lüth JB, Grünherz N, Gross F (1978) Studies on the pathogenesis of spontaneous hypertension in rats. Circ Res Suppl I 43 : 98—106
5. Hamrell BB, Low RB (1978) The relationship of mechanical V_{max} to myosin ATPase activity in rabbit and marmot ventricular muscle. Pfluegers Arch 377 : 119—124
6. Imamura K, Tanijiri H, Ikeda M, Takatsu T, Kashii C, Kawamura K (1976) Further study on cardiac hypertrophy in spontaneously hypertensive rats. Jpn Heart J 17 : 349—351
7. Jacob R, Ebrecht G, Kämmereit A, Medugorac I, Wendt-Gallitelli MF (1977) Myocardial function in different models of cardiac hypertrophy. An attempt at correlating mechanical, biochemical and morphological parameters. Basic Res Cardiol 72 : 160—167
8. Katz AM (1970) Contractile proteins of the heart. Physiol Rev 50 : 63—158
9. Nagoaka A, Kikuchi K, Kawaji H, Matsuo T, Aramaki Y (1972) Life-span, hematological abnormalities, thrombosis and other macroscopical lesions in the spontaneously hypertensive rats. In: Okamoto K (ed) Spontaneous hypertension. Igaku Shoin, Tokyo, pp 149—154
10. Okamoto K, Aoki K (1963) Development of a strain of spontaneously hypertensive rats. Jpn Circ J 27 : 282—293
11. Okamoto K, Yamori Y, Ooshima A, Park C, Haebara H, Matsumoto M, Tanaka T, Okuda T, Hazama F, Kyogoku M (1972) Establishment of the inbred strain of the spontaneously hypertensive rat and genetic factors involved in hypertension. In: Okamoto K (ed) Spontaneous hypertension. Igaku Shoin, Tokyo, pp 1—8
12. Pfeffer JM, Pfeffer MA, Frohlich ED (1971) Validity of an indirect tail-cuff method for determining systolic arterial pressure in unaenesthesized normotensive and spontaneously hypertensive rats. J Lab Clin Med 78 : 957—962
13. Shiverick KT, Thomas LL, Alpert NR (1975) Purification of cardiac myosin. Application to hypertrophied myocardium. Biochim Biophys Acta 393 : 124—133
14. Uchida K, Murakami U, Miratsuka T (1977) Purification of cardiac myosin from rat heart. Proteolytic cleavage and its inhibition. J Biochem 82 : 469—476

Cross Bridge Mechanics in the Heart Muscle of Spontaneously Hypertensive Rats[1]

A. SCHNEIDER AND B.E. STRAUER

Pressure load of the heart in essential hypertension results in left ventricular hypertrophy with contractility of the ventricle in situ being approximately normal (see session C, Strauer). Spntaneously hypertensive rats (SHR, strain Okamoto) represent a widely accepted animal model for essential hypertension. In these rats ventricular function in situ is normal as in human hypertension. Isolated left ventricular papillary muscles show a decrease of isotonic contraction velocity, whereas maximum isometric tension development and contractility parameters not related to velocity are approximately normal or even increased in compensated stages of hypertension of SHR [1 (see session A, Bürger and Strauer)].

The object of the study presented concerns the question whether mechanical properties of isolated contractile proteins — independent of influences from membrane systems or cytosol — are altered in SHR and whether there is a change of these properties with age. The method used was the application of step changes of length to actomyosin fibres and recording the resulting isometric tension course.

Free calcium ions facilitate the interaction of myosin with actin and thus activate muscle contraction [3]. The stretching of an activated muscle fiber up to 1% of its length within 2 — 3 ms yields an increase in tension as a consequence of stretching the myosin cross bridges attached to actin at the moment of stretch. According to Huxley [5], the attached cross bridges are the substrate of series elasticity of muscle. By the quick stretch the elastic structure of the attached cross bridges (HMM — S 2 subunit of myosin) is stretched, resulting in tension increase. This state of extension is unphysiological for the cross bridge; therefore it detaches, resulting in a fall of tension. This detachment disturbs the equilibrum of attached and detached cross bridges. To reconstruct this equilibrum detached cross bridges attach in a synchronous manner, resulting in a delayed tension increase [13, 14].

---

1 Supported by the Deutsche Forschungsgemeinschaft

Methods

Spontaneously hypertensive rats, strain Okamoto, and normotensive Wistar-Kyoto control rats (NR) were used [10]. Functional isolation of myocardial contractile proteins was achieved by incubation of papillary muscles in a glycerol solution, resulting in destruction of cell membranes and removal of cytosol. Thus it was possible to expose the contractile proteins to a controlled chemical environment.

Left heart papillary muscles of rats kept at resting length were extracted in glycerol solution (50% glycerol, 50% water, 20 m*M* Histidine, 10 m*M* NaN_3, pH = 7.0) for 2 days at 4 °C and then stored at −20 °C for at least 1 week in fresh glycerol solution until used. From the glycerol extracted papillary muscels, fiber bundles were dissected measuring 2 − 3 mm in length and about 0.3 mm in diameter. These fiber bundles were washed in ATP-free solution, and their ends were glued to the two glass rods of the apparatus. Resting length was determined in relaxing solution as the biggest length causing no detectable elastic force. All experiments were performed at room temperature (22 °C).

The experimental apparatus (Fig. 1) consisted of a servo motor allowing step movement of a glass rod within 3 ms over variable amplitudes. The other glass rod was fixed to a RCA 5734 force transducer valve (compliance 1μm/100 mg) for isometric tension measurement. The tension was displayed on a Textronix 5103 N oscilloscipe and recorded by a ultraviolet recorder (Honeywell 1858 visicorder).

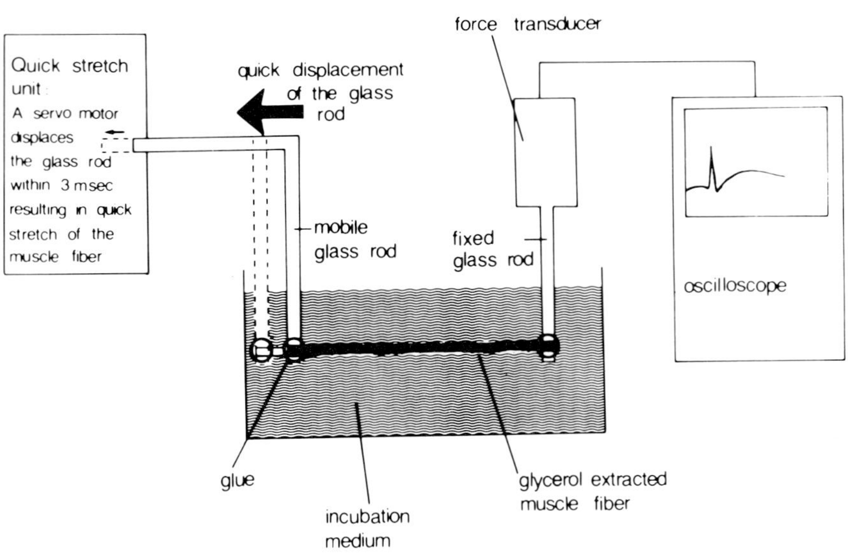

Fig. 1. Diagrammatic representation of the apparatus for stretch experiments on glycerol extracted muscle fibers: the muscle is quickly stretched by the servo motor, and the stretch-reactive isometric tension course is recorded

The amplitude of the initial tension peak following stretch is named "immediate stiffness" T_1. In this paper the term "stiffness" is used according to Huxley [5]. See Fig. 2 for determination of the time constant τ, a measure for the velocity of delayed tension increase.

Incubation media were composed of:

1. Relaxing solution: ATP, 15 m*M*; $MgCl_2$, 15 m*M*; imidazole, 20 m*M*; EGTA, 4 m*M*; and NaN_3, 10 m*M*, with pH = 6.7.

2. Contraction solution: the same constituents as relaxing solution with the addition of $CaCl_2$ 4 m*M*, resulting in a free calcium ion concentration of 5.7×10^{-5} *M*. Free calcium ion concentration was adjusted mixing relaxing and contraction solution.

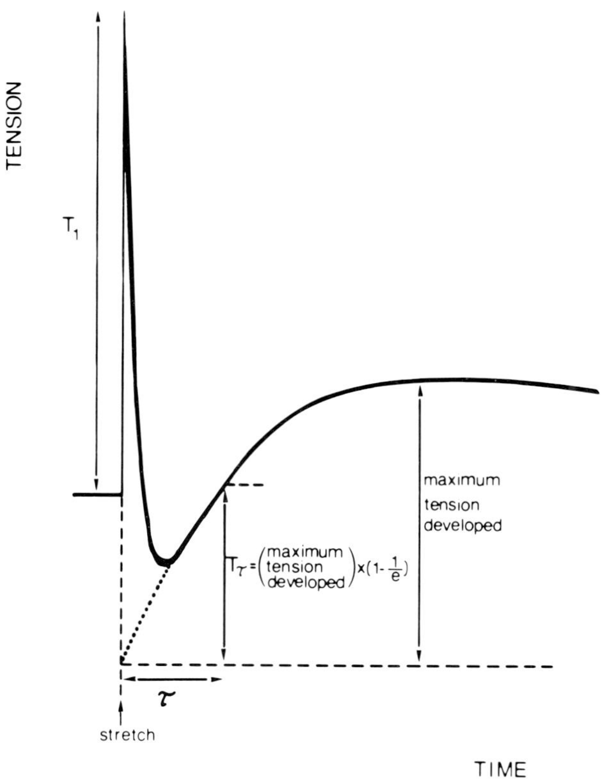

Fig. 2. Determination of the parameters of tension behavior following quick stretch of a glycerol extracted muscle fiber. The curve of delayed tension development is extrapolated (...........) to the beginning of stretch (↑); the time constant τ is the time elapsing until the extrapolated curve of actively developed tension reaches a value that is 1/e smaller than the maximal actively developed tension; this tension value is named T_τ.

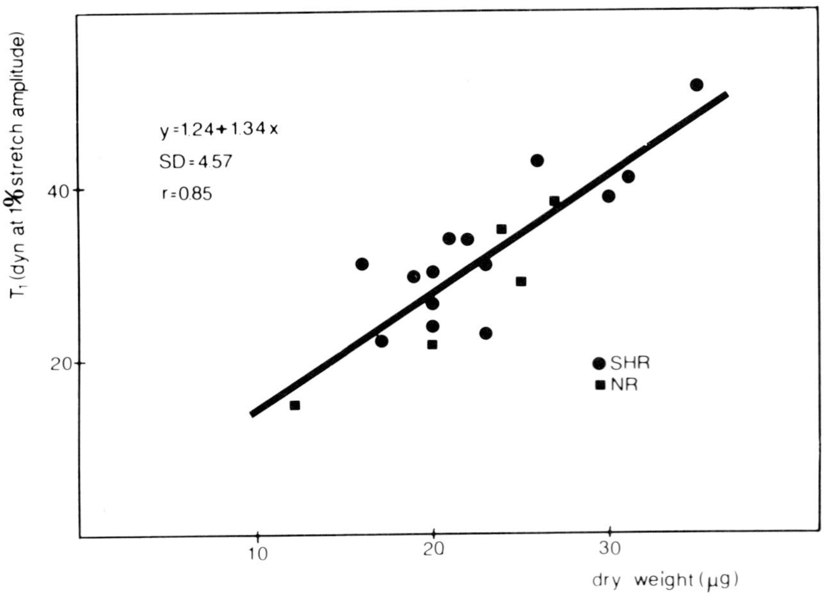

Fig. 3. The relation between stiffness (T_1) at maximum activation and dry weight of the sample. There is a linear relation between stiffness and dry weight. The T_1 values were obtained at a free calcium ion concentration of 5 x 10^{-5} *M* and a stretch amplitude of 1% of the initial length

Washing solution: KCl 20 m*M*; imidazole, 20 m*M*; NaN_3, 5 m*M*; $MgCl_2$, 15 m*M*; and EGTA, 4 m*M*, with pH = 6.7.

Washing the finally prepared fiber bundles with water leaves essentially only contractile proteins. Their dry weight can be used as a measure of contractile protein. This is underlined by a linear relation between stiffness and dry weight (Fig. 3).

Results

Comparison of Immediate Stiffness of Myocardial Fibres from SHR and NR

The amplitude of the immediate stiffness T_1 depends on the amplitude of quick stretch in a linear way. Stiffness increases with increasing concentration of free calcium ions; the concentration effect curve has a sigmoidal shape as shown in Fig. 4.

The free calcium ion concentration, where half of the effect obtainable with calcium is seen (EC 50), differs insignificantly among the six groups examined (SHR and NR; 10, 40, and 80 weeks old) between pCa = 6.06 and pCa = 6.23.

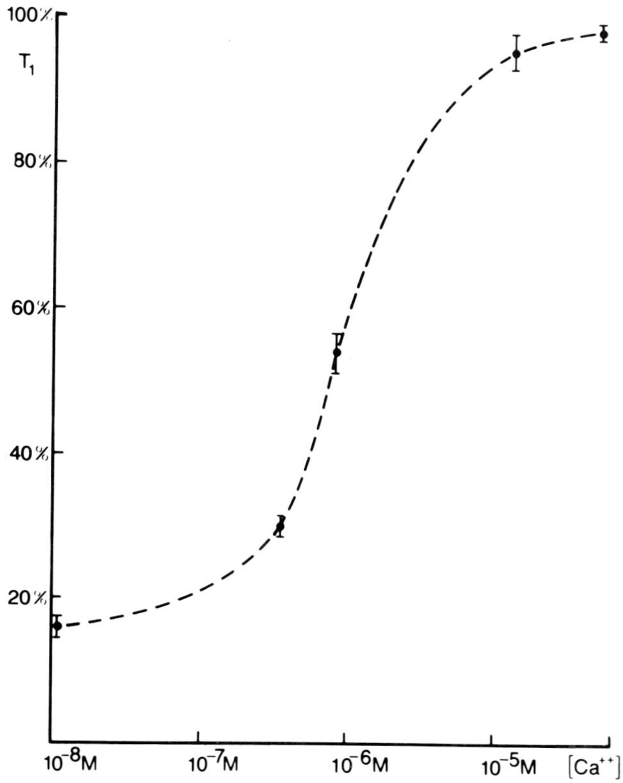

Fig. 4. Concentration effect curve of calcium ion concentration (*abscissa*) on the amplidute of immediate stiffness T_1 (*ordinate*; the maximum value is taken as 100%). 10-week-old normotensive rats, M ± SEM, n = 8

Comparing the stiffness at various calcium concentrations reveals marked differences between SHR and NR. At low Ca^{++} SHR heart fibres show higher stiffness values than heart fibres of NR (stiffness values expressed as percent of the maximum stiffness values at high Ca^{++} concentration; Figs 4, 5).

Comparing the maximum stiffness per unit of dry weight, there are no detectable differences between SHR and NR and no changes with age. There is a linear relation between the amplitude of stiffness and the dry weight of the sample (Fig. 3).

Comparison of Contraction Time Constants of SHR and NR

The time constant τ (see Fig. 6) is significantly longer in SHR than in NR at all ages. Normotensive rats show a slight and continuous increase of τ with increasing age. In SHR there is a slight increase between 10 and 40 weeks of age similar to the course in NR. In 80-week-old SHR, however, the time constant is

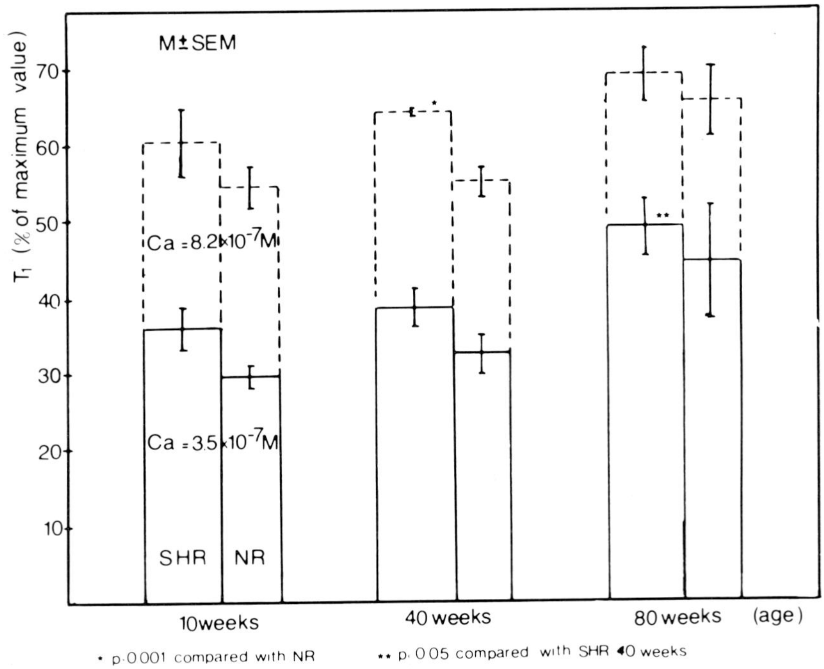

Fig. 5. Stiffness (T_1) values at two different free calcium ion concentrations (3.5 x 10^{-7} *M, continued lines*, and 8.2 x 10^{-7} *M, interrupted lines*) expressed as percent of the respective maximum values (compare Fig. 4). In any case, the percentage is higher in SHR than in NR

much longer. The difference between 40 and 80 weeks of age is more marked in SHR than in NR. The increase of τ is significant at 80 weeks of age in both cases.

Discussion

The immediate stiffness T_1 is caused by stretch of the cross bridges attached to actin at the moment of length change [5]. Therefore, the amplitude of T_1 is a measure for the number of cross bridges attached at the moment of stretch. This explains the correlation between T_1 and dry weight of the preparation, which approximately represents the amount of contractile protein (Fig. 3).

Stiffness rises with increasing concentration of free calcium ions (Fig. 4). Calcium ions facilitate the interaction of myosin with actin by binding to the troponin molecule attached to the actin filament. This binding results in a conformational change within troponin and the tropomyosin molecule linked to troponin. Thus, the binding sites of actin are opended and the myosin cross bridges can attach to them [3].

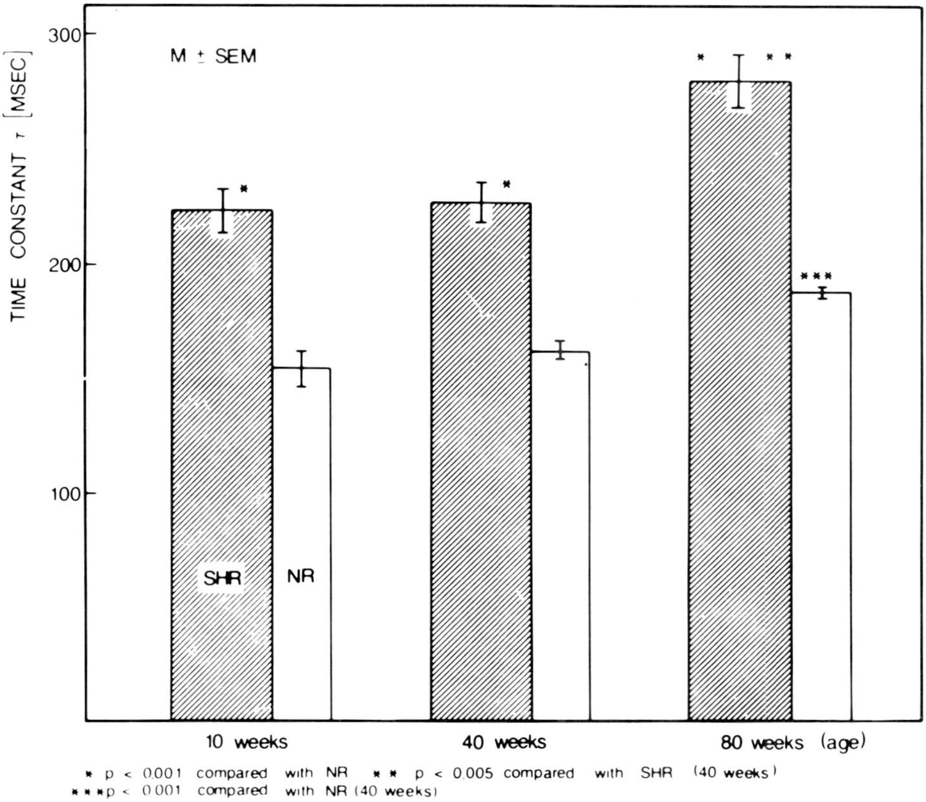

Fig. 6. Time constant τ of delayed tension increase of NR and SHR at different ages. (Free $Ca^{++} = 1.4 \times 10^{-5}$ *M*; all groups n = 8 except NR 80 weeks: n = 5)

The fact that the EC_{50} of calcium is not different between NR and SHR of any age group indicates that the calcium binding to troponin is not different between these groups.

The quantiatative differences in the reaction of stiffness to calcium ion concentration between SHR and NR (Fig. 5) indicate that there are differences in the reactions following calcium binding to troponin. This means there are differences in the troponin at sites other than the calcium binding site, in the tropomyosin, in the actin binding site for myosin, or in the binding site of myosin cross bridges (HMM — S1 subunit of myosin) for actin.

The delayed tension development is caused by a synchronous attachment and rotation of the myosin cross bridges. The velocity of this delayed tension development, expressed by the time constant τ, is a measure of the rotation rate of the cross bridges [15, 16].

The time constant is longer in SHR than in NR already in the stage of early hypertension (10 weeks) and does not change greatly as long as the heart is not failing. This difference either represents a very early hypertrophy — or hypertension — reacitve change or it has a hereditary base; a decision between these alternatives will be made possible by investigating rats younger than 10 weeks. The clear increase of τ in 80-week-old SHR probably must be seen in connection with the beginning cardiac failure appearing at this age.

The system observed in experiments on glycerol-extracted muscle fibres is only the system of isolated contractile proteins. Therefore it is not surprising that one finds marked discrepancies when comparing the reported results to contractility parameters of papillary muscles from SHR and NR [1, (see session A, Bürger and Strauer)].

Many other mechanisms have to be taken into account when comparing myosin cross bridge properties in isolated actomyosin and contractility parameters of the intact papillary muscle and the heart in situ, e.g., (1) influences of nervous or humoral origin, the most important of which is probably the elevated sympathetic tone in SHR [2, 6, 7, 11, 18], and renal factors; and (2) excitation conduction in the heart and electromechanical coupling, e.g., the decreased calcium binding and transport capacity of sarcoplasmic reticulum in SHR hearts [9], possibly resulting in an increased mean intracellular calcium concentration [4, 12]. Calcium release by the sarcoplasmic reticulum has a similar velocity as the time constant τ [17] and may influence contraction velocity.

The fact that the maximum isometric tension development of intact papillary muscle — a parameter not influenced by cross bridge rotation rate [8] — is even higher in SHR in compensated stages than in NR indicates that some of the mechanicms mentioned act to improve contactility and so compensate the reduced contractile properties of isolated actomyosin.

Summary

Mechanical properties of isolated contractile proteins of the heart muscles of normotensive (NR) and spontaneously hypertensive rats (SHR) of different age groups (10, 40, 80 weeks) were investigated. Glycerol extracted preparations from left ventricular muscles were activated in solutions containing different free calcium ion concentrations and were quickly stretched within 3 ms. The amplitude of tension increase synchronous with stretch as a measure for the amount of activated contractile protein revealed no difference at high Ca^{++} concentrations and higher values for SHR preparations at low Ca^{++} concentrations. The time constant of the delayed tension increase following stretch as a measure for actomyosin cross bridge rotation rate showed significantly slower cross bridge rotation in SHR compared with NR at all age groups investigated and decreasing roatation rate with age in both NR and SHR. A very early hypertrophy- or hypertension-reactive change in SHR heart muscle or a hereditary difference between contractile proteins of heart muscles of SHR and NR are discussed.

References

1. Bürger S, Meinardus A, Strauer BE (1978) Hypertrophiegrad and Dynamik des linken Ventrikels bei der spontanen essentiellen Hypertonie der Ratte Klin Wochenschr 56 : 207—209
2. Coote JH, Sato Y (1977) Reflex regulation of sympathetic activity in the spontaneously hypertensive rat. Circ Res 40 : 571—577
3. Ebashi S, Endo M (1968) Calcium ion and muscle contraction. Prog Biophys Mol Biol 18 : 123—183
4. Froehlich JP, Lakatta EG, Beard E, Spurgeon HA, Weisfeldt ML, Gerstenblith G (1978) Studies of sarcoplasmic reticulum function and contraction duration in young and aged rat myocardium. J Mol Cell Cardiol 10 : 427—438
5. Huxley AF, Simmons RM (1971) Proposed mechanism of force generation in striated muscle. Nature 233 : 533—538
6. Iriuchijma J (1973) Sympathetic discharge rate in spontaneously hypertensive rats. Jpn Heart J 14 : 350—356
7. Judy WV, Watanabe AM, Henry DP, Besch HR, Murphy WR, Hockel GM (1976) Sympathetic nerve activity: Role in regulation of blood pressure in the spontaneously hypertensive rat. Circ Res Suppl II 38 : 21—29
8. Katz AM (1972) The force-velocity curve. Cardiol 57 : 2—10
9. Limas CJ, Cohn JN (1977) Defective calcium transport by cardiac sarcoplasmic reticulum in spontaneous hypertensive rats. Circ Res Suppl I 40 : 62—69
10. Okamoto K, Aoki K (1963) Development of a strain of spontaneously hypertensive rats. Jpn Circ J 27 : 282—293
11. Okamoto K, Nosaka S, Yamori Y, Matsumoto M (1967) Participation of neural factors in the pathogenesis of hypertension in the spontaneously hypertensive rat. Jpn Heart J 8 : 168—180
12. Penpargkul S, Bhan AK, Scheurer J (1976) Studies of subcellular control factors in hearts of uremic rats. J Lab Clin Med 88 : 563—570
13. Schädler M, Steiger GJ, Rüegg JC (1971) Mechanical activation and isometric oscillation in insect fibrillar muscle. Pfluegers Arch 330 : 217—229
14. Steiger GJ (1973) Mechanische Experimente an Herzmuskelpräparaten. Habilitationsschrift, University of Bochum
15. Steiger GJ (1977) Tension transients in extracted rabbit heart muscle preparations. J Mol Cell Cardiol 9 : 671—685
16. Thorson J, White DCS (1969) Distributed representations for actin-myosin interaction in the oscillatory contraction of muscle. Biophys J 9 : 360—390
17. Tritthart H, Kaufmann R, Volkmer HP, Bayer R, Krause H (1973) Ca-movement controlling myocardial contractility. Pfluegers Arch 338 : 207—231
18. Yamori Y (1976) Neural and non-neural mechanisms in spontaneous hypertension. Clin Sci Mol Med 51 : 431s—434s

The Utilization of Energy by the Myocardium Hypertrophied Secondary to Pressure Overload[1]

N.R. ALPERT AND L.A. MULIERI
with the technical assistence of R.P. GOULETTE

Introduction

Cardiac hypertrophy is an important well-documented consequence of systemic hypertension in humans and animals. In a simple sense the hypertrophy is compensatory. Without the accretion of new tissue, consisting of contractile [1, 2, 3] as well as noncontractile components [4], dilation and failure would occur.

The problem is not a simple one. Precise analysis of the hypertrophied myocardium indicates that alterations at a molecular level exist. Morbidity and mortality in hypertensive patients increase in direct proportion to the degree of myocardial hypertrophy and age [5]. There is an abnormal response to severe endurance exercise stress at a stage of the disease when other signs of cardiac dysfunction are absent at rest or at low endurance work loads [6]. In hypertrophied human hearts force-velocity curves, calculated from intraluminal pressure changes, geometry, and estimates of series compliance, are depressed [7]. Additional evidence of alterations in the performance of the hypertrophied heart is reflected in the changes observed in systolic electromechanical time intervals which can be interpreted in terms of excitation-contraction (EC) coupling as well as mechanical abnormalities [8, 9]. Finally, in failing hearts enlarged secondary to hypertensive heart disease, there is a depressed contractile protein ATP-ase activity [10].

It is our hypothesis that chronic stress-induced myocardial growth involves fundamental molecular changes in the myocardium. Alterations are present even during the early stages of hypertrophy when gross failure is not apparent. This process is adaptive, in that the increased pressure demands on the heart are met. The process impinges on the cardiac reserve, however, and if rate demands are made or if the alterations progress far enough, failure ensues.

The development of this functional change is a gradual process. Our strategy to study this process involves the use of an animal model, rabbit right ventricular hypertrophy secondary to pulmonary artery banding, where failure is not pre-

1 This work was supported in part by NIH grants 1 R01 HL22845-01, T32 HL07073, and 1 R01 HL17592

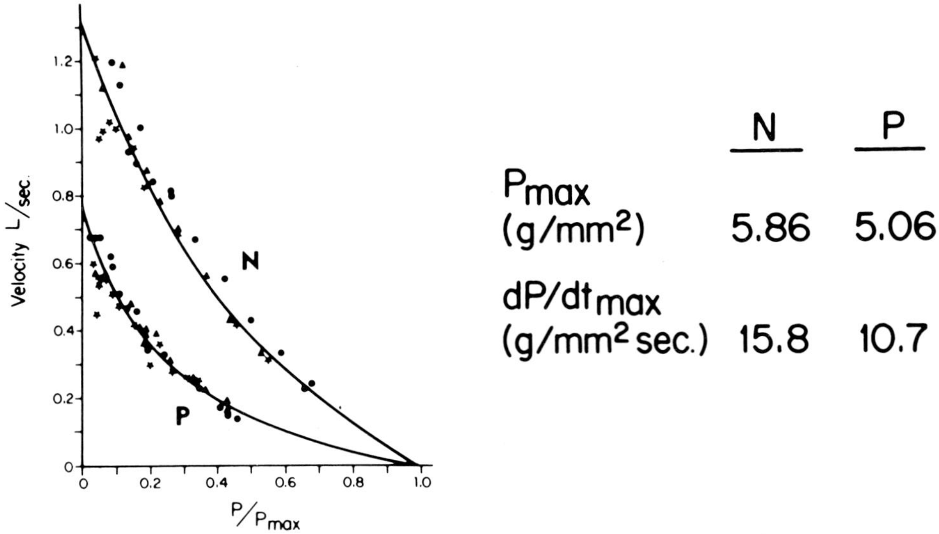

Fig. 1. The force-velocity curve and isometric tension of rabbit right ventricular papillary muscles from normal (*N*) hearts and those hypertrophied secondary to pulmonary artery banding (*P*). Redrawn from Hamrell and Alpert [11]

sent. Alterations known to be present in human hypertrophy are known to exist in this model such as changes in mechanics involving depressed maximum velocity of shortening (V_{max}) and rate of tension development (dP/dt_{max}) (Fig. 1 [11]). There is depressed actin-activated myosin ATPase activity [12, 13] and altered EC coupling as expressed by the increase in time to peak tension (TPT [11]) and the mechanical response to increasing the calcium ion concentration in the incubation medium [14].

It is our plan to use rapid myothermal techniques to evaluate the contribution of the altered myocardial EC coupling and contractile systems to the energetics of tension development in the rabbit heart which is hypertrophied secondary to pressure overload.

Methods

Animal Models. All experiments are performed on right ventricular papillary muscles from male albino rabbits weighing 1.8—2.0 kg. Pressure overload hypertrophy is produced by placing a spiral monel metal constrictor around the proximal pulmonary artery as previously described [11]. These animals are sacrificed 4 — 6 weeks postoperatively, the heart is quickly removed and placed in oxygenated Krebs-Ringer solution, and the papillary muscles are prepared as described below.

Temperature and Force Measurements. The right ventricle is opened, and the papillary muscle is excised and mounted on planar, vacuum-deposited bismuth

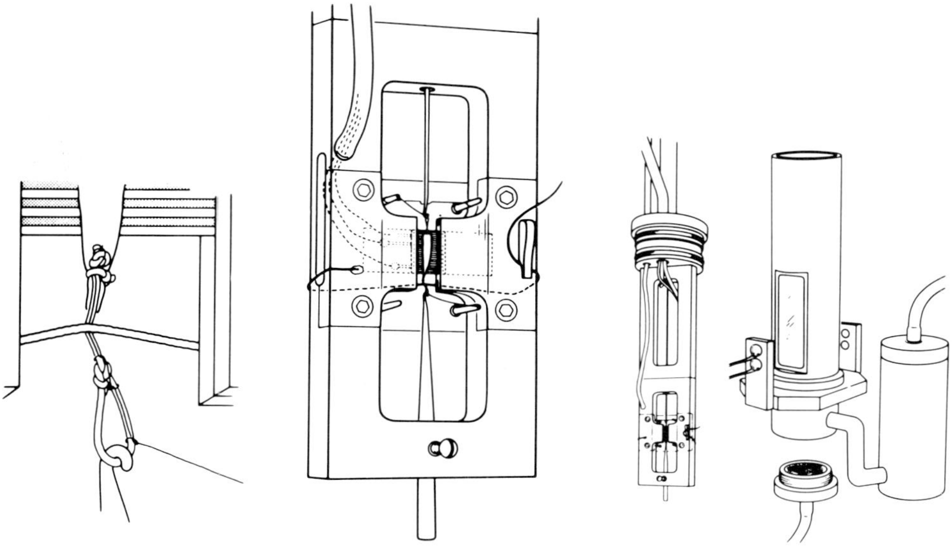

Fig. 2. A planar Hill-type vacuum deposited bismuth and antimony thermopile system. (A) Enlargement of tendinous end of the muscle attached to the stationary hook, with stimulating electrode as an integral part of the silk ligature, and a horizontal tether to insure contact of the papillary muscles with the thermopile junctions. (B) The thermopile mounted in the brass frame with the cut end of the papillary muscle (*upper end*) fixed to a glass link which is connected to the force transducer. (C) The complete thermopile and brass frame as assembly. (D) The incubation chamber with Krebs-Ringer reservoir (*lower right*) and oxygenation system (*lower left*). The window in the chamber and infrared diodes permit in situ calibration. Redrawn from Mulieri et al. [15]

and antimony thermopiles as previously described (Fig. 2 [15]). The cut end of the muscle is attached to an isometric force transducer [16] while the tendinous end is fixed to a stationary hook (Fig. 2B). A horizontal tether forces the lower tendinous end of the muscle into close contact with the active thermopile elements (Fig. 2A). The thermopile assembly (Fig. 2C) is placed inside the thermopile chamber (Fig. 2D), allowing the muscle to be bathed in oxygenated Krebs-Ringer solution or surrounded by moist air. The thermopile has low thermal capacity which permits its use with papillary muscles weighing as little as 1 mg. In addition, this type of thermopile has high sensitivity and low electrical resistance so that it can be matched with a Kipp galvanometer recording system. The frequency response of the system is 60 Hz with a cumulative drift of 0.14 mcal/h. When the muscle is heated externally by the application of a 5 kHz subthreshold sine wave, there is a 6.5 ms delay between the first detectable temperature change and the current onset. When a threshold stimulus is applied to the muscle, the earliest detectable temperature change is noted 19—20 ms after application of the stimulus. With the myothermal delays described above, initial heat measurements associated with each twitch can be made. The entire myothermal assembly is palced in a 70-liter constant temperature bath where equilibration in Krebs-Ringer solution is carried out at 21 °C for 2 h. The muscle is stimulated at 0.2 Hz and the experiments are accepted only if muscle heat and tension performance are stable over the entire experimental period (5—10 h) and twitch tension is at least four times greater than resting tension.

Initial Tension-Dependent and Tension-Independent Heat Measurements. The temperature of a contracting papillary muscle is determined by the evolution of resting, initial, and recovery heats and the associated cool-off characteristics of the system. The steady-state temperature oscillation which occurs with each isometric contraction can be measured with our rapid myothermal techniques

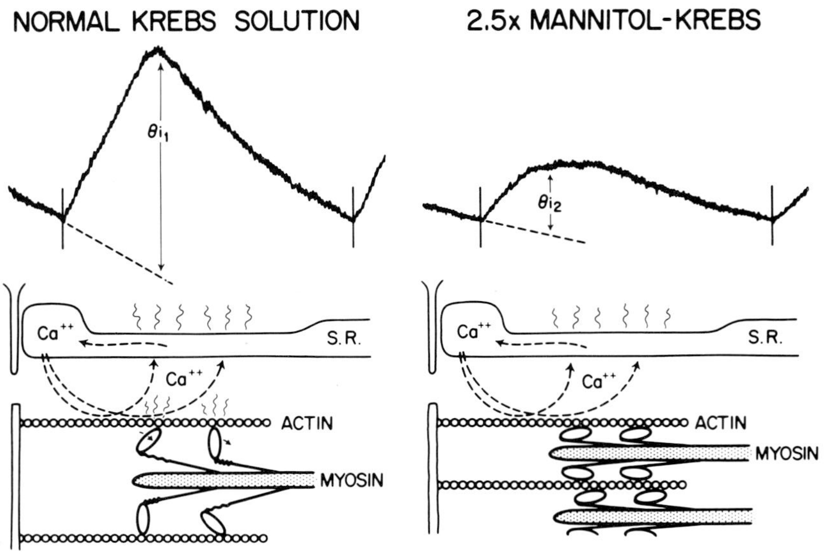

Fig. 3. Initial TDH and TIH measurements. The *upper curve on the left* is the steady-state temperature oscillation of right ventricular papillary muscle during isometric contraction. θ_{i1} is the temperature change corrected for heat loss as described in the text. The diagram *below on the left* represents the major sources of initial heat evolution: cross bridge cycling with ATP hydrolysis and Ca^{++} removal by the SR and the associated ATP hydrolysis. The *upper right hand trace* is the steady state temperature change of the stimulated papillary muscle incubated in 2.5 X hyperosmotic mannitol-Krebs solution where isometric tension is virtually eliminated. The temperature change, θ_{i2}, of the TIH is corrected for heat loss as described. This triggerable heat evolution under these conditions is primarily the result of calcium removal by the SR *(diagram lower right).* The temperature change associated with tension development is the difference between θ_{i1} and θ_{i2}

and consists of the initial heat and recovery heat (Fig. 3 upper trace, normal Krebs solution). Temperature changes associated with the initial heat liberation are corrected for heat loss by the extrapolation procedures shown by the dashed line in Fig. 3 (normal Krebs solution). The dashed line is obtained by translating the cool off curve which occurs upon cessation of stimulation. The corrected temperature change, $\theta i1$, is converted to the corresponding heat evolution by multiplication with the effective heat capacity of the muscle plus adhering Krebs solution as previously described [15]. The initial heat is made up of the tension-dependent and tension-independent heats (Fig. 3, left upper and lower diagram). The former represents cross bridge cycling and ATP splitting during tension development, while the latter represents the energy cost of excitation and the translocation of calcium during contraction and relaxation. Tension-independent heat (TIH) is obtained by measuring the triggerable heat output when tension is eliminated by incubating the muscle in hyperosmotic (2.5 X N) mannitol Krebs solution (Fig. 3, right upper and lower diagrams). The temperature change under these conditions, $\theta i2$, is obtained and corrected for cool off as previously described. The heat production is calculated by multiplying this temperature by the effective heat capacity of the muscle and adhering Krebs solution. The tension-dependent heat (TDH) is the difference between initial heat and TIH.

Results

General. The right ventricular heart-weight — body-weight ratio and papillary muscle cross sectional area increased to 213% and 185%, respectively, in the pressure overload preparations (P) (Table 1). The dry/wet weight ratios of papillary muscle and liver were 104% (NS) and 114% ($P < 0.02$) of normal (N), respectiveley, for the P preparations.

Table 1. Pressure overload hypertrophy (*P*)[a]

	weight RV/Body g/kg	X-Section RV Pap M mm^2	weight Dry/Wet Pap M	Liver
Normal	0.31 ± 0.01	0.57 ± 0.06	0.23 ± 0.006	0.28 ± 0.01
P	0.66 ± 0.02	1.05 ± 0.11	0.24 ± 0.005	0.32 ± 0.02
	$P < 0.001$	$P < 0.001$	N.S.	$P < 0.02$

[a] RV = right ventricle; Pap M = Papillary muscle

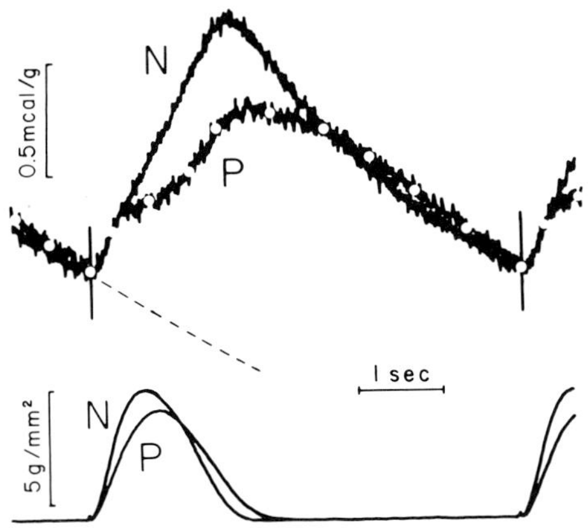

Fig. 4. Steady-state force (*lower*) and temperature (*upper*) changes for the normal (*N*) and pressure overload (*P*) preparations

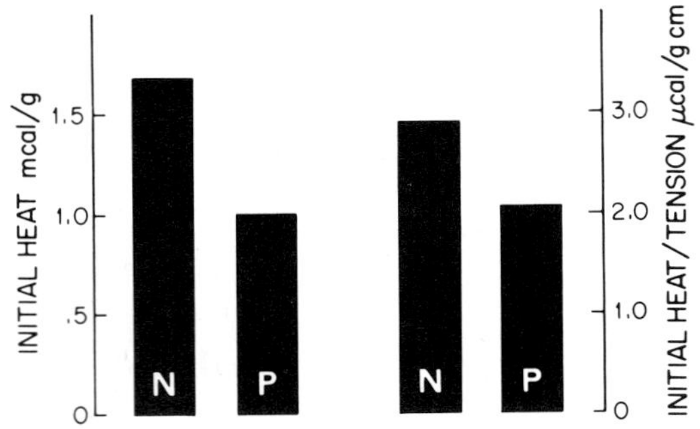

Fig. 5. Initial heat per gram of muscle and per unit tension for the normal (*N*) and pressure overload (*P*) preparations

Mechanical and Thermal Measurements. Peak isometric twitch tension was 5.8 ± 0.3 SEM g/mm^2 for the N muscles. The P preparations had twitch tensions which were 86% of the control (NS) while the initial heat production was lower and was liberated more slowly (Fig. 4). The initial heat per gram of N muscle and per unit tension were 1.71 mcal/g and 2.90 μ cal/g cm, respectively. In the P preparations the initial heat was reduced 41% per gram of muscle and 29% per unit tension (Fig. 5). The TDH and TIH components of the initial heat are 2.15 μ cal/g cm and 0.39 m cal/g, respectively, for the N preparation. These values are reduced by 53% (TIH) and 14% (TDH) for the P preparations.

Discussions

Myocardial hypertrophy which occurs as a result of prolonged pressure overload permits the heart to meet the demands for increased power placed on it. The change in performance is not directly related to the increase in muscle mass. There is an apparent alteration in the performance of the whole heart as well as for each muscle unit. The former expresses itself in terms of a depressed response to severe endurance exercise stress [6], a downward shift in the calculated force-velocity curve [7], changes in the systolic electromechanical time intervals [8, 9], and a decrease in contractile protein ATPase activity [10]. In previous studies of pressure overload hypertrophy, we and others reported a depression in mechanical V_{max} [11, 17], an increase in time to peak tension [11], a depressed myosin ATPase acitvity [10, 18–26], and an altered response to increasing external calcium ion [14]. These changes suggest subtle alterations at the molecular level which influence the quality and limitations of the adaptation. In a preliminary set of experiments, we previously reported a depressed heat production per unit of tension for these preparations [27]. The present studies are an extension of that report with additional experiments and an analysis to place the data in a framework of the molecular events known to occur during contraction and relaxation.

The TIH is considered to be a reflection of the energy cost of calcium cycling. If we assume that every two calcium ions transported from the sacroplasm into the sarcoplasmic reticulum (SR) require the splitting of one ATP [28] and that realease from the SR, initial binding to the SR, binding to troponin, and release from troponin are thermo-neutral in a complete cycle, then the calcium movement can be calculated for a contraction relaxation cycle. Wilkie determined that the contraction-relaxation cycle molar enthalpy for phosphocreatine splitting is 11 kcal/mol [29]. The TIH is thus equivalent to the removal of 0.070 (N) and 0.032 (P) μ moles of Ca^{++} per gram for each contraction-relaxation cycle. According to Solaro and Briggs [30, 31], this would represent over 90% (N) and 60% (P) saturation of the activation system for the two preparations. This apparent high value may be explained by assuming that calcium pumping is a continuous process throughout the contraction relaxation cycle, and therefore the total amount pumped is not directly related to the cytoplasmic calcium concentration. In addition the in vivo stoichiometry may be somewhat different from in vitro measurements.

Although the tension-dependent heat, presumed to represent cross bridge cycling, is depressed only 14% (N.S.) in the P preparations, we believe there may be a significant depression of 21% in the parameter. The latter figure is predicted on the basis of a regression line fit of TDH versus myosin ATPase data from a larger series of experiments, including P animals as well as thyrotoxicosis-induced hypertrophy where oppositely directed changes in heat liberation and myosin ATPase occur [32]. Since the time to peak tension is prolonged in these hearts (128%) and we assume that the major portion of TDH is liberated during contraction time, the actual tension-dependent heat rate is reduced to 64% of normal. This reduction in TDH rate is approximately equal to the reduction in actin-activated myosin ATPase from these hearts which is reduced to 70% of normal. From measurements of fast and slow muscles in the rat [33] one would predict a twofold change in TDH for each onefold change in ATPase acitvity or a reduction of TDH to 40% of normal. That this does not occur may reflect a fundamental difference between fast and slow cardiac and skeletal myosins.

The TDH data can be analyzed in terms of an enzyme kinetic analysis of cross bridge cycling and tension development [34, 35]. The main features of this scheme are that the acitvated contractile system exists in two distinct states, with the actin and myosin associated and disassociated (Fig. 6). The overall rate-limiting step exists in the dissociated or „off“ state between M**ADPPi and M‡ADPPi (Fig. 6, arrow 1). This step probably controls the overall cycling

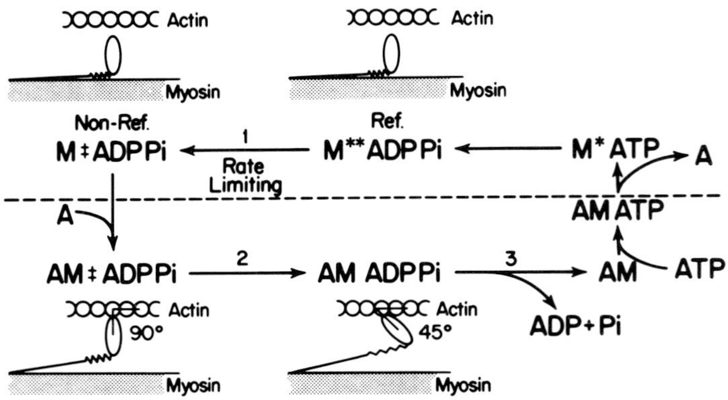

Fig. 6. Actin-acitvated myosin ATPase kinetics and cross bridge behavior. *M*, myosin; *A*, actin; *ATP*, adenosine-triphosphate; *ADP*, adenosine diphosphate; *Pi*, inorganic phosphate; and M‡, *M***, different conformational states of myosin. *Upper portion* of diagram represents "off" state and the *lower portion* the "on" state. Redrawn from Eisenberg and Hill [34]

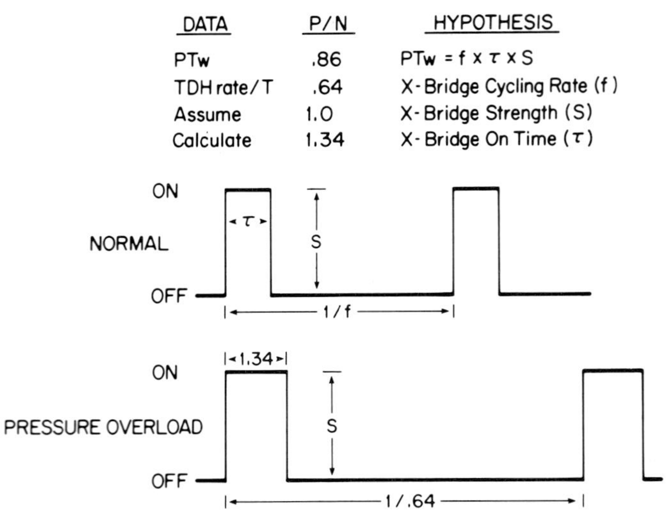

Fig. 7. The "on-off" cycle of cross bridges for the control and pressure overload preparations (see text for discussion)

rate. In the associated or "on" state force is generated when the cross bridge head rotates from the 90° to the 45° position, stretching the compliant elements in the myosin molecule (Fig. 6, arrow 2). Although this step is not rate limiting for the overall cycling, the length of time that the myosin head stays in the "on" position at an angle less than 90° and the compliance of the myosin link determine the force developed per cycle. This "on" positon corresponds to the conformational states $AM^{\ddagger}$ADPPi, AM ADPPi, and AM (Fig. 6, arrows 2 and 3) [34, 35].

Thus the energetics of tension development can be analyzed in terms of the "on" time and the cycling rate (Fig. 7). As a first approximation to quantify the chemomechanical aspects of tension development, consider the following model. Assume that the peak twitch (PTW) is a function of the cross bridge cycling rate (TDH rate) (f), the "on" time (τ), and the average stiffness of the cross bridge (S). Under conditions of pressure overload, if we assume S to be unity for both preparations, the increase in efficiency of tension development results from an increase in "on" time and a decrease in cycling rate (Fig. 7).

The ability of the heart to alter its internal structure in response to pressure overload stress effects the contractile system (myosin) and the EC coupling system (SR). These changes make the pressure overload hypertrophied heart an efficient slow-tension-producing machine. It is adapted to develop higher pressures at a slower rate. The increased efficiency of tension or pressure development results from a decrease in the amount and rate of calcium ion cycling as well as a decrease in the actomyosin cycling rate and an increase in the cross bridge"on" time during the concentration relaxation cycle. Wehen rate demands are made on the heart the adaptation is anticompensatory. Thus, in severe exercise stress where heart rate increases, the demand for developing pressure faster cannot be met by the pressure overload hypertrophied heart. As a result the specific adaptations which facilitate efficient, slow force development in pressure overload hypertrophy prevent rapid force development and may lead to decompensation when such demands are made.

References

1. Morkin E (1971) Myocardial nucleic acid metabolism in experimental cardiac hypertrophy. In: Alpert NR (ed) Cardiac hypertrophy. Academic Press New York, pp 259–271
2. Schreiber SS, Oratz M, Rothschild MA (1971) Initiation of protein synthesis in the acutely overloaded perfused heart. In: Alpert NR (ed) Cardiac hypertrophy. Academic Press, New York, pp 215–245
3. Zak R, Fischman DA (1971) Studies on protein synthesis in heart muscles during development and in experimentally produced hypertrophy. In: Alpert NR (ed) Cardiac hypertrophy. Academic Press, New York, pp 247–258
4. Rabinowitz M, Schenbrenner V, Albin R, Gross NJ, Zak R, Nair KG (1971) Synthesis and turnover of heart mitochondria in normal, hypertrophied and hypoxic rat. In: Alpert NR, (ed) Cardiac hypertrophy. Academic Press, New York, pp 283–299

5. Kannel W, Gordon BT, Offutt D (1969) Left ventricular hypertrophy by electrocardiogram: Prevalence, incidence and mortality in the Framingham study. Ann Internal Med 71 : 89—105
6. Amery A, Julius S, Whitlock LS, Conway J (1967) Influence of hypertension on the hemodynamic response to exercise. Circulation 36 : 231—237
7. Karlinar JS, Gault JH, Eckberg D, Mullins CB, Ross Jr J (1971) Mean velocity of fiber shortening. A simplified measure of left ventricular myocardinal contractility. Circulation 44 : 323-333
8. Weissler A, Harris W, Schoenfeld CD (1968) Systolic time intervals in heart failure in man. Circulation 37 : 149—159
9. Weissler A, Peeler R, Roehll W (1961) Relation between left ventricular ejection time, stroke volume, and heart rate in normal individuals and patients with cardiovascular disease. Am Heart J 62 : 367—378
10. Alpert NR, Gordon MS (1962) Myofibrillar adenosine triphosphatase activity in congestive heart failure. Am J Physiol 202 : 940—946
11. Hamrell BB, Alpert NR (1977) The mechanical characteristics of hypertrophied rabbit cardiac muscle in the absence of congestive heart failure: The contractile and series elastic elements. Circ Res 40 : 20—25
12. Shieverick KT, Hamrell BB, Alpert NR (1976) Structural and functional properties of myosin associated with compensatory cardiac hypertrophy in rabbit. J Mol Cell Cardiol 8 : 837—851
13. Thomas LL, Alpert NR (1977) Functional integrity of the SH1 site in myosin from hypertrophied myocardium. Biochim Biophys Acta 481 : 680—688
14. Kaufmann RL, Homburger H, Wirth H (1971) Disorder in excitation-contraction coupling of cardiac muscle from cats with experimentally produced right ventricular hypertrophy. Circ Res 28 : 346—357
15. Mulieri LA, Luhr G, Trefry J, Alpert NR (1977) Metal film thermopiles for use with rabbit right ventricular papillary muscles. Am J Physiol 233/5 : C146—C156
16. Hamrell BB, Panaanan R, Trono J, Alpert NR (1975) A stable, sensitive, low compliance capacitance force transducer. J Appl Physiol 38 : 190—193
17. Spann FJr, Buccino RA, Sonnenblick EH, Braunwald E (1967) Contractile state of cardiac muscle obtained from cats with experimentally produced ventricular hypertrophy and heart failure. Circ Res 21 : 341—354
18. Galeone A, Dal Santo G (1952) Sull'attivita ATPasica (adenosintrifosfatasica) del cuore negli stati di insufficienza miocardica. Minerva Medica 43/I : 1264—1270
19. Luchi RJ, Kritcher EM, Thyrum PT (1969) Reduced cardiac myosin adenosine trophosphatase activity in dogs with spontaneously occurring heart failure. Cric Res 24 : 513—519
20. Swynghedauw B, Klotz C, Leger JJ, Preteseille M (1973) Heart myosin adenosine triphosphatase and light subunits in experimental chronic aortic insufficiency in the rabbit. J Mol Cell Cardiol 5 : 501—514
21. Oganessyan S, Zaminian T, Bay N, Petrossian V, Koschkarian A, Martirosian I, Eloyan M (1973) Structural and functional changes of the contractile proteins in experimental-induced cardiac hypertrophy in animals and heart failure in man. J Mol Cell Cardiol 5 : 1—24

22. Katagiri T, Morkin E (1974) Studies on the substructure of myosin in cardiac hypertrophy. Characterization of light chains. Biochim Biophys Acta 342 : 262–274
23. Shiverick KT, Hamrell BB, Alpert NR (1976) Structural and functional properties of myosin associated with compensatory cardiac hypertrophy in the rabbit. J Mol Cell Cardiol 8 :837–851
24. Thomas LL, Alpert NR (1977) Functional integrity of the SH_1 site in myosin from the hypertrophied myocardiu. Biochim Biophys Acta 481 : 680–688
25. Raszkowski RR, Welty JD, Peterson MB (1977) The amino acid composition of actin and myosin and Ca^{2+}-activated myosin adenosine triphosphatase in chronic canine congestive heart failure. Circ Res 40 : 191–198
26. Litten III RZ, Brayden JE, Alpert NR (1978) The ATPase acitivity of subfragment I from the hypertrophied heart. Biochim Biophys Acta 523 : 377–384
27. Alpert NR, Mulieri LA (1977) The partitioning of altered mechanics in hypertrophied heart muscle between the sarcoplasmic reticulum and the contractile apparatus by means of myothermal measurements. Basic Res Cardiol 72 : 153–159
28. Weber A, Herz R, Reiss I (1966) Study of kinetics of calcium transport by isolated fragmented sarcoplasmic reticulum. Biochem Z 345 : 329–369
29. Wilkie DR (1968) Heat, work and phosphoryl creatine breakdown in muscle. J Physiol (London) 195 : 157–183
30. Solaro JR, Wise RM, Shiner JS, Briggs NF (1974) Calcium requirments for cardiac myofibrillar activation. Circ Res 34 : 525–530
31. Solaro RJ, Briggs FN (1974) Calcium conservation and the regulation of myocardial contraction. In: Dhalla NS (ed) Myocardial biology. In Recent advances in studies on cardiac structure and metabolism. University Park Press, Baltimore, Vol. 9, pp 359–374
32. Alpert NR, Mulieri LA, Litten RZ (1979) The functional significance of altered myosin ATPase activity in enlarged hearts. Am J Cardiol 44 : 947–953
33. Wendt IR, Gibbs CL (1974) Energy production of mammalian fast- and slow-twitch muscles during development. Am J Physiol 226 : 642–657
34. Eisenberg E, Hill TL (1978) A cross bridge model of muscle contraction. Prog Biphys Mol Biol 33 : 55–82
35. Lymm RW, Taylor EW (1971) Mechanism of adenosine triphosphate hydrolysis by actomyosin. Biochemistry 10 : 4617–4624

Coronary Haemodynamics, and Myocardial Adenosine Release Under the Influence of Digitalis Glycosides (Digoxin)

B.E. Strauer, J. Schrader and S.B. Bürger

Introduction

Digitalis glycosides exert significant inotropic effects on both the normal and failing human heart [4, 22, 23, 27]. Despite the evidence for this, there are no data available concerning cardiac performance of the hypertrophied left ventricle in hypertensive heart disease. Although it may be assumed that digitalis glycosides improve ventricular function in the failing heart, the effects on concentric or irregular left ventricular hypertrophy are presently unknown.

With regard to smooth muscle behavior, especially the coronary vessels, vasoconstriction has been suspected in experimental and clinical conditions using various kinds of digitalis glycoside preparations [5—7, 12, 32, 33]. "Vasoconstriction" might be due to direct smooth muscular effects, to metabolic responses or to both. Accordingly measurement of coronary haemodynamics and of the efflux of reported vasoregulating substances (such as adenosine may be appropriate to differentiate between direct vascular or indirect, metabolically induced effects of digitalis glycosides on the coronary vascular bed.

The present study was therefore designed in order to analyse ventricular function, coronary haemodynamics and the coronary release of vasoactive substances (adenosine, hypoxanthine and inosine). A total of 12 patients with both essential hypertension and concentric or irregular left ventricular hypertrophy but without coronary artery stenoses were utilized in this study.

Methods

Case Material. Studies were carried out during diagnostic cardiac catheterization, coronary angiography and left ventriculography in 12 patients with suspected coronary artery disease without coronary artery stenoses as evidenced by angiographic procedures (Tab. 1). The 12 patients (eight men, four women; mean age, 40) showed cardiac compensation according to the criteria of the New York Heart Association. In nine of the patients the case history was that of

1 Supported by the Deutsche Forschungsgemeinschaft

Table 1. Patient population[a]

Number	$n = 12$
Age (years)	40
Severity degree (WHO Report)	II
EH duration (years)	> 4
Angina pectoris	$n = 9$ (75%)
Dyspnoe[a] at rest	—
Dyspnoe[a] at exercise	$n = 5$ (42%)
Previous myocardial infarction	—
Previous cerebral insult	—
Left heart hypertrophy (chest x-ray)	$n = 8$ (67%)
(ECG)	$n = 11$ (92%)
Left atrial hypertrophy (ECG)	$n = 9$ (75%)
Coronary artery stenosis	—
Regional wall contraction abnormalities	—
Coronary reserve ($R_{cor}/R_{cor}{}^{b}$)	3.1
Irregular left ventricular hypertrophy	$n = 2$ (17%)
Left ventricular muscle mass	149 g/m^2
End-diastolic volume	86 ml/m^2
Mass to volume ratio	1.73

[a] EH, essential hypertension; ECG, electrocardiogram; and R_{cor}, coronary resistance

[b] 0.5 mg/kg dipyridamole IV

occasional attacks of angina pectoris, and five possibly showed slight exertional dyspnoea. Eleven patients exhibited electrocardiographic signs of left ventricular hypertrophy, while in eight the chest X-ray showed left ventricular hypertrophy. With regard to case history, none of the patients exhibited symptoms of a previous myocardial infarction. The mean muscular mass of the left ventricle, which was determined by ventriculography, was 162 g/cm^2 and was 80% above our normal value (Tab. 1). With a mean of 86 ml/m^2 the end-diastolic volume was within the normal range, so that a considerable left ventricular hypertrophy with an increase in the mass-volume ratio to 1.73 was present. Coronary artery disease of the large coronary arteries could be excluded in all patients by selective coronary angiography. There were no regional wall contraction disturbances of the left ventricle (hypo-, a- and dyskinesis). However, two patients exhibited an irregular or asymmetric anterior wall hypertrophy without signs of a ventriculo-arterial pressure gradient or intraventricular abstruction.

Cardiac Catheterization and Angiography. Left ventricular and aortic pressures were measured through catheters (pigtail, Cordis) that were directly connected to pressure transducers (Statham F23 Gb). The catheter system had a natural frequency above 20 Hz and a phase lag linear with frequency in this frequency range.

Left ventriculograms were obtained with multiple hole catheters using power injections (Contrac) and 40—60 ml/76% meglumine sodium diatrizoate. The projection was 30° in the right anterior oblique view. Left ventricular volumes were calculated by: $V = \pi LM^2/6$ (V = volume, L = longest measured chamber axis and M = internal transverse diameter at the mid-point of L). L was taken directly from the ventriculogram and M was derived from the area (F) of the left ventricle ($M = 4.F/\pi L$). In each patient the correction factor was determined considering magnification and distortion. Volume measurements were performed for end diastole as well as for each frame during systole until the peak value of systolic circumferential wall stress was obtained.

Peak systolic wall stress was determined from intraventricular pressure, radius and wall thickness by use of the Laplace equation ($T_{syst} = P.r/2d$; P = peak systolic developed pressure, r = internal left ventricular radius and d = wall thickness) [16, 17]. The left ventricular internal radius has been derived from volume measurements ($r = \sqrt[3]{3.V/4\pi}$). Wall thickness (d) was taken frame by frame as the averaged thickness of a 4-cm segment of the free wall on the anterior projection one-third of the distance from the apex. Each value for (1) intraventricular pressure, (2) ventricular radius and (3) ventricular wall thickness was taken for the instantaneous wall stress calculation until the peak value of systolic cirmumferential wall stress was obtained. The stress calculated by this procedure represents mean values across the thickness of the wall. This mean value underestimates maximal stress, which occurs at the endocardium, and it overestimates minimal stress at the outer layers (epicardium); however, application of the mean value does not lessen the validity of this stress value because it deviates from thin-walled calculations by approximately 10—15% [25—27].

Determinations of left ventricular mass were made from end-diastolic chamber dimensions, that is, from end-diastolic measurements of wall thickness and volume. These calculations were based on the determinations of shell volume created by adding lateral wall thickness to calculated ellipsoidal chamber dimensions and subtracting adjusted chamber volume. Shell volume was converted to mass by multiplying by the specific gravity of heart muscle: left ventricular muscle mass (LVMM) = LVTV − EDV (LVTV = left ventricular total volume; EDV = end-diastolic volume); $LVTV = 4/3 \cdot \pi\ (L/2+d)\ (M/2+d)^2$; $LVMM = 4/3 \cdot \pi\ (L/2+d)\ (M/2+d)^2 - EDV$. Left ventricular mass to volume ratio was obtained by dividing left ventricular mass by the end-diastolic volume.

Coronary Sinus Sampling and Coronary Blood Flow. A Goodale-Lubin catheter (Ch. 7) was inserted through the left cubital vein and introduced into the coronary sinus for coronary sinus blood sampling and for coronary blood flow determinations. Coronary blood flow was measured after right and left heart catheterization and before left ventriculography by means of the argon method with gas chromatogrphic analysis of argon in arterial and coronary venous blood. Details as well as the accuracy of this method, which allows measurements of coronary blood flow up to 400 to 450 ml/min x 100 g, have previously been published in detail [13, 14, 24, 28—30]. The linearity of this method over the whole range of physiologically existing coronary blood flow has been shown using comparisons with flowmeter and coronary sinus sampling techniques [2, 3, 31]. Argon blood concentrations were determined after extraction through a specially designed extraction chamber by gas chromatography (trace gas analyzer 1533 B, Varian, Darmstadt, FRG). Measurements of coronary blood flow were carried out under resting conditions and during maximal coronary vasodilation [31]. The latter was achieved by the intravenous injection of a potent coronary vasodilator (dipyridamole 0.5 mg/kg), which was given to each patient in dosages exerting no major effects an aortic pressure or heart rate. Coronary vascular resistance (mm Hg/ml per min x 100 g) was determined as the ratio between mean diastolic aortic pressure minus mean left ventricular diastolic pressure and coronary blood flow. Myocardial oxygen consumption (ml/min x 100 g) was calculated as the product of coronary blood flow and the arterial-coronary venous oxygen difference (volume percent). Arterial and coronary venous oxygen saturations were measured with carbon monoxide oximetry. Statistical analysis was performed with the Student's t-test.

Determinations of Adenosine, Inosine and Hypoxanthine in Arterial and Coronary Venous Blood. For collection of blood (15 ml), a specially constructed syringe was utilized which permitted rapid mixing of ice-cold Locke solution (NaCl 5 mM, KCl 5 mM, $NaHCO_3$ 6 mM, $CaCl_2$ 2.2 mM, Na_2HPO_4 0.9 mM, NaH_2PO_4 0.1 mM, glucose 5 mM, pH 7.4 mM containing 2×10^{-4} M dipyridamole) with blood (15 ml) during withdrawal from the patient. Addition of dipyridamole, a known inhibitor of the cellular uptake and deamination of adenosine [19], proved to effectively prevent changes of the plasma concentrations of adenosine during and after sampling. Following immediate centrifugation in the cold to remove the erythrocytes, an aliquot of the supernatant was extracted with 2 N perchloric acid, neutralized with KOH and treated with activated charcoal. The procedures for the determination of adenosine, inosine and hypoxanthine have previously been described in detail [18]. In brief, following thin-layer chromatography of the charcoal eluate, adenosine and its degradatives were quantitated spectrophotometrically by enzymatic degradation of all purine compounds to uric acid. Using a dual wavelength, double-beam spectrophotometer (Perkin-Elmer, Model 356), as little as 50—100 pmol of each purine compound could be detected. The concentrations of adenosine, inosine and hypoaxanthine in the plasma (C) were calculated according to the following formula:

$$C = c' \cdot (a + b - (\frac{a \cdot HK}{100}) \cdot d^{-1}$$

where (a) represents the volume of blood drawn, (b) the volume of Locke solution the blood was diluted with, (d) the volume of the supernatant after removal of erythrocytes, which is analyzed for the respective purine compound, (c') the amount of each purine present in (d) and (HK) hematocrit of the venous or arterial side.

After local anaesthesia and introcuction of the required chatheters (left ventricle or aorta, coronary sinus, and right atrium), digoxin (Lanicor, 0.01 mg/kg body wt.) was slowly administered intravenously over a 5-min period. Ten and 5 min before as well as 15, 30 and 50 min after the digitalis injection, heart rate, left ventricular pressure, aortic blood pressure, cardiac output (thermodilution method) and derived parameters were determined. The arteriocoronary venous oxygen saturation (CO-oximetry) was measured simultaneously. Left ventricular coronary blood flow was determined by means of the argon method 5 min before and 50 min after the intravenous digoxin injection. All catheters were introduced using the Seldinger method. Apart from the local anaesthetic (Xylocaine), there was no pre-medication.

Metabolic parameters (adenosine, inosine, etc.) were analysed in eight patients, whereas for the haemodynamic and coronary results, findings of four additional patients could be used.

Results

Ventricular Function. Before digoxin, left ventricular function, which can be derived from isovolumic and auxotonic parameters, was normal (Table 2); 50 min following digoxin, significant increase of the velocity-related contractility was present, as evidenced by a marked increase in the maximum rate of pressure rise (+ 19.4%), independent from pressure and heart rate (Fig. 1).

Table 2. Haemodynamics before and 50 min following 0.01 mg digoxin IV per kg body wt [a]

	Before digoxin	After digoxin	P	%
P_{LV} (mm Hg)	196 ± 23	198 ± 21	n.s.	+ 1.1
P_{LVED} (mm Hg)	15.9 ± 3.8	15.7 ± 3.1	n.s.	−1.2
dp/dt_{max} (mm Hg/s)	2250 ± 287	2687 ± 243	p<0.001	+ 19.4
Heart rate (l/min)	74 ± 13	71 ± 12	n.s.	−5.2
Cardiac index (l/min · m²)	3.67 ± 0.57	3.26 ± 0.58	p<0.001	−11.2
Stroke volume index (ml/beat · m²)	50.9 ± 12.5	47.6 ± 12	n.s.	−6.5
Cardiac work (mm Hg·ml/min·m²)	675 ± 86	610 ± 91	p<0.005	−9.7
~TTI (~P_{syst}·n)	13828 ± 2927	13296 ± 2652	n.s.	−3.8

[a] PLV, left ventricular systolic pressure; PLVED, left ventricular end-diastolic pressure; dp/dt_{max}, maximum rate of ventricular pressure development; TTI, tension time index (pressure-frequency product)

Table 3. Coronary haemodynamics

pt. No.	V_{cor} [ml/min·100 g]			R_{cor} [mm Hg·min·100 g·ml^{-1}]			$avD\text{-}O_2$ [Vol %]			MVO_2 [ml/min·100 g]		
	C	Dig	% C	C	Dig	% C	C	Dig	% C	C	Dig	% C
1	61	42	69	1.42	1.73	122	14.47	14.67	101.4	8.82	6.01	68
2	77	76	101.5	0.89	1.08	121	10.75	11.83	110	9.35	8.16	87
3	66	52	79	1.18	1.48	125	12.45	13.31	107	8.22	6.92	84
4	61	60	98	1.59	1.4	88	13.15	14.09	107	8	8.45	106
5	47.7	47.1	99	1.72	1.87	109	10.59	11.69	110	5.05	5.5	109
6	71	53	75	1.11	1.66	150	11.66	12.99	111	8.28	6.88	83
7	73	56	77	1.13	1.48	131	12.06	12.43	103	8.8	6.96	79
8	66	52	79	1.4	2.07	148	14.19	14.41	102	9.36	7.49	80
x	65.34	54.76	84.69	1.31	1.59	121.25	12.42	13.18	106.43	8.24	7.04	87
SD ±	9.07	10.14	12.69	0.28	0.31	20.13	1.45	1.15	3.85	1.38	0.99	13.85
p		<0.01			<0.02			<0.005			<0.025	

V_{cor}: coronary blood flow; R_{cor}: coronary resistance; $avD\text{-}O_2$: arterio-coronary venous oxygen difference, and MVO_2 : myocardial oxygen consumption

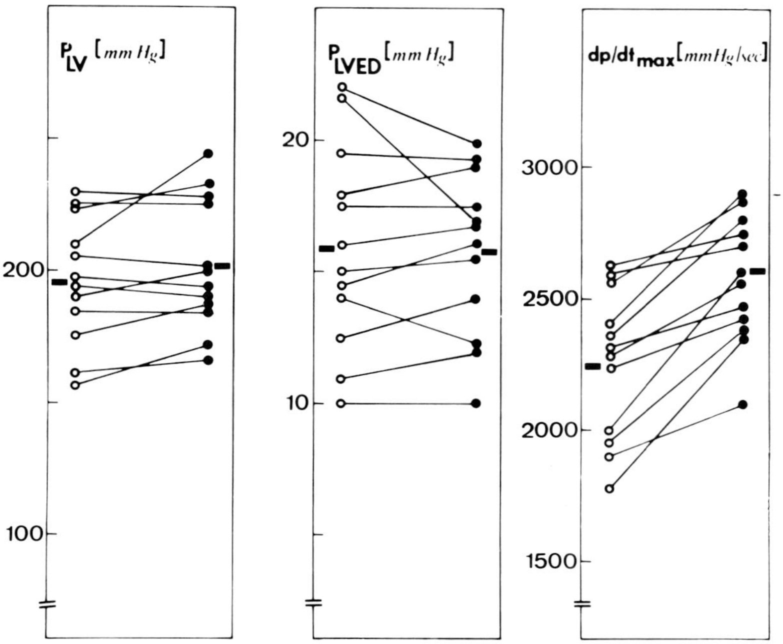

Fig. 1. Left ventricular systolic pressure, P_{LV}, left ventricular end-diastolic pressure, P_{LVED}, maximum rate of left ventricular pressure development (dp/dt_{max}) before (○) 0.01 50 min following (●) 0.01 mg digoxin IV per kg body wt

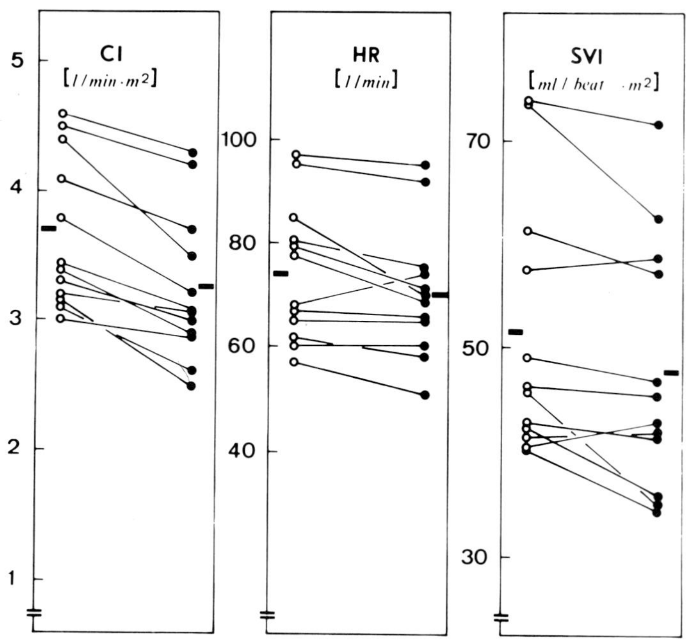

Fig. 2. Cardiac index (*CI*), heart rate (*HR*), stroke volume index (*SVI*) before (○) and 50 min following (●) 0.01 mg digoxin IV per kg body wt

Cardiac index decreased (by 11.2%) and — resulting from the changes in the mean systolic pressure and cardiac index — a reduction in the external cardiac work by 9.7% was found (Fig. 2). Heart rate and stroke index were reduced by 5.2 and 6.5%, respectively, which were without statistical significance. Left ventricular-end diastolic pressure remained unchanged. Corresponding to the arterial pressure elevation and the reduction in the cardiac index, total peripheral resistance was significantly increased (by 14.9.%).

Coronary Haemodynamics and Myocardial Oxygen Consumption (Table 2). The coronary vascular resistance was markedly increased due to arterial hypertension associated with an elevation of coronary perfusion (Table 3). Fifty min after the digoxin injection, coronary blood flow was significantly reduced, whereas the coronary vascular resistance and arteriocoronary venous oxygen difference increased (Table 3). Left ventricular oxygen consumption fell significantly in these patients.

Release of Adenosine, Inosine and Hypoxanthine. As demonstrated in Fig. 3, adenosine and its degradative product inosine are continuously realeased from the human heart, while no consistent changes were found for hypoxanthine. Rate of release of adenosine and inosine as calculated from the respective AV

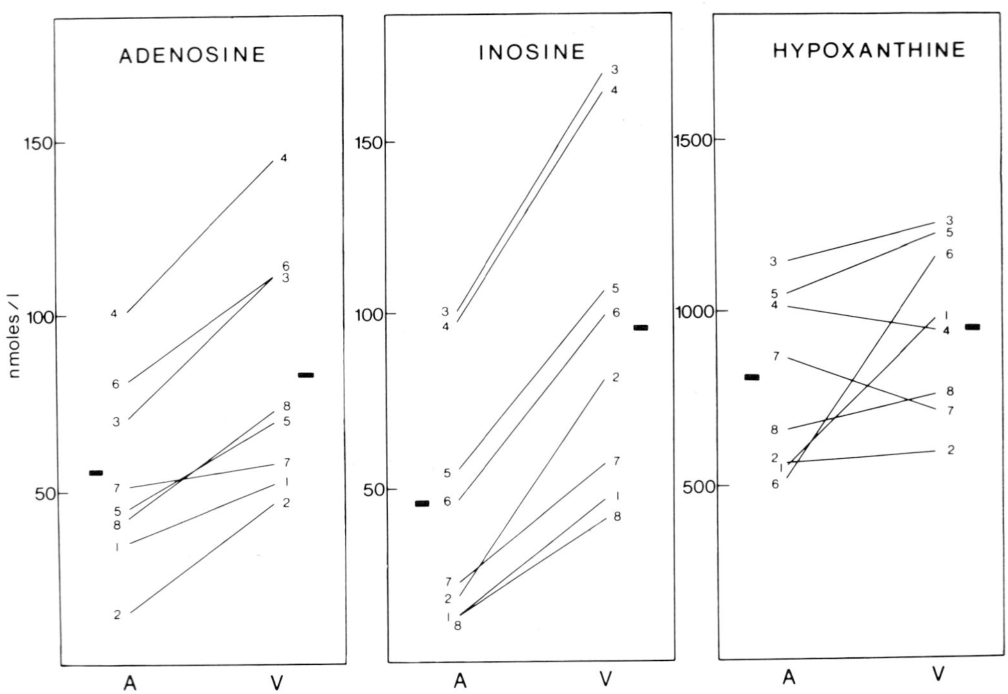

Fig. 3. Concentrations of adenosine, inosine and hypoxanthine in arterial (*A*) and coronary venous (*V*) human blood

differences proved to be 1.8 n mol/min per 100 g and 3.47 n mol/min per 100 g, respectively.

Arterial and venous concentrations of adenosine and inosine were in the same range; values for hypoxanthine, however, were about one order of magnitude higher and are similar to values previously reported in the literature [34].

After administration of digoxin, rate of release of adenosine and inosine was considerably diminished. Values decreased to 0.2 n mol/min per 100 g and 1.58 mol/min per 100 g, respectively. Under these conditions coronary flow was diminished and this was associated with a decrease in myocardial oxygen consumption. As shown in Fig. 4, the rate of release of adenosine correlated well with respective changes in coronary flow and/or coronary resistance (Table 4).

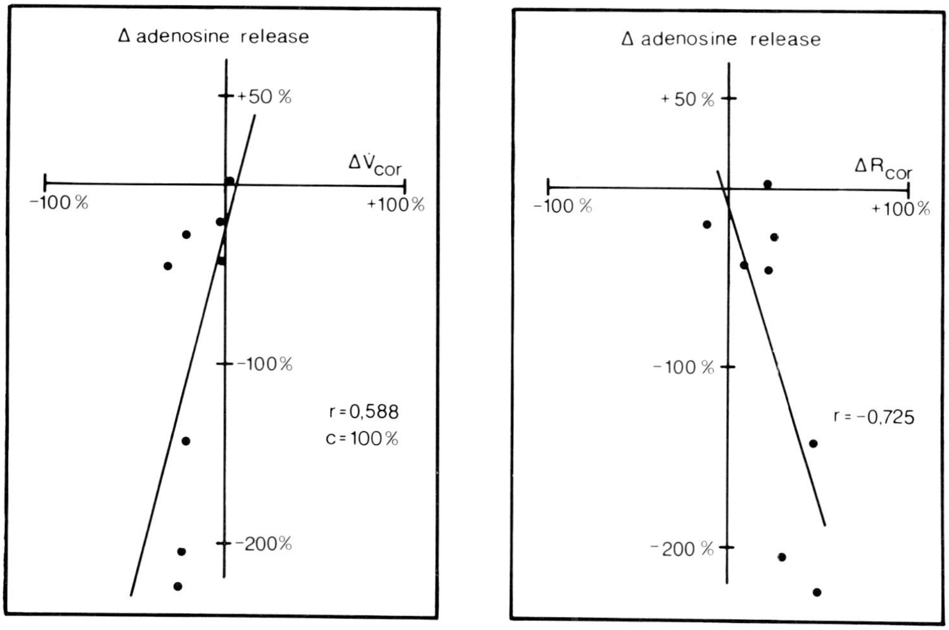

Fig. 4. Relationships between the changes in adenosine release and the alterations in both coronary blood flow (*left*) and coronary resistance (*right*)

Discussion

The investigations show that a considerable increase in inotropism and a slight decrease in the pumping values (cardiac index, stroke volume index and cardiac work) represent the main effects of intravenously administered digoxin (0.01 mg/kg body wt.) on the ventricular function in essential hypertension with cardiac compensation and at normal coronary angiogram. The changes in coronary haemodynamics were characterized by a marked decrease in coronary blood flow and an increase in coronary vascular resistance and arteriocoronary venous

Table 4. Arteriocoronary venous concentrations and differences of adenosine, inosine and hypxanthine before and 50 min following 0.01 mg digoxin IV per kg body wt

Pt.	Adenosine Controls avd n mol/l	Adenosine Controls Release/ 100 g p mol × 100 g/min	Digoxin avd n mol/l	Digoxin Release/ 100 g p mol × 100 g/min	Inosine Controls avd n mol/l	Inosine Controls Release/ 100 g p mol × 100 g/min	Digoxin avd n mol/l	Digoxin Release/ 100 g p mol × 100 g/min	Hypoxantine Controls avd n mol/l	Hypoxantine Controls Release/ 100 g p mol × 100 g/min	Digoxin avd n mol/l	Digoxin Release/ 100 g p mol × 100 g/min
1	39.9	2434	31.4	1319	168.1	10254	100.9	4240	101	6161	126	5292
2	30.8	2371	31.7	2473	60.8	4682	51.8	4092	29.9	2302	65.3	5159
3	17.2	1131	15.9	827	35.2	2323	25.3	1316	428.1	28254	− 75.8	− 3942
4	28.9	1760	23.5	1407	52.4	3206	18.2	1094	583.1	35587	169	10140
5	24.5	1169	14.2	668	52.7	2514	31.8	1516	166.1	7923	121.3	5713
6	42.5	3017	−70.1	−3747	67.9	4821	37.7	1998	−102.3	− 7263	350.6	18581
7	4.1	295	− 5.5	− 308	33.1	2416	− 2.2	− 123	−163.4	−11928	− 82.5	− 4620
8	28.3	1867	−15.5	− 806	28.2	1861	− 15.7	− 816	87.5	5775	88.1	4581
x	27.0	1756	3.1	229	62.3	4010	31.0	1665	141	8351	95.2	5113
SD±	12.3	871	34.2	1902	45.0	2751	35.5	1791	252.8	16218	138.4	7407
P			N.S.	$P<0.05$			$P<0.05$	$P<0.05$				

cvd = arteriocoronary venous difference

oxygen difference, while the myocardial oxygen consumption decreased. As a result there was an increase in oxygen extraction associated with a decrease in coronary blood flow.

The increase in the maximum rate of left ventricular pressure generation associated with largely unchanged end-diastolic and systolic pressure shows that digoxin has a positive inotropic action on the hypertensive heart with concentric hypertrophy. This finding is consistent with the digitalis-induced inotropic changes in the normotensive left ventricle. However, this left ventricular inotropic increase was paralleled by fall in the parameters of the pumping function (cardiac index, stroke index, and cardiac work). This is partly frequency-related, but can also be explained by the coexistent increase in left ventricular impedance, which can be assessed on the basis of the changed total peripheral restistance having increased by 14.9%. Digoxin causes a further increase in the peripheral resistance, which already is increased in essential hypertension, and it seems that this increase can suffice to cause a decrease in left ventricular pumping function despite increased inotropism. This implies that the positive inotropic action of digoxin on the hypertensive heart with cardiac compenstion is rather a "luxus inotropism" and is not suited to compensate for an afterload-dependent decrease of the pumping function. As left ventricular end-diastolic pressure and stroke ly unchanged, the fall in the stroke index and the external cardiac work, i.e. the stroke work of the left ventricle, imply that with digoxin the left ventricular function curve, i.e. the relationship between end-diastolic pressure and stroke work, has been shifted downwards to lower ejection volumes. In the insufficient heart such a reduction in ventricular function can be improved or normalized by drugs with a positive inotropic action.

In the compensated hypertensive heart an opposite effect has to be expected on the basis of present findings, which indicate that digoxin, despite a considerable positive inotropic action, does not improve ventricular function in essential hypertension with cardiac compensation. Contrary to decompensated essential hypertension, digoxin cannot transform the considerable increase in inotropism into an improved ventricular pumping function which is effective and therapeutically useful.

Corresponding to the ventriculodynamic determinants of myocardial energy demand, an increased oxygen consumption of the left ventricle would have to be expected as a result of the digoxin-induced inotropic increase. However, the findings show that after digoxin the myocardial oxygen consumption fell despite significant increase in inotropism. Accordingly, it can be assumed that a change in the maximum rate of left ventricular pressure development does not exert an equally pronounced influence on myocardial oxygen consumption or that the balancing effects of other parameters on oxygen consumption have to be considered in these patients. This primarily concerns the reductions in heart rate, cardiac index, stroke index and external cardiac work. There is little probability of a balance change of the systolic and/or diastolic wall stress as a result of digoxin because systolic and end-diastolic pressure in the left ventricle remained merely constant.

Corresponding to the reduced coronary blood flow, the increased coronary vascular resistance and the increased arteriocoronary venous oxygen difference, a moderate decrease in oxygen supply of the myocardium may be present. As there is no simultaneous metabolic relief of the left ventricle, the unchanged myocardial oxygen consumption is compensated for by an increased oxygen extraction of left ventricular coronary blood flow. It is conceivable that in essential hypertension the increased coronary vascular resistance and the decreased coronary blood flow may cause a decrease in the oxygen supply of the myocardium, which is already more sensitive to ischaemia due to left ventricular hypertrophy. In this context stenosis of the large coronary arteries need not be present because — as has been shown in our studies — the hypertensive heart with no pathological findings revealed by coronary angiography, of normal size and with cardiac compensation can already show a marked impairment of the coronary reserve and thus of the coronary capacity. Irrespective of whether there is a coronary macroangiopathy, a coronary microangiopathy or a normal coronary arterial system with attendant ventricular hypertrophy associated with essential hypertension, digoxin would not be suited for improving left ventricular function and coronary flow as well as the oxygen availability to the concentrically hypertrophic myocardium.

The present study provides the first evidence that the human heart normally continuously releases vasoactive adenosine into the coronary circulation. Release of adenosine from the normoxic heart has already been described in animal experiments [11, 15, 19, 21], and in man adenosine release was demonstrated during pacing-induced angina [8].

From the values obtained in the present study some comparison is possible with respective figures reported in the literature. Threshold concentration for the vasodilatory effect of adenosine in many species is between $5 \times 10^{-9} - 5 \times 10^{-8}$ M [22]. In the present study venous plasma concentration was 7×10^{-8} M and thus falls within this range.

The rate of release of adenosine from the human heart was calculated to be 1.7 n mol/min per 100 g. A value similar to this was also determined in the guinea-pig heart [18, 20].

Furthermore, we found a good correlation between coronary flow (resistance), myocardial oxygen consumption and adenosine release after administration of digoxin. Therefore, our findings are constistent with the hypothesis [1, 10] that adenosine may be involved in the regulation of coronary blood flow. It remains to be elucidated, however, to what extent changes in coronary flow as in the present study may have influenced the release of adenosine into the coronary system.

Several other possibilities, however, must also be considered participating in the digoxin-induced vasoconstriction. It is well established that digitalis has a direct constrictor effect in several vascular beds [7, 32, 33]. In addition, evidence is available that the coronary effects of digoxin may be neurally mediated via alpha adrenergic fibres [9]. Thus, available evidence indicates that most likely multiple mechanisms rather than a single factor may be responsible for the observed changes in coronary resistance after digoxin.

Summary

In hypertensive heart disease with concentric (regular or irregular) hypertrophy the effect of intravenously administerd digoxin (0.01 mg/kg body wt.) is reflected by a marked, velocity-related inotropic increase of the left ventricle by 19.4%, whereas the pumping function parametes (cardiac index, cardiac work and stroke index) decreased by between 6.5% and 11.2%. Left ventricular coronary blood flow was reduced by 15%, whereas coronary vascular resistance and arteriocoronary venous oxygen difference increased by 21.4% and 5.9%, respectively. The oxygen consumption fell by 13% in these patients. In untreated patients, the rate of release of adenosine, inosine and hypoxanthine was measured from AV differences to be 1.94, 3.47 and 9.7 n mol/min. 100 g, respectively. Under the influence of digoxin (0.01 mg/kg I/V), the release of adenosine decreased by 51%. Similar changes were also observed for inosine and hypoxanthine. Thus, the human heart releases adenosine in measurable quantities. The rate of adenosine release is comparable to values determined by us in animal experiments. The digoxin-induced decrease in coronary flow correlated with the concept that adenosine may be involved in the regulation of coronary flow in the human heart. From the clinical point of view, the inotropic increase caused by the intravenous administration of digoxin in essential hypertension with cardiac compensation cannot only be transformed into an improved left ventricular pumping function for therapeutic use but also, in addition, a moderate decrease in coronary flow and oxygen availability to the myocardium occurs. Therefore, the use of digoxin in essential hypertension associated with concentric hypertrophy should be recommended with reservation.

References

1. Berne RM (1963) Cardiac nucleotides in hypoxia: Possible role in regulation of coronary blood flow. Am J Physiol 204 : 317–322
2. Bretschneider HJ (1967) Aktuelle Probleme der Koronardurchblutung und des Myokardstoffwechsel. Regensburg Aerztl Fortbild 1 : 11
3. Bretschneider HJ, Cott L, Hilgert C, Probst R, Rau G (1966) Gaschromatographische Trennung und Analyse von Argon als Basis einer Fremdgasmethode zur Durchblutungsmessung von Organen. Verh Dtsch Ges Kreislaufforsch 32 : 267
4. Covell JW, Braunwald E, Ross JrJ, Sonnenblick EH (1966) Studies on digitalis. XVI. Effects on myocardial oxygen consumption. J Clin Invest 45 : 1535
5. Daggett WM, Weisfeldt ML (1965) Influence of the sympathetic nervous system on the response of the normal heart to digitalis. Am J Cardiol 16 : 394

6. De Mots H, Rahimtoola SH, Kremakau EL, Bennett W, Mahler D (1976) Effects of ouabain on myocardial oxygen supply and demand in patients with chronic coronary artery disease. J Clin Invest 58 : 312
7. Fleckenstein A, Fleckenstein G (1975) Further studies on the neutralisation of glycoside-induced contractures of coronary smooth muscle by Ca-antagonistic compounds. Naunyn Schmiedebergs Arch Pharmacol 287 : R38
8. Fox AC, Reed GE, Glassman E, Kaltman AJ, Silk BB (1974) Release of adenosine from human hearts during angina induced by rapid arterial pacing. J Clin Invest 53 : 1447—1457
9. Garan H, Smith TW, Powell J (1974) The central nervous system as a site of action for the coronary vasoconstrictor effect of digoxin. J Clin Unvest 54 : 1365—1372
10. Gerlach E, Deuticke B, Dreisbach RH (1963) Der Nukleotidabbau im Herzmuskel bei Sauerstoffmangel und seine mögliche Bedeutung für die Koronardurchblutung. Naturwissenschaften 50 : 228—229
11. Gerlach E, Schrader J, Nees S (1979) Sites of action of adenosine in the heart. I Coronary system. In: Baer HP, Drummond GJ (eds) Physiological and regulatory functions of adenosine and adenine nucleotides. Raven, New York, pp 127—136
12. Gracey DR, Brandfonbremer M (1963) The effect of lantoside C on coronary vascular resistance. Am Heart J 66 : 88
13. Kochsiek K, Heiss HW, Tauchert M, Strauer BE (1971) Koronarreserve und Sauerstoffverbrauch bei hypertrophischer obstuktiver Kariomyopathie. Verh Dtsch Ges Inn Med 77 : 880
14. Kochsiek K, Larbig D, Harmjanz D (1971) Die hypertrophische obstuktive Kardiomyopathie. Springer, Berlin Heidelberg New York (Experimentelle Medizin. Pathologie und Klinik, vol 35)
15. Rubio R, Berne RM (1969) Release of adenosine by the normal myocardium in dogs and its relationship to the regulation of coronary restistance. Circ Res 25 : 407—415
16. Sandler H, Dodge HT (1963) Left ventricular tension and stress in man. Circ Res 13 : 91
17. Sandler H, Dodge HT (1968) The use of single plane angiocardiograms for the calculation of left ventricular volume in man. Am Heart J 75 : 325
18. Schrader J, Gelach E (1976) Compartmentation of cardiac adenine nucleotides and formation of adenosine. Pfluegers Arch 367 : 129—135
19. Schrader H, Berne RM, Rubio R (1972) Uptake and metabolism of adenosine by human erythrocyte ghosts. Am J Physiol 223 : 159—166
20. Schrader J, Haddy FJ, Gerlach E (1977) Release of adenosine, inosine and hypoxanthine from the isolated guinea pig heart during hypoxia, flow-autoregulation and reactive hyperemia. Pfluegers Arch 369 : 1—6
21. Schrader J, Gerlach E, Baumann G (1979) Sites and mode of action of adenosine in the heart. II. Ventricular myocardium. In: Baer HP, Drummond GJ (eds) Physiological and regulatory function of adenosine and adenine nucleotides. Raven, New York, pp 137—144

22. Sonnenblick EH, Williams JF, Glick G, Mason DT, Braunwald E (1966) Studies on digitalis. XV. Effects of cardiac glycosides on myocardial force-velocity relations in the nonfailing human heart. Circulation 34 : 532
23. Strauer BE (1975) Digitalis and Myokardinfarkt. Med Klin 48 : 1937
24. Strauer BE (1977) Ventrikelfunktion und koronare Hämodynamik bei der essentiellen Hypertonie. 43rd Meeting Deutsche Gesellschaft für Kreislaufforschung. Verh Dtsch Ges Kreislaufforsch 43 : 91
25. Strauer BE (1979) Ventricular function and coronary hemodynamics in hypertensive heart disease. Am J Cardiol 44 : 999
26. Strauer BE (1979) Myocardial oxygen consumption in chronic heart disease: Role of wall stress, hypertrophy and coronary reserve. Am J Cardiol 44 : 731
27. Strauer BE (1980) Hypertensive heart disease. Springer, Berlin Heidelberg New York
28. Strauer BE, Tauchert M, Cott L, Kochsiek K, Bretschneider HJ (1970) Simultane Bestimmung des Sauerstoffverbrauches und der Koronardurchblutung des linken Ventrikels bei Mitral- und Herzklappenfehlern mit einem neuen hämodynamischen Parameter und der Argon-Fremdgasmethode. Verh Dtsch Ges Inn Med 76 : 217
29. Strauer BE, Tauchert M, Heiss HW, Kochsiek K, Bretschneider HJ (1972) On the relations between coronary blood flow, oxygen consumption and cardiac work in patients with and without angina pectoris. In: Maseri A (ed) Myocardial blood flow in man. Methods and significance in coronary disease. Minerva Medica, Torino, pp 465–475
30. Strauer BE, Brune J, Schenk H, Knoll D, Perings E (1976) Lupus cardiomyopathy. Cardiac mechanics, hemodynamics and coronary blood flow in uncomplicated systemic lupus erythematosus. Am Heart J 92 : 715
31. Tauchert M (1973) Koronarreserve und maximaler Sauerstoffverbrauch des menschlichen Herzens. Basis Res Cardiol 68 : 183
32. Vatner SF, Higgins CB, Franklin D, Braunwald E (1971) Effects of digitalis glycoside on coronary and systemic dynamics in conscious dogs. Circ Res 28 : 470
33. Vatner SF, Higgins CB, Franklin D, Braunwald E (1971) Effects of a digitalis glycoside on coronary and systemic dynamics in conscious dogs. Circ Res 28 : 470–479
34. Verdouw PD, Stam H, Remme WJ (1980) Fundamental validity and clinical usefulness of myocardial lactate balance during ischaemia. A comparison with other biochemical markers. In: Moret PR, Weber J, Haissly JC, Denolin H (eds) Lactate. Springer, Berlin Heidelberg New York, pp 207–223

Part II: Microscopic Pathology of the Myocardium and Coronary Arteries

Microscopic Pathology of Heart Muscle and of Coronary Arteries in Arterial Hypertension

W. Hort

In hypertension the heart develops structural changes at the macroscopic, the light microscopic, and the ultrastructural level. I will try to give you a brief report concerning the morphology of heart muscle fibers and its muscle nuclei, the adrenergic nerves and the blood supply of the myocardium in response to arterial hypertension. Additionally, I shall discuss whether structural adaptive processes in the myocardium of laboratory animals are the same ones as in human pathology.

Let me begin with the muscle cells in hypertrophied hearts. The basis for understanding the quantitative changes in heart muscle cells during hypertension is given by the fundamental finding of Linzbach [20, 21] that the heart is an organ with a nearly constant number of heart muscle cells. In some animal species a constant number of heart muscle cells was found, too, e.g., in guinea pigs and rats. In dogs it differs from breed to breed.

During physiologic growth the muscle fibers get thicker and longer without an increase in number. The same mechanism occurs during physiologic hypertrophy up to the critical heart weight of 500 g. The critical heart weight is surpassed under pathologic conditions, e.g., in severe forms of hypertension. Beyond this critical point a new mechanism appears. The number of fibers increases, resulting in hyperplasia. This augmentation of muscle fibers is probably due to longitudinal cleavages. The principle of the constant number of heart muscle cells allows one to calculate the thickening of muscle fibers during hypertrophy and to compare these accounts with the measurements. Regarding the thickness of heart muscle fibers in rats with experimental hypertension, we were surprised by the large increase in diameters compared with the moderate increase of heart weight. I think this discrepancy is due to a destruction of muscle fibers resulting from a sudden increase in pressure and from vascular lesions. Therefore these findings are not directly transferable to the human heart with its slow increase in weight corresponding with a gradual increase in pressure in essential hypertension.

The growth of muscle fibers raises the question of whether the lengthening of fibers is caused by a lengthening of sarcomeres. Today we know that the lenght of a sarcomere is nearly a natural constant with a length of 2.0 μ in the diastolic state. This length is maintained during physiologic and pathologic growth.

Hence it follows that there must be a new formation of sarcomeres according to the elongation of the heart. Until now it is very difficult to decide where the insertion of new sarcomeres arises. Probably the region of intercalated disks is of great importance to this mechanism. A new formation of filaments near the sarcolemma is significant to the thickening of muscle fibers.

The new formation of contractile filaments is not the first structural alteration in growing heart muscle cells. Ten min after aortic bending to produce experimental hypertrophy in the dog large accumulations of polyribosomes appear and the growth of rough sarcoplasmic reticulum starts [3]. Another early cytoplasmic response is mitochondrial hypertrophy with an increase of the ratio of mitochondria to myofibrils. In late stages of hypertrophy with commencing insufficiency there is a decrease in this ratio. In the end stages of hypertrophy, myofibrillar lysis with preferential loss of thick myofilaments may occur [4].

Now let us consider the nuclei of heart muscle cells (Fig. 1). Nearly 100 years ago in 1886 Goldenberg [7] described hypertrophied nuclei in hypertrophied muscle fibers. With increasing size, deformations of nuclei may occur partly due to impressions of enlarged myofibrils. In cross sections nuclei may appear wing shaped. Fifteen years ago Sandritter and Scomazzoni [31] described polyploid nuclei in normal human hearts. Beyond diploid nuclei adult human hearts contain tetraploid and octoploid nuclei, too. Under pathologic conditions, for example in hypertension, the degree of polyploidization increases with advanced enlargement of muscle fibers and with continuous overload. But the size of nuclei is not absolutely correlated with the DNA contained.

Experimental studies on hypertension are generally performed in laboratory animals. In contrast to the hearts of human beings and primates under normal conditions, polyploid nuclei do not occur in the hearts of laboratory animals,

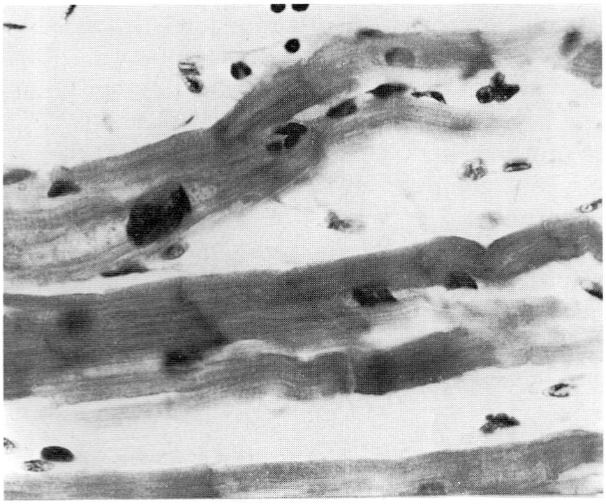

Fig. 1. Hypertrophied nuclei in hypertrophied muscle fibers of a human heart (400 x)

for example, rats, rabbits, and dogs. In myocardial hypertrophy there are similar differences concerning the DNA content of heart muscle nuclei. In rats Kuhn et al. [18] induced hypertension by constricting one renal artery and removing the other kidney. A marked increase of muscle fiber thickness appeared, but a pronounced increase of polyploidization did not occur. In laboratory animals myocardial hypertrophy results without an essential increase of the DNA content of heart muscle. In the heart of the turkey — a species with physiologic hypertension — no essential polyploidization develops within the thick left ventricular wall [29].

These findings emphasize that there are marked differences in nuclear reactions of the heart between laboratory animals and man. Therefore, results concerning the DNA content are not transferable from these animals species to human beings.

Up to now our knowledge concerning the sympathetic myocardial innervation in cardiac hypertrophy due to hypertension is very limited. There are only a few quantitative studies of the adrenergic nerves of the myocardium. Borchard [2] from our Department of Pathology reported that in hypertrophied human auricles with an increasing diameter of muscle fibers a highly significant widening of ground plexus and a less pronounced transmitter depletion occurred. Furthermore severe pathologic changes in cardiac nerves in cases of simultaneous hypertrophy and scarring were observed. In recent animal experiments Borchard and Völker (unpublished work) studied the noradrenaline content and the adrenergic nerves in the myocardium of rats with experimental renal hypertension. They found a significant decrease of noradrenaline concentration, a reduction of specific fluorescence, and ultrastructural degenerative changes of the adrenergic nerves.

In opposition to these findings Unge et al. [33] described an increase in the density of adrenergic nerves in relation to small vessels in the left ventricular wall in rats trained to swim and to a much less extent in hypertensive rats. Further investigations are necessary to clarify these interesting problems.

Now let us discuss the time course of development and regression of myocardial hypertrophy induced by hypertension. In human beings with acute glomerulonephritis, left ventricular hypertrophy is well developed within about 3 weeks. In animal experiments in rats with constriction of one renal artery the structural cardiovascular adaptation to hypertension was largely completed within 3 to 4 weeks [24].

After reversal of hypertension regression of myocardial hypertrophy occurs, provided that there are no irreversible changes in the ventricular wall, e.g., extensive scars. There is a physiologic example of regression of myocardial hypertrophy after reversal of hypertension. In the newborn a physiologic atrophy of the right ventricular wall occurs after the postnatal closure of the ductus arteriosus. Keen and I [11, 17] observed at the same time that the weight of the right ventricular wall falls rapidly during the 1st month of life. This weight decrease follows the decrease of pressure in the pulmonary circulation after a very short latent period.

In cases of rapidly decreasing blood pressure a more rapid decrease of ventricular weight occurs, for example, in declipped renal hypertensive rats. In these animal experiments a rapid decrease of left ventricular weight occurred during the 1st week. After about 3 weeks nearly complete regression was maintained [23].

What are the structural changes in the myocardium during regression of hypertrophy? After treadmill exercises the number of muscle fibers in the ventricular wall remained constant [10]. Up to now our knowledge concerning the ultrastructural changes during regression of myocardial hypertrophy has been limited. Hatt et al. [9] described in short-term experiments myofilaments irregulary mixed with Z-material and T-tubules filled with hyalin and dense material. They concluded that, at the cellular level, regression of hypertrophy occurs slower than its induction.

In our own experiments together with Frenzel [14] we observed in rats after swimming exercise during the phase of rapid regression, which occurs within the first 10 days, an accumulation of mitochondria under the sarcolemma and an increase of degenerative changes, especially of the mitochondria. But until now we cannot explain the mechanism of structural muscle fiber shortening during regression of myocardial hypertrophy. The length of sarcomeres remains constant but, despite this fact, up to now we have never seen sarcomeres being broken up. But our investigations are not finished as yet.

The blood supply of the enlarged hypertrophied heart which has adapted to hypertension is of main importance. The question arises whether there is a harmonious growth of the heart and its blood vessels or if a narrow pass develops with increasing myocardial weight.

Let us begin with the microcirculation. In the heart of infants four to six muscle fibers are enclosed in each mash of the capillary network (Fig. 2). Under physiologic conditions the distances between the capillaries remain constant in the adolescent and adult. Increasing thickness of muscle fibers during physiological growth implies a capillary to muscle fiber ratio of 1:1 in the adult heart. In cases of physiologic hypertrophy there is a mild increase of muscle fiber diameters and, accordingly, the capillary distances as well. Beyond the critical heart

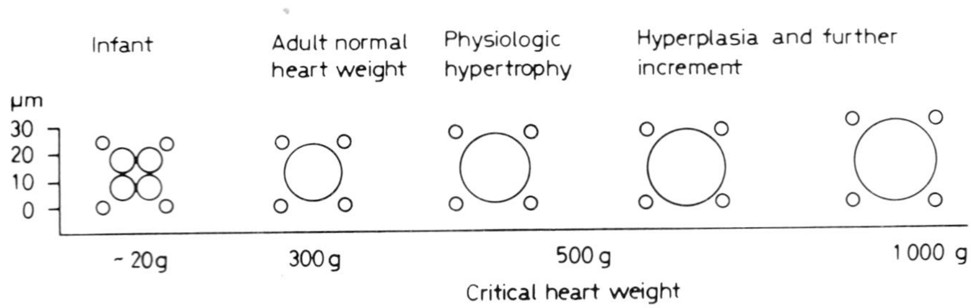

Fig. 2. Scheme of the capillarization of the human heart. The *small circles* signify capillaries, the *larger ones* signify muscle fibers. From Hort [12]

weight, hyperplasia of muscle fibers occurs, and a corresponding augmentation of capillaries results. The ratio 1:1 remains constant [12].

Until now it has not been finally decided if in animal experiments the structural changes of the microcirculation are completely the same ones as in human hearts. Ljungquist and Unge [22] for example, concluded from microangiogra-investigations that a neoformation of myocardial capillaries in swimming exercised rats occurs in contrast to rats with aortic stenosis [25]. There are, however, contradictory findings, too. To illuminate these questions further investigations with combined quantitative methods should be done.

Until now there has been a lack of quantitative investigations concerning the number of arterioles and small intramural arteries in correlation to cardiac hypertrophy. Some qualitative changes have been described concerning these vessels. Dr. Rahlf (see session B) will report about this subject and therefore I will make only a few comments. Technical details are important in estimating the degree of sclerotic changes in small intramural vessels. In our postmortem material we have injected arteries under pressure and we only rarely observed severe stenosis of these vessels. In opposition to Ratcliff and Redfield [30] we missed a positive correlation between the severity of atherosclerosis of large epicardial coronary arteries and arterioles. On the contrary, several times we have seen, together with Wilkat [12] an inverse correlation and we suppose that there could exist a protective influence of severe arterial stenosis against arteriolosclerosis.

To summarize: In hypertrophied hearts as a rule there is no significant narrow pass in the capillaries or the arterioles. Is there one in the large coronary arteries? Vogelberg [34], for example, missed a growth of the coronary ostia beyond the critical heart weight and Schoenmackers [32] described a slowdown in the growth of the coronary arteries beyond this critical level, but there are also contradictory findings.

Comparing the growth of coronary arteries and of myocardium, it is important to consider that the cross-sectional area of an artery and the mass of the myocardium have various dimensions. Therefore, in our material we have compared the diameter of the coronary arteries and the diameter of the myocardium, calculated from the cube root of the heart weight. Under these conditions we found a nearly harmonious growth of coronary arteries and heart muscle mass from birth to adulthood. Beyond the critical heart weight we observed a further growth of unchanged coronary arteries in a nearly harmonious manner, too. But there are a large scattering of measurements. Hutchins et al [15] employed a very similar method and also described a proportional increase in coronary arteries size and myocardial mass.

I think that in general a reduced blood supply to the myocardium is not due to a decreased growth of the coronary arteries during the development of hypertrophy but is mainly due to stenosis and obstructive coronary atherosclerosis. The distribution pattern of atherosclerotic lesions in coronary arteries is well known. Generally, atherosclerosis prefers the proximal part of the two left coronary arteries. In the right coronary artery a smoother peak exists and a second mild peak occurs 7—10 cm distal to the ostium [14, 26]. Within the branches of the coronary arteries sclerotic changes are much less frequent than in the arteries themselves. We found them most frequently within the first centimeter of the branches. The pattern of distribution was similar to the pattern in the coronary arteries. There was a rather good correlation between the frequency of sclerotic lesions and the diameter of the vessels [27].

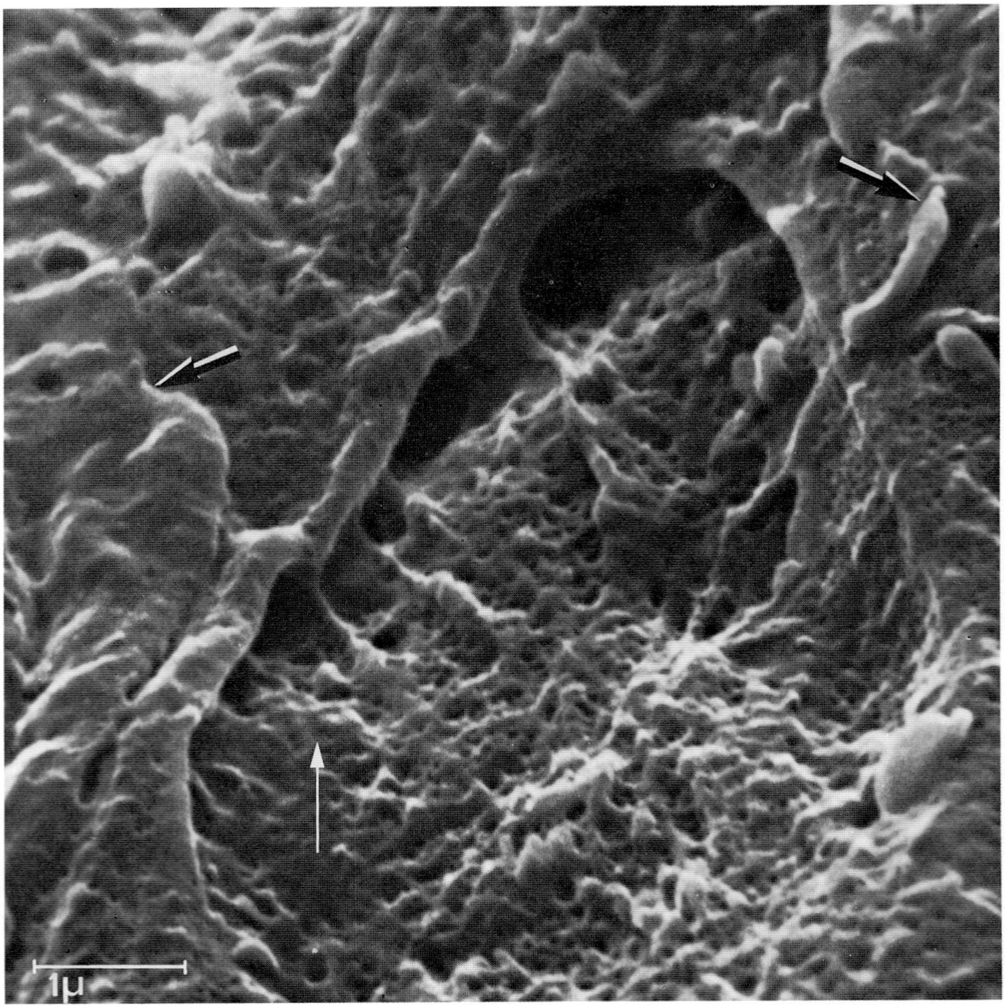

Fig. 3. Scanning electron micorgraph of a coronary artery of a rat with experimental hypertension. Formation of gaps. The *thin arrow* indicates the direction of the blood flow; the *thick arrows* indicate the boundaries of endothelial cells. 12620x. Courtesy W. Lenz, Pathologisches Institut, Universität Düsseldorf

Hypertension is one of the most important risk factors in the development of coronary atherosclerosis. In postmortem examination of patients with hypertension Freudenberg et al. [5] observed diffuse intimal thickenings. Bäuerle [1], for example, described a preference of sclerotic plaques for the distal parts of coronary arteries. In our own observations we could not recognize a special pattern of distribution of severe coronary atherosclerosis in cases of hypertension [14]. We believe that the risk factors favor the progression of atherosclerotic lesions in its areas of predilection.

In discussing the natural history of atherosclerosis, one of the most interesting problems concerns the early lesions. In experimental hypertension marked changes arise in the endothelial cells. My co-worker Lenz [19] studied these alterations after experimental hypertrophy, formation of gaps, and a subendothelial accumulation of granular material. These gaps are an important cause of the increased permeability of the arteries in hypertension [6, 8, 16, 28].

The arterial lesions in the coronary arteries of rats are not completely identical with atherosclerosis in human beings. Probably, experimentally induced changes in coronary arteries of primates would be a better model. I hope that I can demonstrate that structural changes induced by hypertension offer a large field for further morphological investigations.

References

1. Bäuerle W (1950) Die Koronarsklerose bei Hypertonie. Beitr Pathol Anat 111 : 108
2. Borchard F (1978) The adrenergic nerves of the normal and the hypertrophied heart. Biochemical, histochemical, electron microscopic and morphometric studies. Thieme, Stuttgart (Normal and pathological anatomy vol 33)
3. Büchner F, Onishi S (1970) Herzhypertrophie und Herzinsuffizienz in der Sicht der Elektronenmikroskopie. Cardiac hypertrophy and cardiac failure in electron microscopy. Urban & Schwarzenberg, München Berlin Wien
4. Ferrans VJ, Maron BJ, Jones M, Thiedemann KU (1976) Ultrastructural aspects of contractile proteins in cardiac hypertrophy and failure. Recent Adv Stud Card Struct Metab 12 : 129
5. Freudenberg H, Knieriem HJ, Möller C, Janzen C (1974) Quantitative morphologische Untersuchungen zur Koronarsklerose und Koronarinsuffizienz. Basic Res Cardiol 69 : 161
6. Gabbiani G, Elemer G, Badonnel MC, Hüttner I (1977) Morphological functional changes of aortic endothelium during different types of hypertension. Prog Biochem Pharmacol 14 : 1
7. Goldenberg B (1886) Über Atrophie und Hypertrophie der Muskelfasern des Herzens. Virchows Arch Pathol Anat 103 : 88
8. Greditzer HG, Fischer VW (1978) A sequential ultrastructural study of different arteries in the hypertensive rat. Exp Mol Pathol 29 : 12

9. Hatt PY, Jouannot P, Moravec J, Perennec J, Laplace M (1978) Development and reversal of pressure-induced cardiac hypertrophy. Light and electron microscopic study in the rat under temporary aortic constriction. Basic Res Cardiol 73 : 405
10. Hort W (1951) Morphologische und physiologische Untersuchungen an Ratten während eines Lauftrainings und nach dem Training. Virchows Arch Pathol Anat 320 : 197
11. Hort W (1953) Quantitative histologische Untersuchungen an wachsenden Herzen. Virchows Arch Pathol Anat 323 : 223
12. Hort W (1955) Quantitative Untersuchungen über die Kapillarisierung des Herzmuskels im Erwachsenen- und Greisenalter, bei Hypertrophie und Hyperplasie. Virchows Arch Pathol Anat 327 : 560
13. Hort W (1971) Quantitative morphology and structural dynamics of the myocardium. Methods Archiev Exp Pathol 5 : 3
14. Hort W, Moosdorf R, Kalbfleisch H, Köhler F, Milzner-Schwarz U, Frenzel H (1977) Site and shape of the most severe stenoses in coronary arteries and their relationship to the risk factors. Postmortem findings. Z Kardiol 66 : 333
15. Hutchin GM, Bulkley BH, Miner MM, Boitnott JK (1977) Correlation of age and heart weight with tortuosity and caliber of normal human coronary arteries. Am Heart J 94 : 196
16. Jellinek H (1977) Surface changes after various types of endothelial injury. Prog Biochem Pharmacol 14 : 208
17. Keen, EN (1955) The postnatal development of the human cardiac ventricles. J Anat 89 : 484
18. Kuhn H, Pfitzer P, Stoepel K (1974) DNA content and DNA synthesis in the myocardium of rats after induced renal hypertension. Cardiovasc Res 8 : 86
19. Lenz W, Stoepel K (1978) Ultrastrukturelle Veränderungen am Endothel und an der übrigen Intima der Kranzarterien von Ratten mit experimenteller Hypertonie unterschiedlicher Dauer. Verh Dtsch Ges Pathol 62 : 339
20. Linzbach AJ (1947) Mikrometrische und histologische Anlayse hypertropher menschlicher Herzen. Virchows Arch Pathol Anat 314 : 534
21. Linzbach AJ (1960) Heart failure from the point of view of quantitative anatomy. Am J Cardiol 5 : 370
22. Ljungquist A, Unge G (1972) The finer intramyocardial vasculature in various forms of experimental cardiac hypertrophy. Acta Pathol Microbiol Scand [A] 80 : 329
23. Lundgren Y (1974) Regression of structural cardiovascular changes after reversal of experimental renal hypertension in rats. Acta Physiol Scand 91 : 275
24. Lundgren Y, Hallbäck H, Weiss L, Folkow B (1974) Rate and extent of adaptive cardiovascular changes in rats during experimental renal hypertension. Acta Physiol Scand 91 : 103
25. Mandache E, Unge G, Ljungquist A (1972) Myocardial blood capillary reaction in various forms of cardiac hypertrophy. Virchows Archiv [Cell Pathol] 11 : 97

26. Montenegro MR, Eggen DA (1968) Topography of atherosclerosis in the coronary arteries. Lab Invest 18 : 586
27. Nauth HF, Hort W, Hubinger R (1979) Untersuchungen über die Lokalisation sklerotischer Veränderungen in den Koronararterien und ihren großen epikardialen Ästen. Z Kardiol. 68 : 832
28. Olsen F (1978) Acute hypertensive damage of arterial vessels of the heart. Acta Pathol Microbiol Scand [A] 86 : 199
29. Pfitzer P (1971) Der DNS-Gehalt der Zellkerne im Herzmuskel des Truthahns. Virchows Arch [Cell Pathol] 8 : 175
30. Ratcliffe HL, Redfield E (1972) Atherosclerotic stenosis of the extramural and intramural coronary arteries of man. Virchows Arch [Pathol Anat] 357 : 1
31. Sandritter W, Scomazzoni G (1964) Desoxyribonucleic acid content (Feulgen photometry) and dry weight (interference microscopy) of normal and hypertrophical heart muscle fiber. Nature 202 : 100
32. Schoenmackers J (1949) Die Herzkranzschlagadern bei der arteriokardialen Hypertrophie. Z Kreislaufforsch 38 : 321
33. Unge G, Mandache E, Ljungquist A (1973) The sympathetic myocardial innervation in various forms of experimental cardiac hypertrophy. Acta Pathol Microbiol Scand [A] 81 : 366
34. Vogelberg K (1957) Die Lichtungsweite der Koronarostien an normalen und hypertrophen Herzen. Z Kreislaufforsch 46 : 101

Microscopic Pathology of Intramural Coronary Arteries and Arterioles of the Left Ventricle in Arterial Hypertension[1]

G. Rahlf

Introduction

Pathological alterations in the small intramyocardial arterial or venous vascular tracts are often called small vessel disease of the myocardium. In its narrower sense, the term "small vessel disease of the heart" is often used synonymously for intramyocardial arterial vascular lesions of degenerative origin. Other terms for such vascular alterations are "arteriolosclerosis of the myocardium" [28, 44], "intramural coronary arteriosclerosis" [26], "intramyocardial arteriopathy" [35] or "small coronary disease" (James 1976, personal communication). It is precisely in this area of arterial vascular lesions of a degenerative type that our knowledge is still inadequate. The nature, localization, frequency, aetiology and functional significance of these pathological vascular alterations, which we understand as intramyocardial microarteriopathy, receive very different treatment in a long series of morphological investigations [3, 13, 14, 24, 29, 42, 44]. Hypertension has been one of the most researched factors in discussing the occurence of intramyocardial microarteriopathy, and some authors believe that there exists a typical hypertension-dependent type of vascular damage in the myodardium [3, 20, 33, 37].

Material and Method

Tissue samples covering the complete wall cross-section of the ventricle from 1000 hearts in rigor mortis, taken from men and women of ages between 4—100 years, were systematically investigated. The heart muscle tissue was fixed in a 4% formalin solution. Frozen and paraffin sections were stained with Oil-Red-O, hematoxylin and eosin, PAS, Elastica, Congo red, Methyl violet, van Gieson stain and Goldner's Trichome method. In some cases fibrin staining was additionally carried out using the Ludewig and Lendrum method or phosphotungstic acid hematoxylin (PTAH).

1 With the support of German Research Society under the terms of Special Research Project 89 — Cardiology Göttingen —

The intramyocardial arteries were classified into:

1. Arterioles (with one muscle layer of the media),
2. Small arteries (with two to three muscle layers), and
3. Arteries (with more than three muscle layers).

The evaluation of the degenerative alterations was made according to the differing degrees of vascular damage cited in Table 1.

In grading the degree of stenosis of the great extramural coronary arteries we followed the WHO recommendation [45].

Nil:	No stenosis:
< 50%	Stenosis of less than half the lumen and
> 50%	Greater degree of stenosis

The risk factor hypertension was collated from clinical records. Advanced concentric pressure hypertrophy (in the absence of aortic stenosis) and severe arteriosclerosis of the kidneys (in the absence of diabetes mellitus) were also attributed to hypertension (239 cases). As a control group we took a sample of hearts from 240 men and women in which no factors seemed to be present which might have led to pathological vascular alterations in the arterial intramyocardial vascular system.

In a second series, we investigated 427 well-contracted hearts and tried to correlate the degree of degenerative intramyocardial microarteriopathy with the muscular weight of the left ventricle including the septum.

Table 1. Differing degrees of vascular damage

Negative	No vascular alterations
Slight	< 25% of the vessels with pathological wall alterations without stenosis of the lumen
Medium	25%–50% of the vessels with pathological wall alterations without significant stenosis of the lumen < 25% of the vessels with stenosis of more than half the lumen
Severe	> 50% of the vessels with pathological wall alterations without significant stenosis of the lumen > 25% of the vessels with stenosis of more than half the lumen

Results

Normal Anatomy of the Small Intramural Coronary Arterial System

In the myocardium two basic types of arterial vessels can be distinguished.

1. The compacta type is an arterial vessel with a thin intima and a well-formed single layered elastica interna. The media contains smooth muscle cells arranged in a circle or flat spiral, so that the media possesses a layer of ring muscle which is seen in cross section. The adventitia is thin and consists of only slightly collagenous fibrous tissue. This type of vessel is most commonly found in the ventricular wall and the atria (Fig. 1).

2. The papillary muscle type is an arterial vessel with an intima of varying breadth, and a single or double layered elastica interna. The media is very broad with bundles of smooth musculature bunched into steep spirals or running lengthways. The adventitia contains dispersed collagenous fibrous tissue. This vessel type is found mainly in the papillary muscles and less often in the trabecularis or in the compacta of the ventricles or atria (Fig. 2).

Mixed forms of these two basic types can be observed in the trabecularis. They often have a broad intima with smooth muscle cells running lengthways are lo-

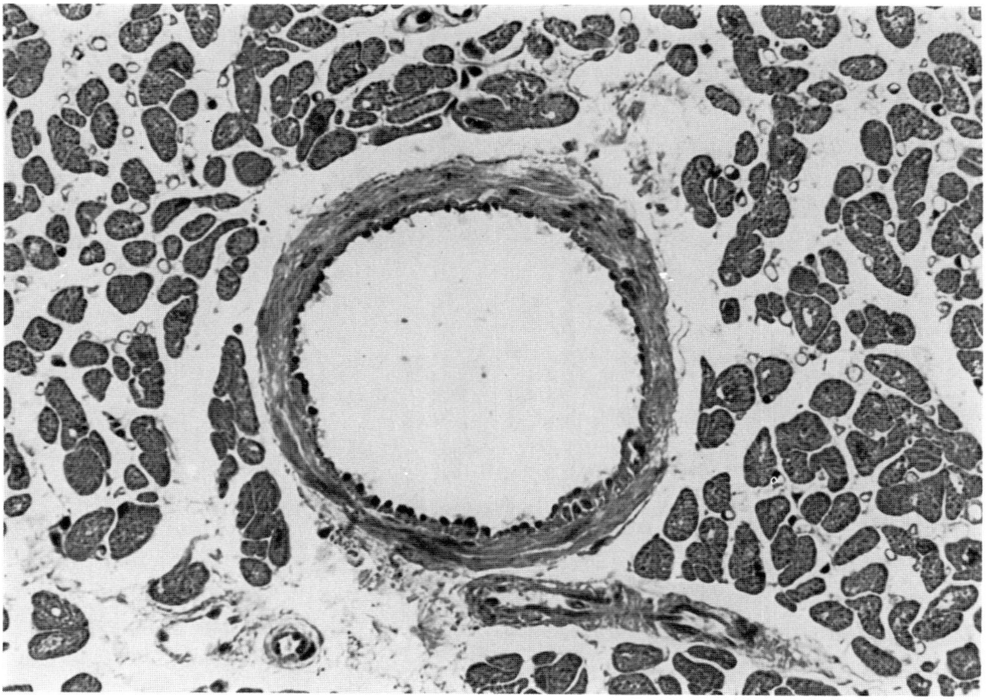

Fig. 1. Compacta type with ring musculature of the media. x 266, Hematoxylin and Eosin

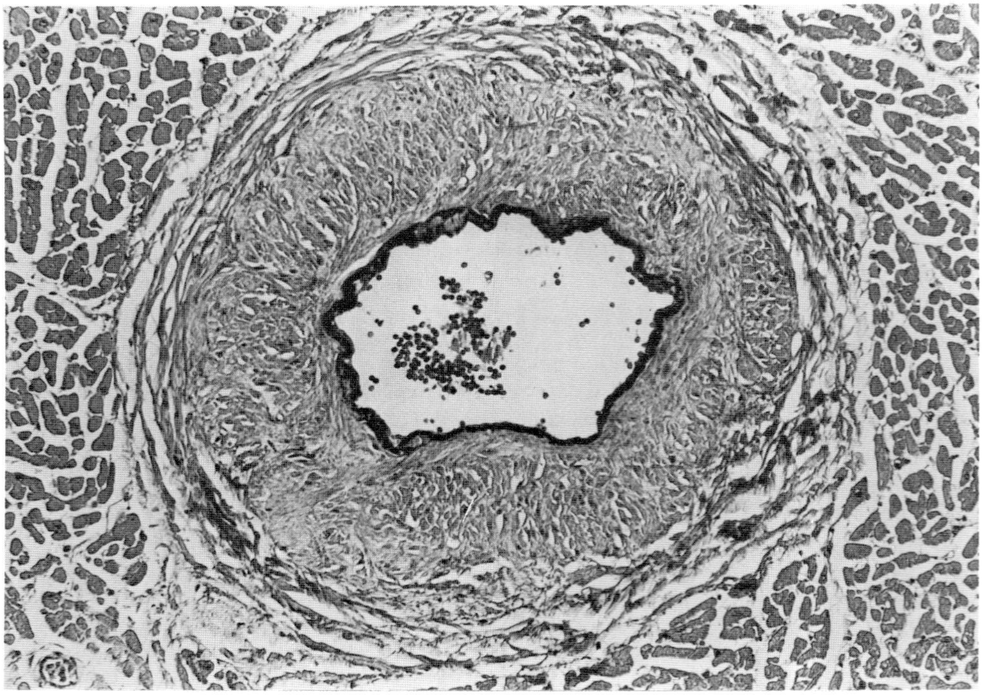

Fig. 2. Papillary muscle type with longitudinal musculature arranged as bundles in the broad media. x 140, Elastica-Goldner

cated in patches or concentrically around the lumen and are surrounded by elastica lamina. Vessels also occur which show a more or less well-developed double layered media in an inner circular and outer longitudinal musculature. We believe that most of these vessels are wall types in different stages of contraction.

Degenerative Vascular Lesions in the Small Intramural Coronary Artery Branches

Degenerative Vascular Lesions in the Compacta Type

In the compacta type, excentric or concentric hyaline homogeneous areas of thickening can be found subendothelially in the intima. These areas develop partly in circular or undulating form. The hyaline PAS-positive deposits can develop into button-, cushion- or pad-shaped growths that lead to considerable displacement of the lumen (Fig. 3). These pads can be shown with elastica staining, revealing thickening of the elastica interna and also sometimes merging or lumpy deterioration and local fragmentation (Fig. 4). Fibrin staining using the

Fig. 4. Thickening and fragmentation of the elastica interna in a cushion pad of ▸ the compacta-type arteries. x 475, Elastica

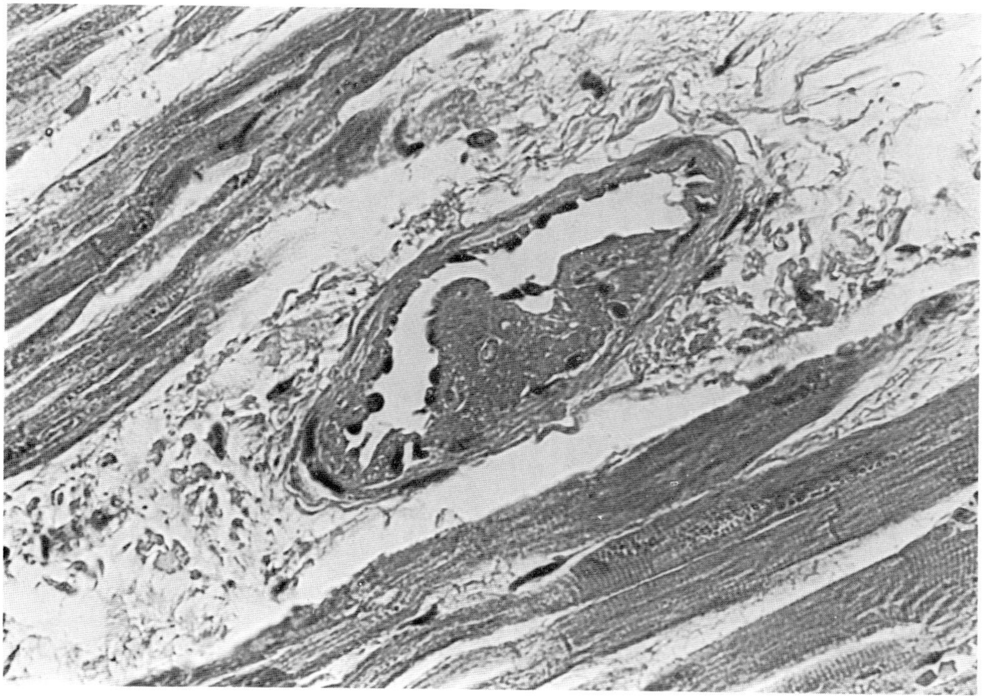

Fig. 3. PAS-positive cushion-like thickening of the intima in the compacta type arteries. x 450

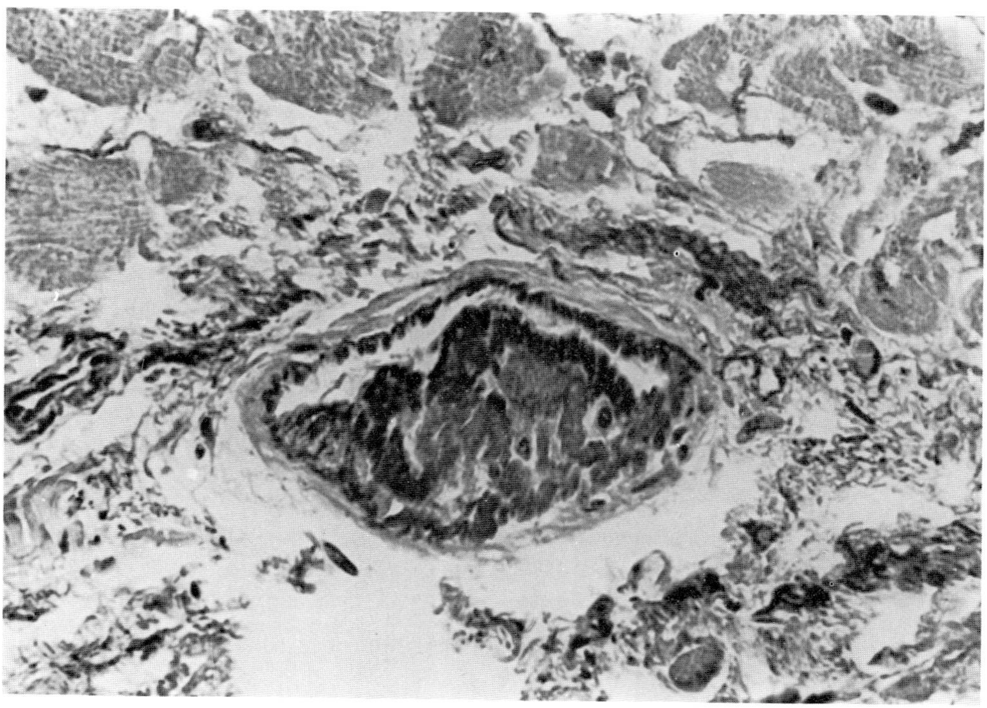

Ladewig and Lendrum method is usually negative. Fat staining reveals only occasional pieces of fat-positive material in these pads. Spreading of the pads leads to narrowing and degeneration of the media. Occasionally cellular elements can be seen in large pads with round or oval nuclei, which partly resemble monocytes or lymphoid cells. The vascular alterations are only of a local character and the pad formation commonly develops at or near vascular branching areas.

Hyaline pads can also be found in the compacta type; here, the elastica interna runs over the pad-like thickening of the intima without any distension, fragmentation or multiplication of the elastic material. These pads are rare, and fat staining is usually positive.

Degenerative Vascular Alterations in the Papillary Muscle Type

In the papillary muscle artery type, disintegration of the elastic lamina in the intima can be seen even in young persons. With increasing age, destruction of the smooth muscle cells occurs in the variably braoad media and is accompanied by local fibrosis. Besides hyperelastosis, the intima can also reveal simultaneous or separate edema (Fig 5). Increasing fibrosis accompanied by continual narrow-

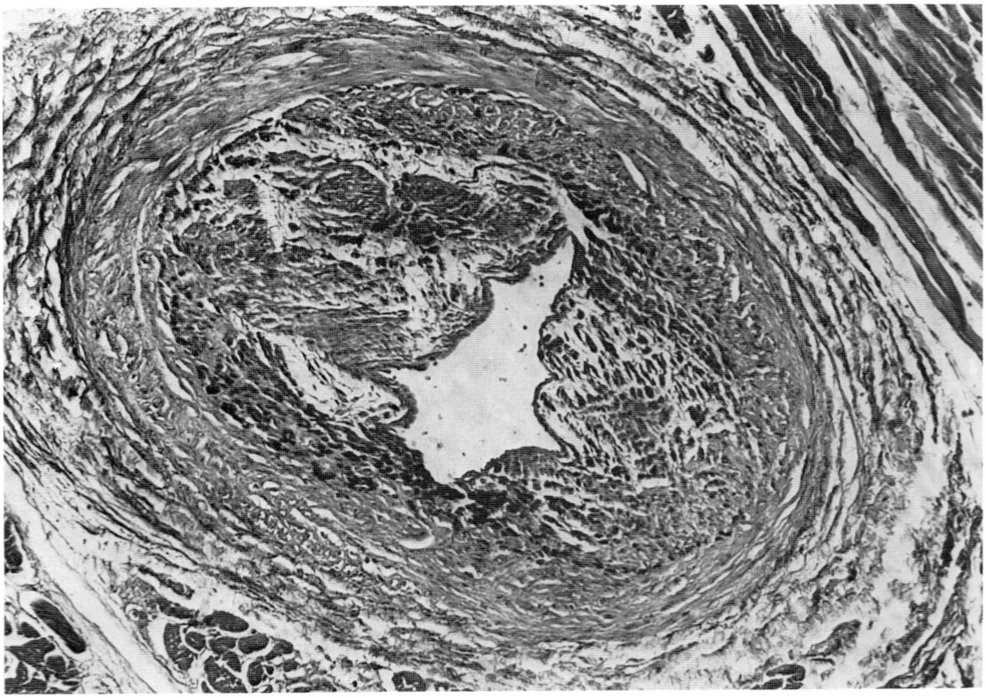

Fig. 5. Hyperelastosis and intimal edema in a papillary muscle type artery. x 76, Elastica-Goldner

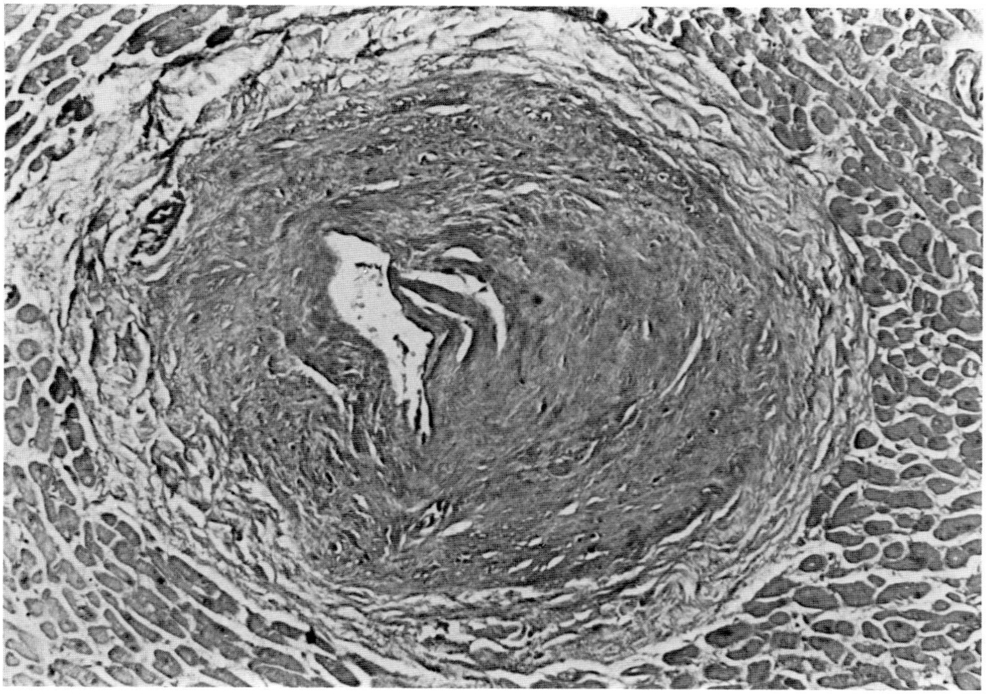

Fig. 6. Complete replacement of intima and media by connective tissue with narrowing of the lumen of a papillary muscle type artery. x 91, Hematoxylin-Eosin

ing of the lumen can lead to a practically complete replacement of the intima and media by connective tissue (Fig. 6). At the same time fibrous tissue increases in the adventitia. Fibrosis and hyperelastosis of the whole vascular wall can develop so severely that intima and media become practically indistinguishable. The boundaries between intima and media can still be reconstructed by means of elastica staining which shows up fragments of the elastica interna.

In the papillary muscle artery type, finely distributed fatty deposits are seen in the intima, media and adventitia. This fat lies in the smooth muscle cells and partly also in the collagenous fibrous tissue. Finely distributed fatty deposits are also found in the surrounding scarred tissue of the myocardium. The typical changes that take place in papillary muscle arteries with hyperfibroelastosis are usually much more severe in the vessels of the left papillary muscles than in those of the right ventricle. Vascular lesions are usually more severe near the tip than the bottom of the papillary muscles.

Frequency and Severity of Vascular Damage

Pathological vascular lesions in the compacta and papillary type increase with age (Fig. 7). The vascular alterations in the papillary muscles occur even during

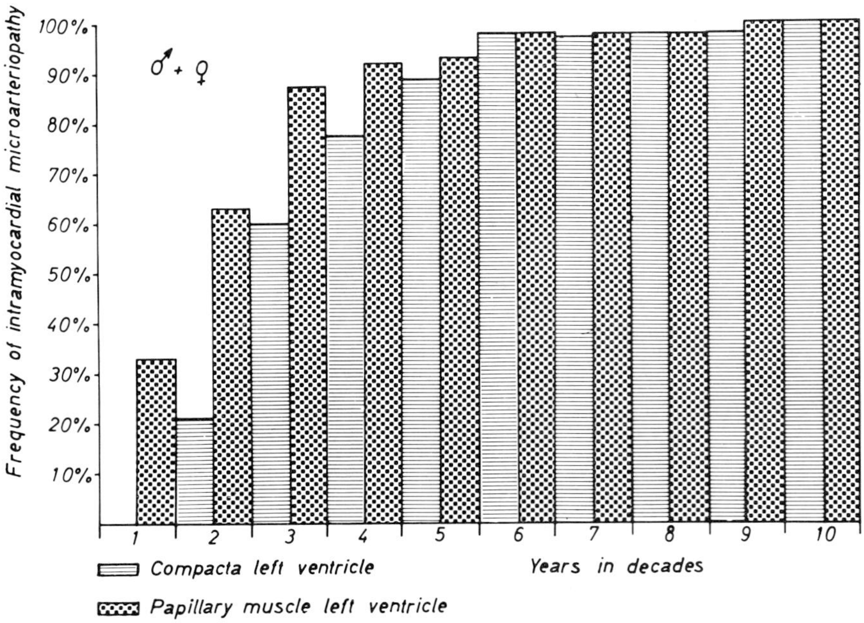

Fig. 7. Frequency of pathological changes in intramyocardial arteries of the compacta and papillary muscle type

the first 10 years of life with a frequency of about 30%. It is not until the 2nd decade that in 21% of the cases pathological lesions in the compacta type appear. From the 6th decade onwards it is hard to find a heart that reveals no pathological vascular changes. In the compacta type it is almost without exception vessels with two to three circular muscle layers of the media that are affected. Arterioles with one muscle layer do not show any pathological alteration until the 4th decade of life (4%). With advancing age, we find that alongside the pathological damage to vessels with two to three muscle layers, an increasing percentage of lesions in arterioles and vessels with more than three muscle layers take place. The pathological vascular alterations in the compacta type vessels occur in men earlier and more extensive than in women.

When one categorizes the degree of severity of intramyocardial microarteriopathy, it is evident that slight lesions are in the majority (Fig. 8). The changeover to medium and severe impairment in the papillary muscle arteries is completed both sooner and more severely than in the wall arteries. Men and women in 7th to 9th decade of life show, in about 5%—10% of cases severe pathological vascular lesions in the compacta type, while in the papillary muscle type the figure lies between 30% and 35%.

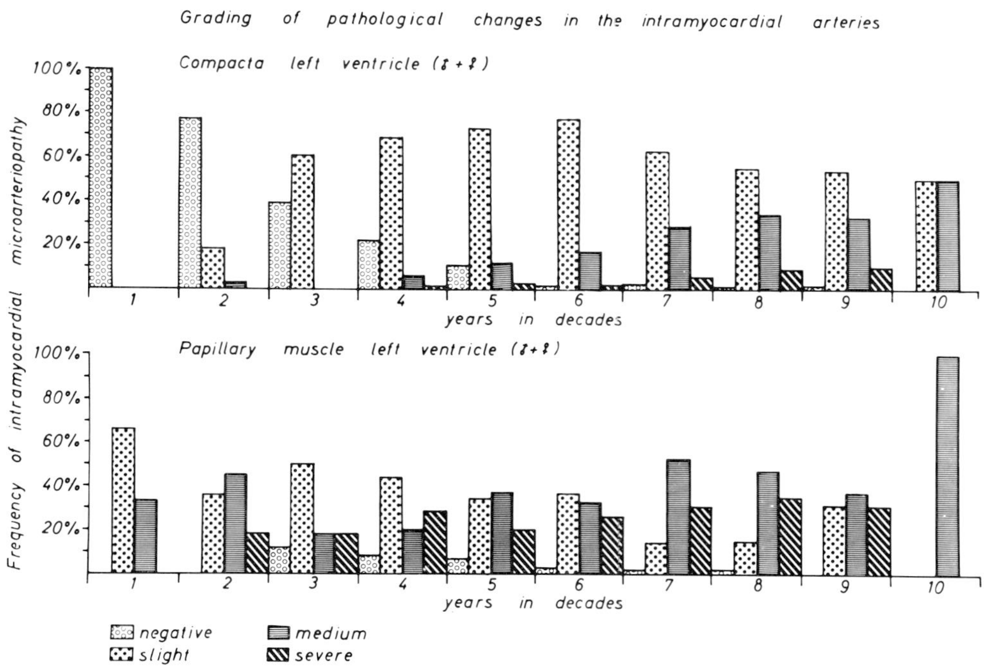

Fig. 8. Grading of pathological changes in the intramyocardial microarteries of the compacta type and papillary muscle type

Influence of Hypertension on the Occurence of Intramyocardial Microarteriopathy

We were able to use for our investigation the hearts of 239 hypertensive patients. There exists no special type of hypertension-dependent vascular damage in the intramyocardial microarteries. It can be seen from Fig. 9 that in the 4th and 5th decades slight vascular damage occurs in the compacta type more frequently in the hypertension than in the control group. This remains valid for medium lesions, especially in the 6th and 7th decade of life. Comparisons are harder to make between older age groups, since fewer subjects are available for random sampling.

In the papillary muscle the influence of hypertension on the occurrence of vascular alterations is more difficult to explain with the evidence collected by us. It seems that the typical changes in papillary muscle arteries with hyperfibroelastosis are rather stronger in hypertension cases. The transition from slight or medium to severe impairment is completed in the papillary muscle arteries not only at the top but also at the bottom of the left papillary muscles.

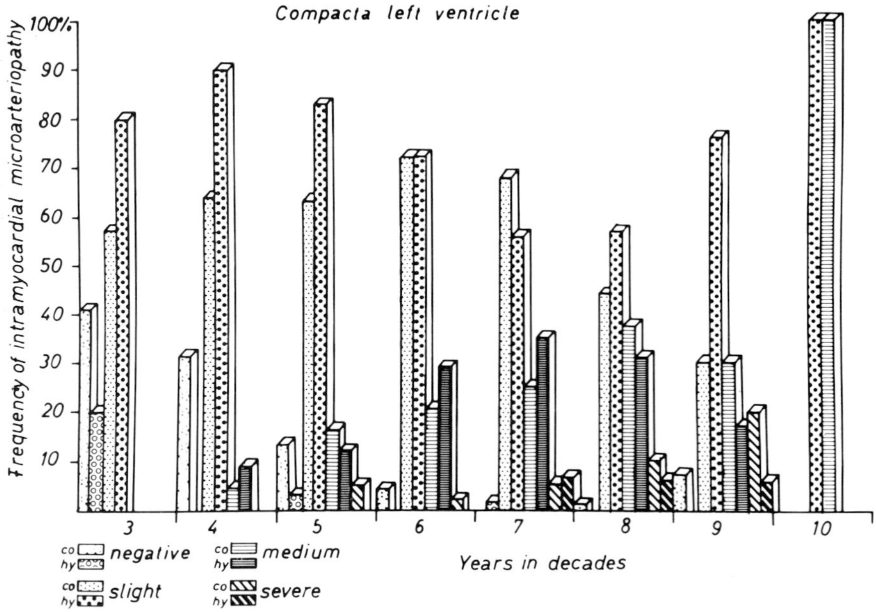

Fig. 9. Comparison of the degree of intramyocardial microarteriopathy (compacts type) in cases of hypertension with controls. *co* control; *hy* hypertension

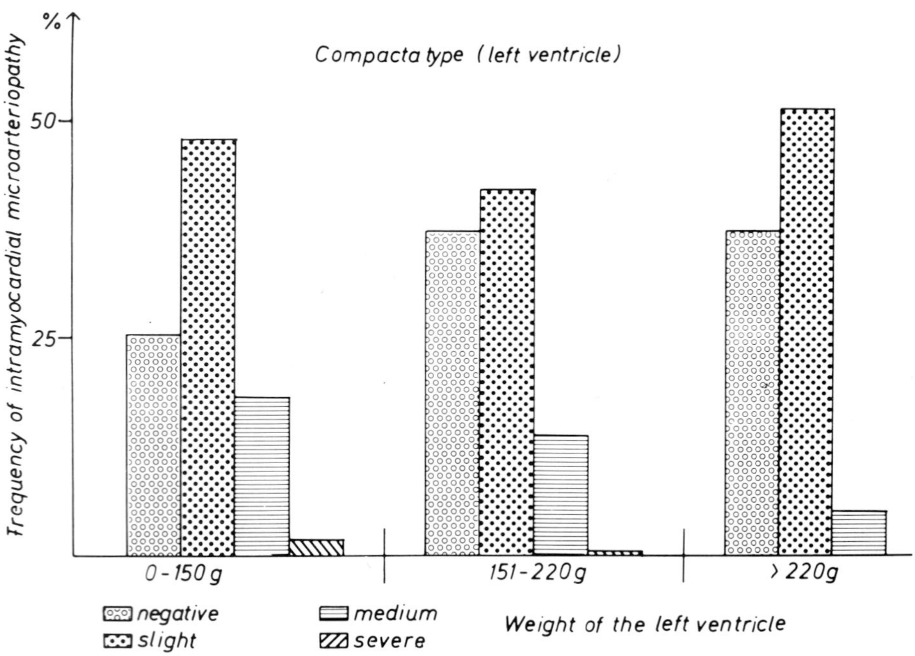

Fig. 10. Correlation of the degree of intramyocardial microarteriopathy with left ventricles grouped according to weight (compacta type)

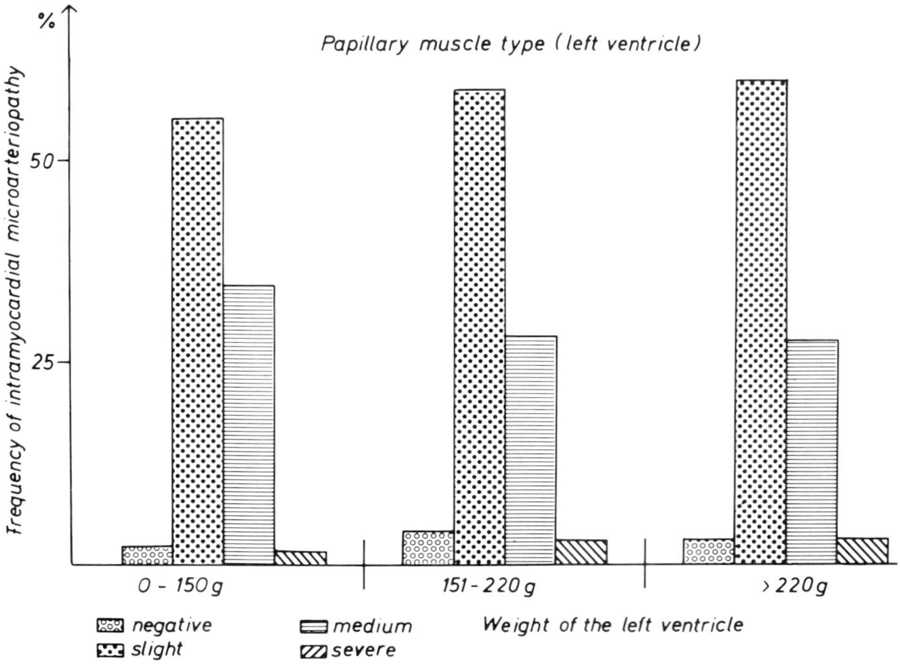

Fig. 11. Correlation of the degree of intramyocardial microarteriopathy with left ventricles grouped according to weight (papillary muscle type)

If we compare the severity of intramyocardial microarteriopathy with left ventricles grouped according to weight we see that there is no strong correlation between increasing muscular weight of the left ventricle and progressive damage of the intramural arterial vessels (Figs. 10, 11).

The most impressive result of our investigations into the influence of hypertension or hypertrophy on microarteriopathy is the following: We found that a greater degree of myocardial micronecrosis or scarring occurred in cases of hypertension or advanced concentric hypertrophy and severe microarteriopathy.

Discussion

Our investigations shwo that statements concerning the incidence of pathological alterations to the small intramyocardial coronary arteries can only be made if the pathological lesions in the compacta and papillary muscle type vessels are analysed separately. The percentage of pathological changes increased with age in both basic vessel types. In the 8th decade of life they occur in the left ventricle in over 90% of all cases. Hypertension is associated with a rise in the frequency of slight and medium lesions in the vessels of the compacta type in the 4th — 7th decades.

In experimentally — induced acute hypertension Olsen [34] has demonstrated an increase of permeability of small intramyocardial arteries and arterioles. The small arteries showed distinct deposits of plasma components in the intima and media as well.

In the papillary muscle arteries the transition from slight or medium to severe impairment is completed in hypertension cases not only at the top but also at the bottom of the left papillary muscles. Hypertension is the chief predisposing factor in the spread of the lesions.

According to our results there exist no specific hypertensive lesions in the intramyocardial microarteries. In nearly all research finding an important causal connection between hypertension and the occurrence of intramural vascular damage, it is predominantly papillary muscle type vessels and their degeneration that are described [3, 15, 32, 33, 38—40]. We believe that hyperfibroelastosis of small intramyocardial arteries is a characteristic degenerative lesion of a special vessel type which normally develops in the papillary muscels. Hypertension only has the effect of reinforcing these lesions. We never found so-called glomoid or plexiform lesions in intramyocardial coronary arteries as described by Salyer and Hutchins [37] in cases of malignant hypertension.

Haerem [14] mentioned hypertension as possible reinforcing factor in the occurrence of intramural vascular lesions, without being able to produce any statistical evidence. He investigated mainly the lesions of the compacta type vessels. Other authors have found no correlation between the severity of the lesions of small intramyocardial arteries and the presence of hypertension [1, 11, 22, 24, 42—44].

Wegelin [44], Baroldi [1, 2] and Volkova [43] consider that vascular alterations are of little significance in the function and maintenance of the myocardium. We disagree with this. In the regulation of blood-flow resistance, and thus in the supply of blood to the heart, an important role is played by the intramural small coronary vessels. It is not only the compacta-type vessels but also the papillary muscle type that shows narrowing of the lumen and degeneration of the intima, elastica interna and media.

It is therefore to be supposed that these changes, particularly when they take on a severe form, can lead functionally to irregular disturbances in the supply of blood to the myocardium. This is supported by the fact that in cases of non-narrowing extramural coronary sclerosis and obvious severe degeneration of the small intramural branches micronecrosis and scarring can be found in the myocardium of the left papillary muscles. Also found are disseminated micronecrosis and scars in the compacta and papillary muscles of the left ventricle, predominantly in cases where a co-occurrence of both microarteriopathy and hypertrophy or hypertension existed. The presence of pressure hypertrophy of the ventricles serves to further lessen the supply of blood to the heart.

Intramyocardial vascular lesions have been held to be one of the causes of functional disturbances of the heart, in particular in cases where the coronary arteriogram has revealed no stenosis in the major extramural coronary arterial system [4—7, 10, 12, 21, 23, 25, 27, 41].

Ueda [42] and Donomae et al. [8, 9] believe that severe intramural damage can lead to chronic heart insufficiency without attacks of angina pectoris, i.e. to so-called silent heart failure or chronic cardiac failure. Similar views are held by Ratcliffe and Redfield [35] and Naeye and Liedtke [31]. James [16—18] regards small vessel disease as a possible cause of heart rhythm disturbance, heart attacks or heart insufficiency. Linzbach [30] believes that intramyocardial microarteriopathy assumes functional importance, particularly in old age. Severe microarteriopathy of the myocardium can, according to Linzbach [28], lead to manifest coronary insufficiency, even in the absence of sclerosis of the extramural arteries.

Summary

1. At least two basic types of arterial vessels can be distinguished in the myocardium.
   a) *Compacta type:* Intramyocardial microarteries with ring musculature of the media.
   b) *Papillary muscle type:* Arteries with longitudinal musculature which are arranged as bundles in the broad media.
2. The manifestations of intramyocardial microarteriopathy are different in these vessel types. PAS positive cushion-like thickening of the intima mainly occurs in the compacta type. The degenerative lesions of the papillary muscle type are characterized by hyperfibroelastosis of intima and media.
3. Pathological vascular lesions in the compacta and papillary muscle type occur more frequently with increasing age.
4. Slight and medium lesions are well in the majority. Severe vascular changes are seen in the 7th to 9th decade in about 5%—10% (compacta type) and in 30%—35% (papillary muscle type), respectively.
5. Hypertension seemed to raise the frequency of slight and medium lesions in compacta type vessels. In the papillary muscle type, the degenerative lesions are spread over the whole area from the top to the bottom of the papillary muscles.
6. There exists no definite positive correlation between intramyocardial microarteriopathy and weight of the left ventricle including the septum.
7. Impairment of the quality of myocardial circulation is only encountered in the presence of severe pathological vascular lesions.
8. Pressure hypertrophy serves to further lessen the supply of blood to the heart, especially in cases with severe intramyocardial microarteriopathy.

References

1. Baroldi G (1962) Histopathological study of the intramural artery vessels in the relation to the pathology of extramural coronary arteries and myocardial damage. Cardiologia 41 : 364–380
2. Baroldi G, Scomazzoni G (1967) Coronary circulation in the normal and in the pathologic heart. Office of the Surgeon General; Department of the Army, Washington DC
3. Blumenthal HT, Alex M, Goldenberg S (1960) A study of lesions of the intramural coronary artery branches in diabetes mellitus. Arch Pathol 70 : 27–42
4. Brest AN, Wiener L, Kasparian H, Duca P, Rafter JJ (1974) Myocardial infarction without obstructive coronary artery disease. Am Heart J 88 : 219–224
5. Bruschke AVG, Bruyneel KJJ, Bloch A, Herpen G (1971) Acute myocardial infarction without obstructive coronary artery disease demonstrated by selective cinearteriography. Am Heart J 33 : 585–594
6. Campeau L (1970) Myocardial infarction with normal selective coronary arteriograms. Am Heart J 79 : 139–141
7. Cheng TO, Bashour T, Singh BK, Kelser GA (1972) Myocardial infarction in the absence of coronary arteriosclerosis. Am J Cardiol 30 : 680–682
8. Donomae I, Matsumoto Y, Kokubu T, Koide RJ, Kobayashi R, Ikegami H, Ueda E, Fujisawa T, Fujimoto S (1962) Pathological studies of coronary artherosclerosis especially of sclerosis of intramuscular coronary arteries. Japn Heart J 3 : 423–441
9. Donomae I, Matsumoto Y, Ueda E (1965) Significance of coronary arteriosclerosis in the intramuscular coronary arteries. Geriatrics 20 : 179–193
10. Engel HJ, Lichtlen P (1976) Angina pectoris und Myocardinfarkt ohne Koronarsklerose. Ther Umsch 33 : 75–86
11. Fishberg AM (1925) Anatomic findings in essential hypertension. Arch Intern Med 35 : 650–668
12. Fouchard J, Caramanian M, Cabrol C, Ecoiffier J, Leduc G, Rasolomampiononа M (1971) Infarctus du myocarde avec coronarographie normale. Lésions histologiques d'endartérite fibreuse. Arch Mal Coeur 64 : 1711–1733
13. Haerem JW (1969) Cushion-like intimal lesions and platelet aggregates in intramyocardial arteries of man. Acta Pathol Microbiol Scand 77 : 73–89
14. Haerem JW (1969) Cushion-like intimal lesions in intramyocardial arteries of man. Acta Pathol Microbiol Scand 77 : 598–608
15. Höpker WW, Nüssel E, Weiler J (1975) Ausbreitungsmuster der Arteriosklerose: Alter und Risikokriterien bei epicardialen und intramuralen Veränderungen der Coronargefäße bei Patienten mit Herzinfarkt. Verh Dtsch Ges Pathol 59 : 348–354
16. James TN (1965) Anatomy of the coronary arteries in health and disease. Circulation 32 : 1020–1033
17. James TN (1967) Pathology of small coronary arteries. Am J Cardiol 20 : 679–691
18. James TN (1968) Diseases of small coronary arteries. JAMA 203, 977–978
19. Jonáš V, Chlumská A, Kozák P (1966) Změny intramurálních koronárních cev u diabetiku. Acta Univ Carol]Med] (Praha) 12 : 379–384

20. Kathke N (1955) Die Veränderungen der Koronararterienzweige des Myokards bei Hypertonie. Beitr Pathol 115 : 405—422
21. Khan AH, Haywood LJ (1974) Myocardial infarction in nine patients with radiologically patent coronary arteries. Engl J Med 291 : 427—431
22. Knežević M, Knežević-Krivak Š, Rode B (1970) Beitrag zur Kenntnis der Pathologie der intrapapillären Koronararterienästchen am linken Herzen. Verh Dtsch Ges Pathol 54 : 348—355
23. Kübler W, Zebe H (1975) Die diabetische Kardiomyopathie. Internist (Berlin) 16 : 520—523
24. Ledet T (1968) Histological and histochemical changes in the coronary arteries of old diabetic patients. Diabetologica 4 : 268—272
25. Lenègre J, Himbert J, Froment R, Normand J, Perrin A (1961) L'infarctus myocardique sans occlusion des artères coronaires. Actual Cardiol Angeiol Int 10 : 357—361
26. Liebegott G (1958) Die intramurale Coronarsklerose bei Hypertonie. Med Klin 35 : 1465—1466
27. Likoff W, Segal BL, Kasparian H (1967) Paradox of normal selective coronary arteriograms in patients considered to have unmistakable coronary heart disease. N Engl J Med 276 : 1063—1066
28. Linzbach AJ (1947) Mikrometrische und histologische Analyse hypertropher menschlicher Herzen. Virchows Arch 314 : 534—594
29. Linzbach AJ (1956) Das Greisenherz. In: Deutscher Internistentag 1955, Leipzig. Volk & Gesundheit, Berlin
30. Linzbach AJ, Akuamoa-Boateng E (1973) Die Altersveränderungen des menschlichen Herzens. II. Die Polypathie des Herzens im Alter. Klin Wochenschr 51 : 164—175
31. Naeye RL, Liedtke AJ (1976) Consequences of intramyocardial arterial lesions in aortic valvular stenosis. Am J Pathol 85 : 569—580
32. Neubuerger KT, Denst J (1955) Les lésions artériolaires des piliers du coeur au cours du rhumatisme cardiaque chronique. Arch Anat Cytol Pathol 31 : 76—81
33. Odel HM (1940) Structural changes in the arterioles of the myocardium in diffuse arteriolar disease with hypertension group 4. Arch Intern Med 66 : 579—602
34. Olsen F (1978) Acute hypertensive damage of arterial vessels of the heart. Acta Pathol Microbiol Scand [A] 86 : 199—200
35. Ratcliffe HL, Redfield E (1972) Atherosclerotic stenosis of the extramural and intramural coronary arteries of man. Virchows Arch 357 : 1—10
36. Rider AK, Billingham ME, Harrison DC (1974) Small vessel coronary disease: Biopsy evidence of intramyocardial arteriopathy. Circulation [Suppl III] 59/50: 109
37. Salyer W, Hutchins GM (1974) Glomoid lesions in systemic arteries in malignant hypertension. Arch Pathol 97 : 104—106
38. Saphir O, Ohringer L, Wong R (1956) Changes in the intramural coronary branches in coronary arteriosclerosis. Arch Pathol 62 : 159—170

39. Schwartz CJ, Mitchell JRA (1962) The relation between myocardial lesions and coronary artery disease. Br Heart J 24 : 761—786
40. Sósnierz M, Wieczorek M (1968) Morphological lesions of intramyocardial arteries in 100 cases examined post mortem. Pol Med J 7 : 839—844
41. Strauer BE (1978) Das Hochdruckherz; II. Koronardurchblutung, Koronarreserve und Sauerstoffverbrauch des linken Ventrikels. Z Kardiol 67 : 452—459
42. Ueda E (1962) Pathological studies of coronary atherosclerosis especially of sclerosis of intramuscular coronary arteries. Med J Osaka Univ 13 : 117—137
43. Volkova KG (1961) The arterioles of the myocardium in hypertension. Exerpta Med Sect 18 5 : 688—689
44. Wegelin C (1944) Über Arteriolosklerose im Myocard. Schweiz Med Wochenschr 74 : 57—60
45. World Health Organization (1958) W H O Techn Rep Ser 143

Reduced Coronary Reserve and Ultrastructural Changes of the Myocardium in Patients with Angina Pectoris, Arterial Hypertension, and Normal Coronary Arteries[1]

D. OPHERK, E. WEIHE, H. ZEBE, G. MALL, H.C. MEHMEL, B. STOCKINS, U. RYAN AND W. KÜBLER

Several recent studies have presented the paradox of patients who suffer from typical stress-induced anginal pain but have normal coronary and left ventricular angiograms [1, 3, 9, 14, 15]. Patients with essential hypertension were excluded in these studies, although they often have symptoms of ischemic heart disease despite normal coronary arteries.

In order to further examine these patients with essential hypertension in addition to left ventricular and coronary angiography the following investigations were performed:

1. Using the Argon method [2, 10, 17], coronary blood flow at rest and after application of dipyridamole (0.5 mg/kg i.v.) was determined for the estimation of coronary reserve and

2. Biopsy specimens were taken from left ventricular myocardium for light and electron microscopic evaluation of arterioles, capillaries, venules, and myocardial cells.

Materials and Methods

Studies were carried out in nine patients with essential hypertension (history of hypertension varied from 4 to more than 20 years, average 8.5 ± 6 years). All patients had a history of typical stress-induced angina pectoris promptly relieved by nitroglycerin and a pathological ECG at rest or during exercise (Table 1). Congestive heart failure or valvular heart disease were not present. Echocardiography revealed no signs of hypertrophic cardiomyopathy and/or asymmetric septal hypertrophy.

Selective coronary arteriography was performed with multiple views of the right (at least three projections) and left (at least five projections) coronary artery (including hemiaxial projections). Pressures in the left ventricle were ob-

1 Supported by a grant from the Deutsche Forschungsgemeinschaft/Germany-SFB 90, Kardiovaskuläres System of the University of Heidelberg

Table 1. Clinical data obtained in nine patients with essential hypertension

Patient No.	Sex and age (yr)		History of Hypertension (yr)	Pathological ECG Rest	Pathological ECG Exercise	Angina Pectoris
1	F	56	5	+		+
2	F	40	12	+		+
3	M	55	4	—	+	+
4	M	52	6	+		+
5	F	49	5	+		+
6	M	46	9	—	+	+
7	M	50	8	—	+	+
8	M	43	5	—	+	+
9	M	56	25	+		+

tained by means of a fluid-filled catheter pressure transducer system. Left ventricular volumes and wall thickness were determined from the monoplane angiogram in a 30^0 RAO projection. Using the Argon method, coronary blood flow at rest and after application of dipyridamole (0.5 mg/kg) was determined for the estimation of coronary reserve (ratio of coronary resistance at rest to coronary resistance during maximal pharmacologic coronary vascodilatation). The Argon technique is suitable for the determination of coronary reserve in patients. According to animal experiments with electromagnetic flowmeters as the reference method, even high coronary flowrates up to more than 300 ml/100 g min could be measured accurately using the Argon method [13].

Biopsy specimens were taken from left ventricular myocardium using the S. Thomas' shield and the King's College bioptome. The heart muscle tissue obtained by biopsy was cut into cylinders of less than 1 mm diameter and immediately fixed by immersion with a formaldehyde-gluturaldehyde solution at room temperature. The composition of the fixative solution was 1.5% glutaraldehyde, 1.5 % formaldehyde, and 0.1 *M* phosphate buffer, pH 7.35 [4]. After a fixation time of at least 1 h and rinsing overnight in 0.1 *M* Na-cacodylate buffer, the specimens were either postfixed with ferrocyanide-reduced osmium [8] or osmium tetroxide in 0.1 *M* Na-cacodylate buffer and dehydrated with ethanol and prophylene oxide. The tissue cylinders were embedded in Epon [11]. The blocks were trimmed so that the total tissue cylinder could be cut into semithin sections. Areas exhibiting appropriately fixed tissue were selected for light and electron microscopic evaluation. The first two or three subendocardial cell layers were omitted from the analysis in order to avoid possible inclusion of Purkinje cells in the morphological examination. The Toluidine blue stained semithin sections were analyzed in a Zeiss axiomat microscope. The ultrathin sections were stained with uranyle acetate and lead citrate and examined in a Zeiss EM 10 electron microscope. The morphometry of muscle fiber diameter was either carried out on projected light microscopic negatives or directly in the light microscope utilizing a MOP 3 (Kontron) morphometric device. The fiber diameter was determined on cross sections. To quantify the degree of cardiac hypertrophy, cell diameters of more than 300 cross-sectioned cardiac muscle cells were measured in each sample.

Results

All patients had a typical stress-induced angina pectoris promptly relieved by nitroglycerine (Table 1). The electrocardiogram revealed abnormalities in all cases, with evidence of left ventricular hypertrophy and descending ST-segments at rest or exercise. In one case (Pt no. 4) a left bundle branch block was observed.

The hemodynamic data are summarized in Table 2. As compared with normal values obtained in control subjects, patients with essential hypertension had a normal left ventricular end-diastolic and end-diastolic volume index and a normal ejection fraction. The left ventricular end-diastolic pressure was significantly ($P < 0.001$) increased. Wall thickness observed in left ventricular angiogram was, with one exception (Pt no. 8), in the upper normal range, the mean value being 11.6 ± 2.5 mm. Resting coronary blood flow was slightly increased. This difference was not significant. After application of dipyridamole, however, maximal coronary blood flow in patients with essential hypertension was markedly ($P < 0.001$) reduced to 165 ml/100 g min. This value corresponds only to 60% of that obtained in normals with maximal coronary flow rate of approximately 300 ml/100 g min. As a consequence, in the hypertensive patients minimal coronary resistance was significantly ($P < 0.001$) augmented and coronary reserve was significantly ($P < 0.01$) reduced to 230 ± 64.9% compared with 424 ± 74.5% in normals (Table 2).

The biopsy specimens from all patients were suitable for light and electron microscopic evaluation except that from patient no. 5.

Light Microscopy

In all patients the light microscopic evaluation did not reveal abnormalities of myocardial muscle fibers, interstitium, and microvascular segments. The values of muscle fiber diameters are shown in Fig. 1. No lesions of small vessels ranging in external diameter from 4 to 30 μ were found. From each patient about 10–15 arterioles, metarterioles, capillaries, and venules could be analyzed. Small arteries exhibiting a media with more than two muscle cell layers were only occasionally encountered. None of the biopsies presented significant interstitial fibrosis.

Table 2. Hemodynamic data obtained in patients with essential hypertension (pat. no. 1—9) and in controls (n = 12) Mean values ± SD [a]

Patient No.	LVEDP mm Hg	AOP A mm HG	AOP B	$\dot{V}_{cor}$ A ml/100 g min	$\dot{V}_{cor}$ B	R_{cor} A mm Hg/ ml/100 g · min	R_{cor} B	Coronary Reserve %	EDVI ml/m²	ESVI ml/m²	EF %
1	22	117	100	108	144	0.95	0.61	156	51	9	83
2	20	108	102	74	172	1.01	0.51	198	49	8	84
3	17	97	92	55	173	1.60	0.47	353	77	29	69
4	12	103	95	92	139	1.01	0.60	168	52	17	68
5	12	110	107	111	208	0.84	0.45	187	99	27	73
6	13	83	79	69	163	0.91	0.37	245	51	14	73
7	15	113	92	73	185	1.27	0.41	310	55	10	82
8	18	103	97	100	162	0.93	0.51	182	125	44	65
9	14	120	113	63	141	1.79	0.66	271	48	16	67
$\overline{X}$	15.9	106	97	83	165	1.15	0.51	230	67	19	74
± SD	3.4	10.6	9.2	19.3	21.2	0.32	0.09	64.9	25.9	11.1	7.0
Controls	(n = 12)										
$\overline{X}$	7.0	90	81	80	290	0.98	0.24	424	76	20	74
± SD	3.0	7.5	11.7	7.3	54.1	0.14	0.05	74.5	20.0	7.0	5.0

[a] LVEDP, left ventricular end-diastolic pressure; AOP, mean aortic pressure; $\dot{V}_{cor}$, coronary blood flow; R_{cor}, coronary resistance; EDVI, left ventricualr end-diastolic volume index; ESVI left ventricular end-systolic volume index; EF, ejection fraction; A, values at rest; and B values after application of dipyridamole

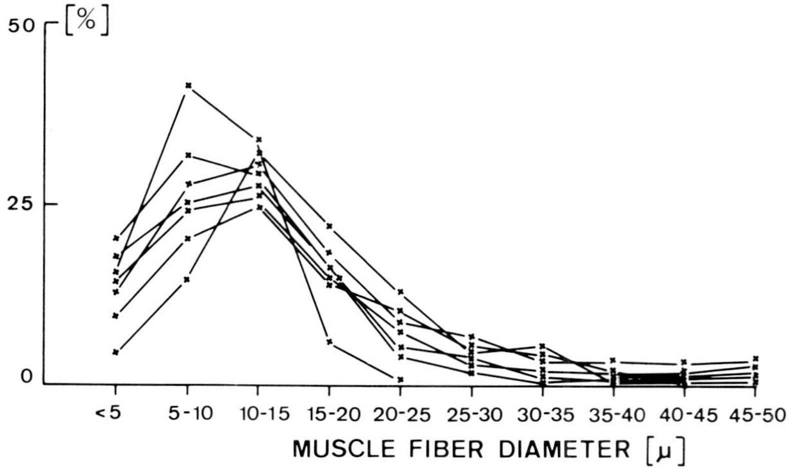

Fig. 1. Histogram of muscle fiber diameters, based on the evaluation of more than 300 cross-sectioned muscle fibers in seven patients with essential hypertension

Electron Microscopy

In all examined patients the myocardial cells contained nomally arranged myofibrils, mitochondira, and sacrotubular system (Fib. 2). Occasionally single damaged mitochondria exhibiting cristolysis were observed (Fig. 2). The most prominent finding in all patients was a more or less severe disorientation and splitting of myofilaments (Figs. 3, 4). The arteriolar microvascular segments showed no pathological changes such as intimal proliferation, medial dissection, or mural deposites (Figs. 5, 6). The capillary and venular segments had also a normal appearance (Figs. 8, 9). There was no thickening of the basal laminas.

Discussion

The nine patients with essential hypertension selected for endocardial catheter biopsy and determination of coronary reserve suffered from typical angina pectoris despite normal coronary angiograms. It can be suggested that the marked reduction in coronary reserve by 60% of the value obtained in normals is responsible for the stress-induced anginal pain and the pathological ECG findings. A similar reduction of coronary reserve has been described in patients with essential hypertension [16] and in patients with left ventricular hypertrophy due to aortic stenosis and insufficiency [5] as well as in animal experiments with left ventricular hypertrophy [6]. A possible and often discussed explanation for this finding is a structural change of the small intramyocardial vessels not visualized by coronary angiography, i.e., small vessel disease [7]. If disease of small vessels

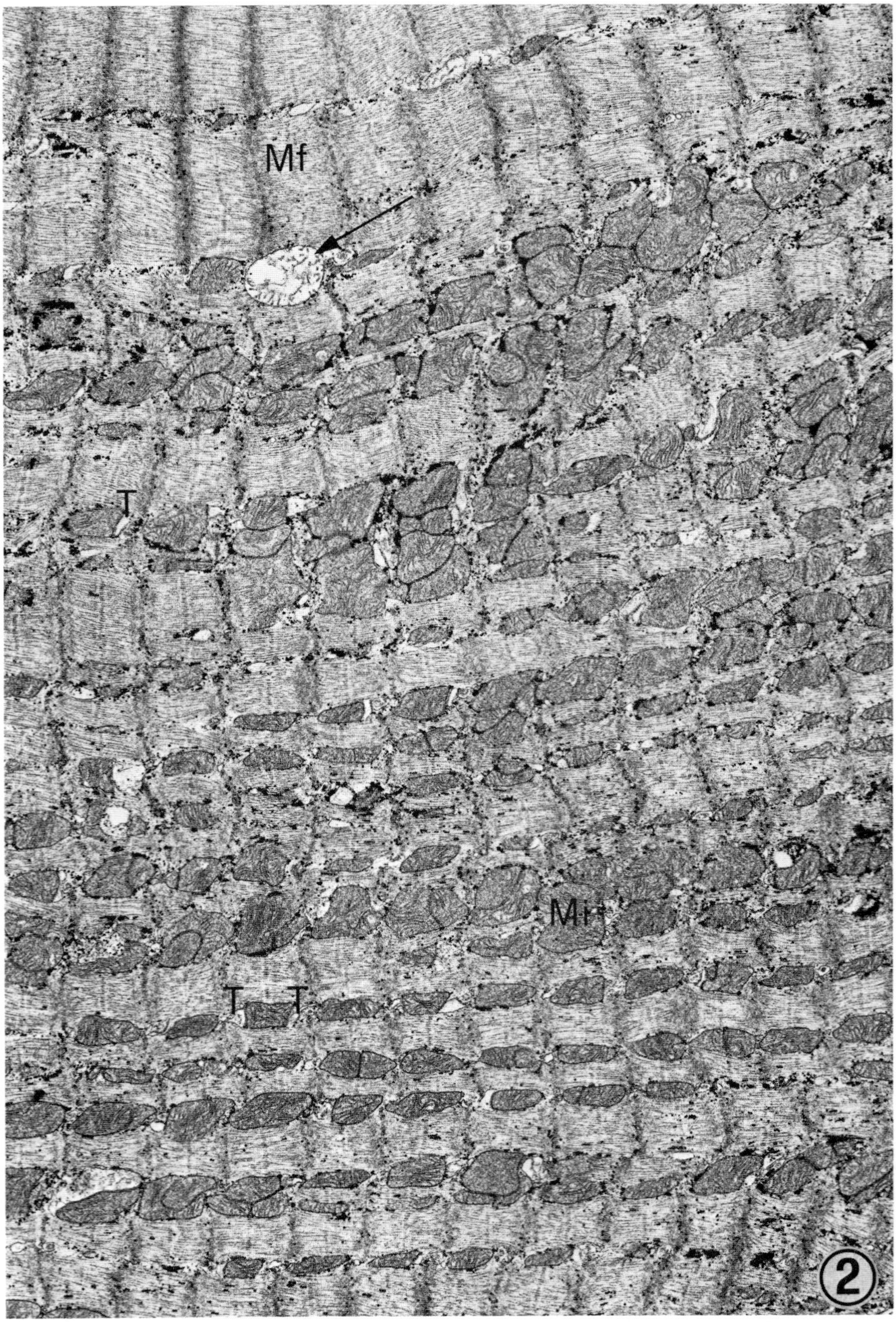
Mf
T
Mi
T
T
2

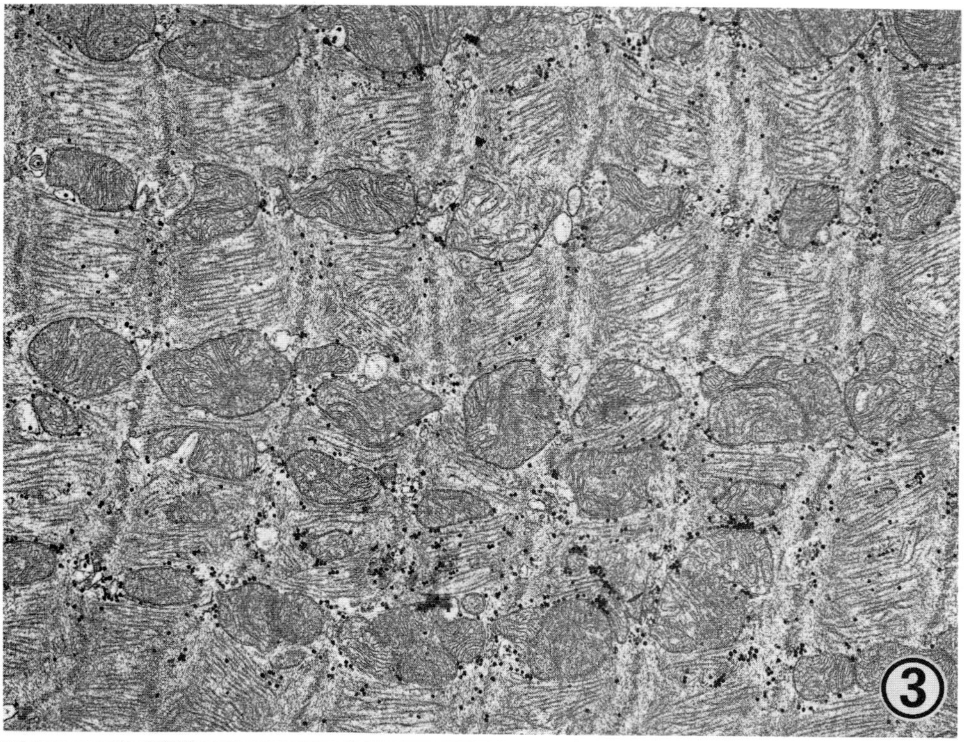
3

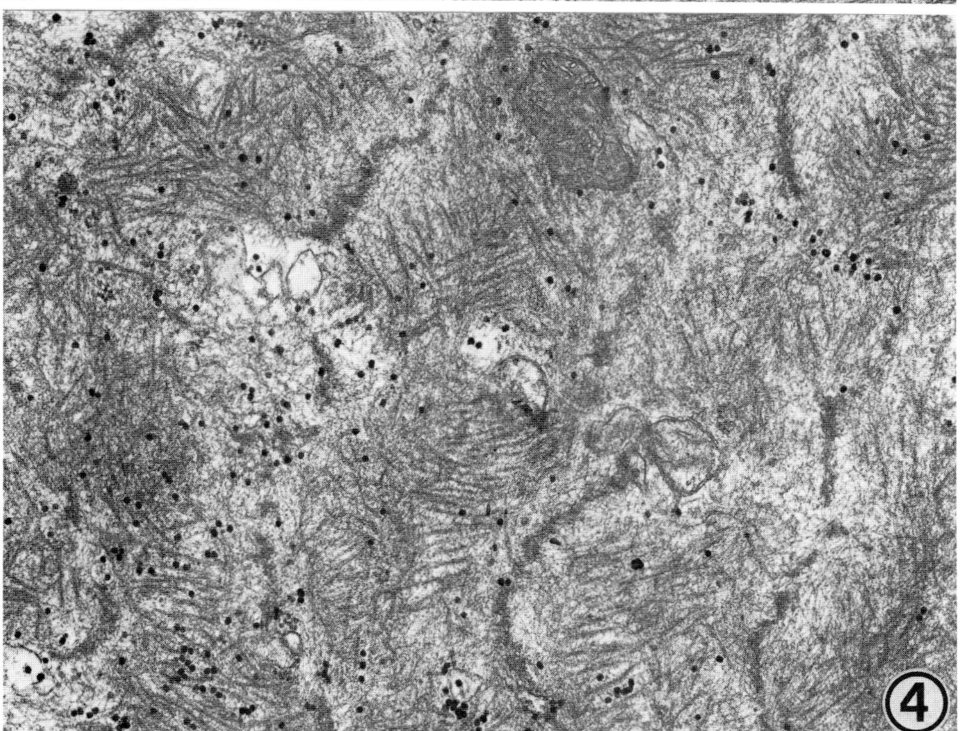
4

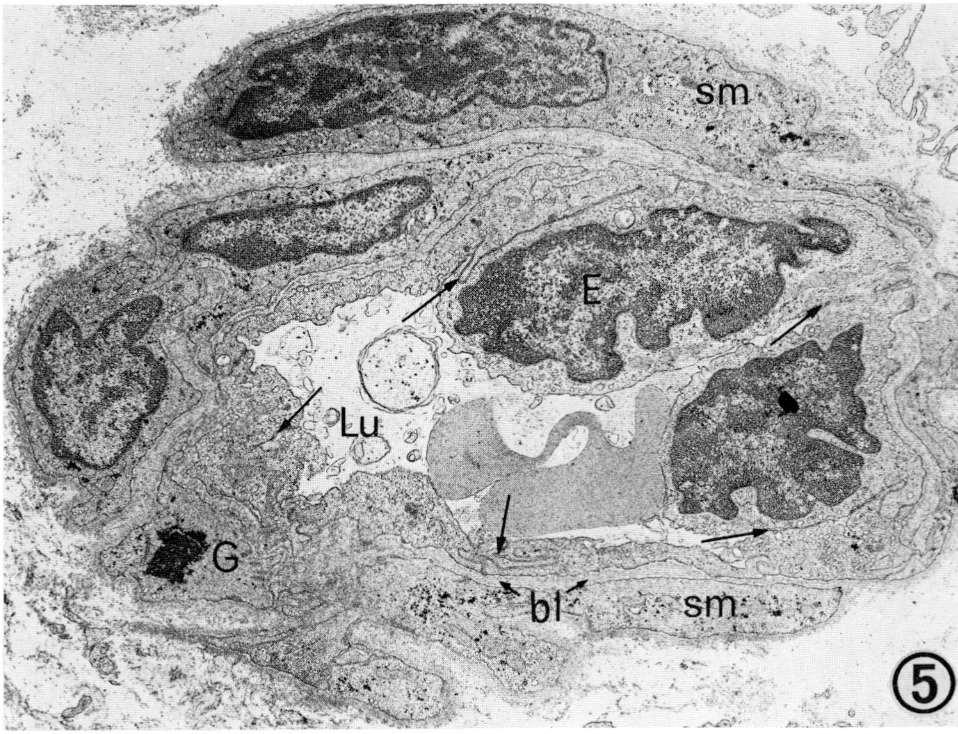

sm
E
Lu
G
bl
sm
5

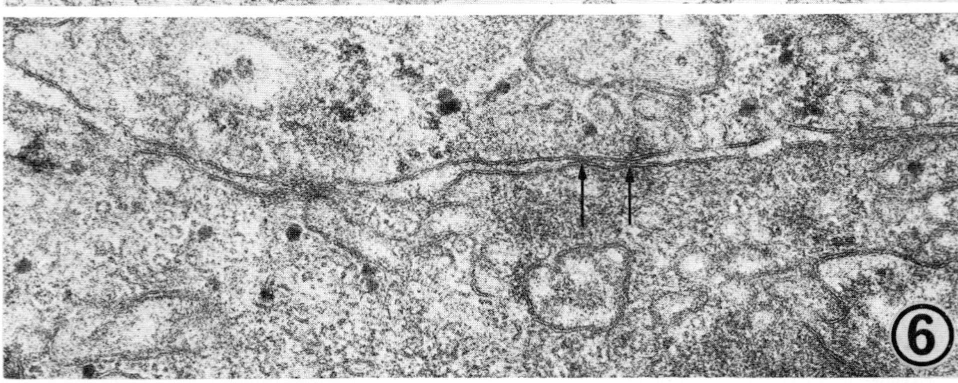

6

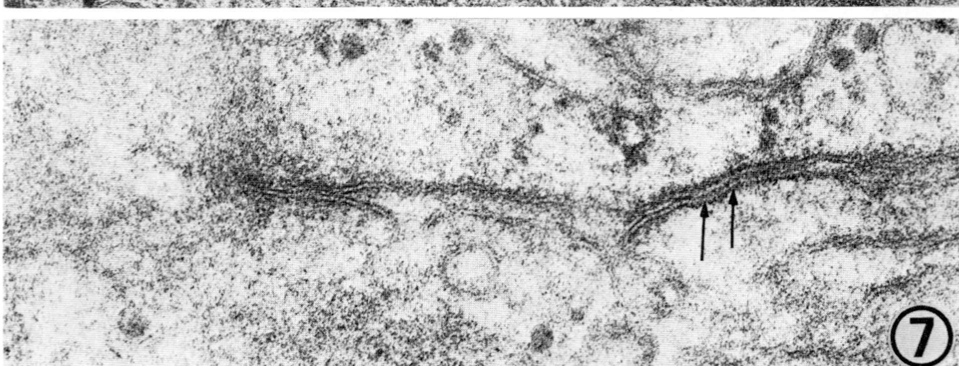

7

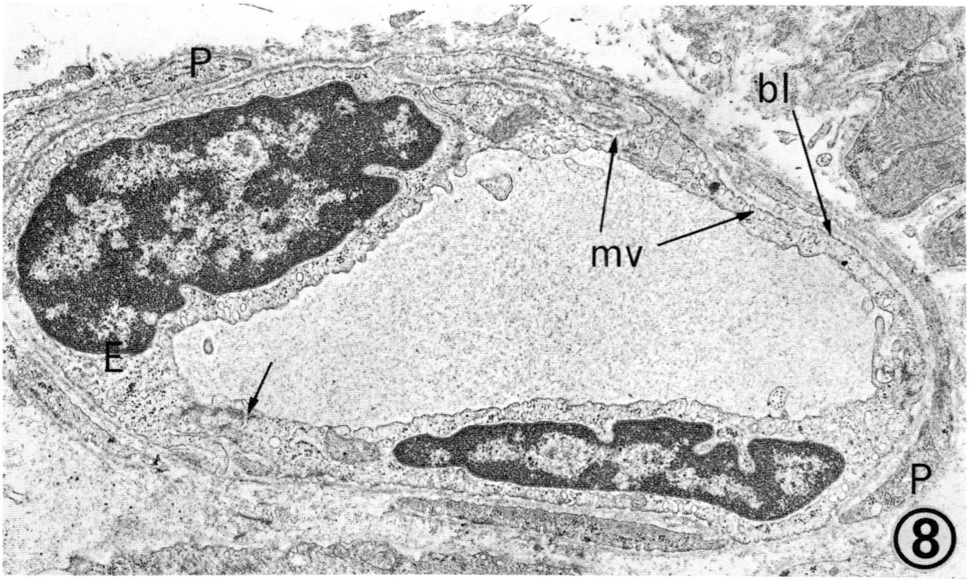
P
bl
mv
E
P
8

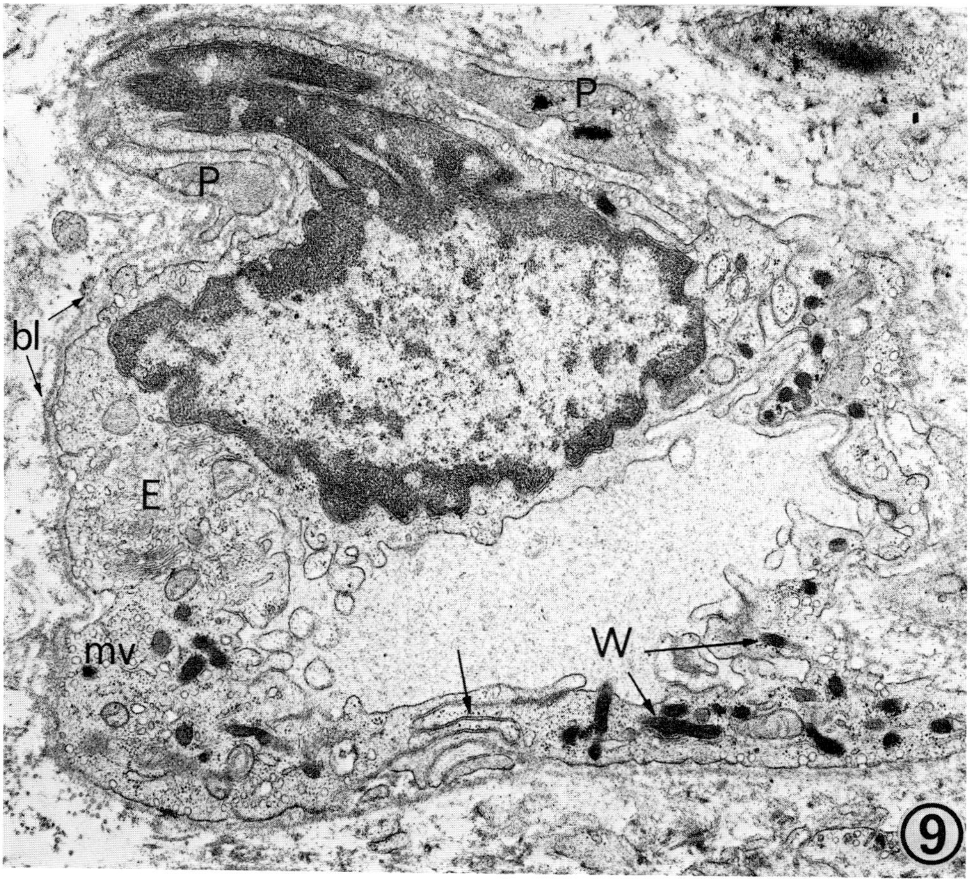
P
P
bl
E
mv
W
9

was sufficiently diffuse to produce anginal symptoms and to reduce coronary reserve, such structural changes should be revealed by examination of the biopsy specimens from the subendocardial region of the myocardium. Our observations do not support this hypothesis. The myocardial biopsy specimens obtained in the patients of this study revealed in all cases normal metarterioles, capillaries and venules. It must, however, be considered that vessels ranging from 30μ to at least 100 μ are technically unavailable for microscopic as well as for angiographic evaluation.

It has been argued that the compressive component of coronary resistance representing the compression of intramyocardial vessels by the intramyocardial pressure, i.e., the myocardial component of coronary resistance, could be increased in patients with essential hypertension as compared with normal subjects. Hemodynamic data listed in Table 2 do not support this hypothesis. This is in agreement with earlier results [16]. The most prominent findings of the morphological examination were a moderate hypertrophy of the myocardial cells and severe disorientation and distortion of myofilaments and Z-bands.

Figs. on p. 214—217:

Fig. 2. Low power electron micrograph showing a relatively unchanged part of a myocardiocyte. Longitudinal orientation of myofibrils (*Mf*) and normal mitochondria (*Mi*), mitochondrium exhibiting cristolysis (*arrow*), normal T-system (*T*). Pt no. 2 (x 6200)

Fig. 3. Electron micrograph showing severe myofilament disorientation. Normal mitochondria. Pt. no. 2 (x 13 200)

Fig. 4. Electron micrograph showing extreme disorientation and distortion of myofilaments and Z-bands. Pt. no. 4 (x 32 300)

Fig. 5. Electron micrograph showing a normal metarteriole, vessel lumen (*Lu*), containing an erythrocyte, endothelium (*E*), interendothelial clefts (*arrows*), vascular smooth muscle cells (*sm*), basal lamina (*bl*), and glycogen (*G*) in a smooth muscle cell of the media. Pt. no. 2 (x 7300)

Fig. 6. Electron micrograph showing the detail of an arteriolar interendothelial cleft with a normal zonula occludens (*arrows*). Pt. no. 2 (x 78 300)

Fig. 7. Electron micrograph showing a normal gap junction (*arrows*) of an arteriolar interendothelial cleft. Pt no. 2 (x 140 000)

Fig. 8. Electron micrograph showing normal capillary with numerous micropinocytotic vesicles (*mv*). Capillary endothelium (*E*), pericytes (*P*), basal lamina (*bl*), and interendothelial cleft (*arrow*). Pt. no. 1 (x 10 700)

Fig. 9. Electron micrograph showing a part of a normal pericytic venule. Venular endothelium (*E*), pericytes (*P*), Weibel-Palade bodies (*W*), interendothelial cleft (*arrow*), micropinocytotic vesicles (m.v.), and basal lamina (bl). Pt. no. 6 (x 17 100)

These alterations seem to be more pronounced in patients with a long history of hypertension. It is interesting to note that based on experimental results in patients with myocardial hypertrophy and normal coronary arteries angina pectoris and reduced coronary reserve could be related to a decrease of capillary density [12]. An alternative explanation would be a defect in local metabolic regulation of coronary blood flow affecting either transmitter formation or receptor response.

Acknowledgment

The authors wish to thank Charlotte Dürr, Carola Frey and Beate Stahl for technical assistance and Steven Meairs for preparing the manuscript.

References

1. Arbogast R, Bourassa MG (1973) Myocardial function during atrial pacing in patients with angina pectoris and normal coronary arteriograms. Comparison with patients having significant coroanary artery disease. Am J Cardiol 32 : 257
2. Bretschneider HJ, Cott L, Hilgert G, Probst R, Rau G (1966) Gaschromatographische Trennung und Analyse von Argon als Basis einer neuen Fremdgasmethode zur Durchflußmessung von Organen. Verh Dtsch Ges Kreislaufforsch 32 : 267
3. Dwyer EM, Wiener L, Cox JW (1969) Angina pectoris in patients with normal and abnormal coronary arteriograms. Am J Cardiol 23 : 639
4. Forssmann WG, Ito S, Weihe E, Aoki A, Dym M, Fawcett DW (1977) An improved fixation method for the testis. Anat Rec 188 : 307
5. Heiss HW, Tauchert M, Strauer BE, Sonntag H, Kochsiek K (1972) Koronare Hämodynamik and myokardialer Sauerstoffverbrauch bei Patienten mit linksventrikulärer Hypertrophie. Z Kreislaufforsch 61 : 260
6. Holtz J, Restorff W von, Bard P, Bassenge E (1977) Transmural distribution of myocardial blood flow and of coronary reserve in canine left ventricular hypertrophy. Basic Res Cardiol 72 : 286
7. James TN (1977) Small arteries of the heart. Circulation 56 : 2
8. Karnovsky MJ (1971) Use of ferrocyanide-reduced osmium tetroxide in electron microscopy. J Cell Biol 51 : 146
9. Kemp HG, Vokonas PS, Cohn PF, Gorlin R (1973) The anginal syndrome associated with normal coronary arteriograms. Report of a six year experience. Am J Med 54 : 735
10. Kochsiek K, Cott LA, Tauchert M, Neubaur J, Larbig D (1970) Measurement of coronary blood flow in various conditions using the argon-technique. In: Kaltenbach M, Lichtlen P (eds) Coronary heart disease. Thieme, Stuttgart, pp 137–153

11. Luft JH (1961) Improvement in epoxy resin embedding methods. J Biophys Biochem Cytol 9 : 409
12. Lund DD, Tomanek RJ (1978) Myocardial morphology in spontaneously hypertensive and aortic-constricted rats. Am J Anat 152 : 141
13. Opherk D, Finke R, Mittmann U, Müller JH, Wirth RH, Schmier J (1977) The influence of the size of acute ischaemic myocardial lesions on coronary reserve and left ventricular function in the dog. Basic Res Cardiol 72 : 402
14. Opherk D, Zebe H, Weihe E, Mäurer W, Mehmel HC, Kübler W (1978) Syndrome X: Results of coronary reserve and myocardial biopsy. Trans Eur Soc Cardiol 1 : 189
15. Richardson PJ, Livesly B, Oram S, Olsen EGJ, Armstrong P (1974) Angina pectoris with normal coronary arteries. Lancet II : 677
16. Strauer BE (1979) Das Hochdruckherz. Springer, Berlin Heidelberg New York
17. Tauchert M, Kochsiek K, Heiss HW, Strauer BE, Kettler D, Reploh HD, Rau G, Bretschneider HJ (1972) Measurement of coronary blood flow in man by the argon method. In: Maseri A (ed) Myocardial blood flow in man, Torino, pp 139–144

Session C: Cardiac Function and Metabolism in Clinical Hypertension

Chairmen: G. Riecker/München (FRG), J. Cohn/Minneapolis (USA)

Part I: Pathogenetic Implications, Ventricular Wall Dynamics and Coronary Circulation

Left Ventricular Hypertrophy in Hypertension: Prognostic and Pathogenetic Implications (The Framingham Study)

W.B. KANNEL AND P. SORLIE

Abstract

The prevalence, incidence, determinants, and prognosis of ECG evidence of left ventricular hypertrophy (ECG-LVH) was examined in the Framingham cohort of 5209 subjects aged 30—62. In the course of 20 years of follow-up 957 subjects in the age range 45—74 developed cardiovascular disease and 856 died and the risk of cardiovascular disease and mortality in persons who developed ECG-LVH was compared to that of those who remained free of it.

The prevalence of ECG-LVH rose with age and one in ten developed some evidence of it in the first 12 years of follow-up. Only 16% with X-ray cardiac enlargement went on to develop ECG-LVH. The higher the blood pressure, the more likely was ECG-LVH to occur, and at pressures exceeding 180 mm Hg. systolic pressure, 50% developed some evidence of ECG-LVH.

ECG-LVH was an extremely lethal phenomenon, associated with an eight fold increased cardiovascular mortality, a risk triple that of hypertension alone. Within 5 years 35% of the men and 20% of the women with ECG-LVH were dead, a relative risk comparable to that associated with overt coronary heart disease (CHD).

The association of ECG-LVH with cardiovascular morbidity and mortality was not accounted for by age, blood pressure, or other associated cardiovascular risk factors. The ECG abnormality appears to identify those with a poor cardiovascular risk profile who have progressed to a compromised coronary circulation and cardiac damage. Associated risk of cardiac failure was three times higher than that of hypertension alone. Risk of strokes, coronary events, and occlusive peripheral arterial disease were all increased three fold or more. ECG-LVH must be regarded as a grave prognostic sign for mortality and an indication of serious cardiovascular disease soon to develop.

The ECG pattern of ECG-LVH has long been recognized as an important clinical finding of great diagnostic value. More recent epidemiological data have indicated that it is also a finding of serious prognostic importance. Estimates of the incidence of ECG-LVH and of the prognosis with which it is associated are based on modest amounts of data. This report extends previous findings from the Framingham Study on this subject, taking advantage of 20 years of follow-up [1—3].

The prevalence and incidence of ECG-LVH and its relation to blood pressure and cardiac enlargement on X-ray will be examined. Also, the risk of developing cardiovascular events, including CHD, strokes, peripheral arterial disease, and cardiac failure, in relation to ECG-LVH will be assessed. The net and joint effect of the ECG abnormality will be determined taking age, sex, hypertension, and other cardiovascular risk factors into account. Also, mortality will be compared in those who develop ECG-LVH versus overt coronary heart disease and versus those who remain free of the abnormality.

Methods

The Framingham Study has been in continuous operation since 1949, following 2336 men and 2873 women aged 30—62 for development of cardiovascular disease in relation to a variety of suspected risk factors. For this report, 20 years of follow-up are available to examine the incidence of cardiovascular morbidity and mortality in the cohort in relation to prior development of ECG-LVH. Mortality and cardiovascular disease outcomes have been ascertained through routine biennial cardiovascular examinations and daily surveillance of hospital admissions and death certification. The examination procedure included a routine 13 lead ECG at each biennial examination with the subject supine. Three standard, seven unipolar precordial leads, and three augmented unipolar leads were obtained. Criteria for "definite" ECG-LVH consisted of: an increased R-wave amplitude in leads reflecting potentials from the left ventricle associated with S-T and T-wave depression and inversion, deep S-waves over the right precordial leads, left axis deviation, and slight prolongation of ventricular activation time (Fig. 1). "Possible" or borderline ECG-LVH was designated when trac-

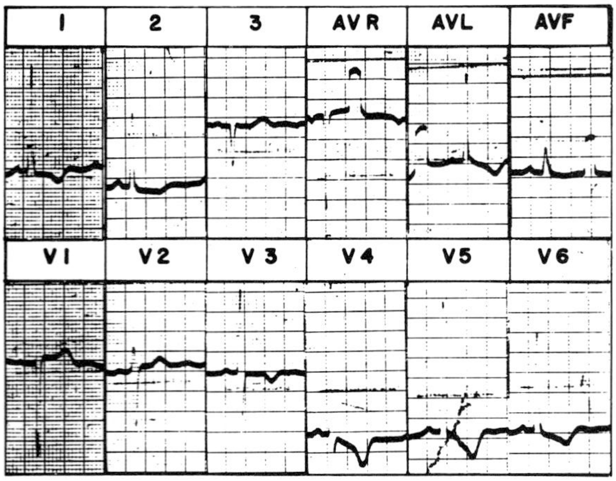

Fig 1. Example of ECG criteria for left ventricular hypertrophy. Definite left ventricular hypertrophy

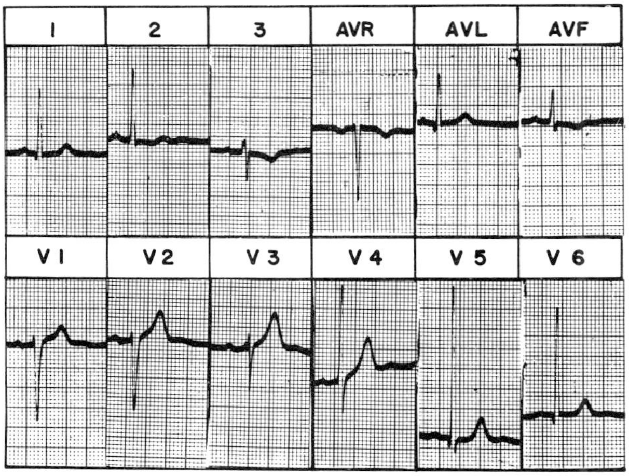

Fig. 2. Example of ECG criteria for left ventricular hypertrophy. Possible left ventricular hypertrophy

ings exhibited an increase in R-wave potential without prominent S-T and T-wave abnormality (Fig. 2). ECG's were interpreted without consideration of any clinical information, with the exception of use of digitalis. Samples of tracings labeled ECG-LVH have been scrutinized in two international comparisons and another NHLBI investigation, and no doubts were raised. About 25% of the abnormal tracing were reviewed by three Boston electrocardiographers with little disagreement. Some tracings read as "definite" ECG-LVH were reread and tested against various commonly accepted ECG criteria for LVH. According to these criteria, "abnormal voltage" was present in 94.5%, and S-T and T-wave changes in 97.4%. Fully 94.8% of tracings fulfilled criteria of Sokolow and Lyon, and an identical percentage met the criteria of Gubner and Ungerleider. Also, 98.3% met the criteria of Katz. Application of the point score system of Romhilt and Estes classified 59% with a score of 4 or more and 46% with a score of 5 or more. Those designated as "definite" ECG-LVH had the findings given in Table 1.

Detailed criteria for each of the major cardiovascular endpoints under consideration have been published elsewhere [3]. Descriptions of the sampling, procedures used, and analytical techniques employed have also been given elsewhere [3]. Follow-up has been reasonably complete, with only 2% completely lost after 20 years.

All subjects with evidence of cardiovascular disease were excluded from the population at risk at the time of initial examination. Also, at each examination, those found to have developed a cardiovascular endpoint were excluded and the rest placed at risk in relation to their ECG-LVH status at the start of each biennium. Average annual incidence of cardiovascular morbidity and mortality was computed in relation to person-years exposure to risk at a given ECG status. In the evaluation of the short term incidence between one biennial exam and

Table 1. ECG characteristics of tracings designated as "definite" ECG-LVH

R_1 & S_3 > 25 mm	35%
Ravl > 11 mm	34%
Single precordial deflection > 30 mm	35%
SV_1 & RV_5 > 35	85%
Left axis deviation (− 30° +)	15%
QRS > 0.09 − 0.10	32%
R-terminal > 0.04	16%
RV_6 > RV_5	8%
Ventricular activation time > 0.05	6%

the next, persons are recharacterized according to ECG status and disease status at each subsequent biennial exam and shifted from one age group to the next as they grow older. The sum of this experience in the ten biennial follow-up intervals is expressed as an overall annual incidence rate. This allows an expansion of the age-specific incidence experience using re-examination as a substitute for a larger cohort.

In the course of follow-up used in this report 957 subjects aged 45—74 developed some form of cardiovascular disease: 732 developed CHD, 138 brain infarctions, 219 cardiac failure, and 179 occlusive peripheral arterial disease. There were 856 deaths, of which 451 were cardiovascular deaths.

Determinants of ECG-LVH

Prevalence

Based on cross-sectional data the prevalence of ECG-LVH over the period of observation was observed to rise steeply with age from a relatively uncommon condition at age 35 to one which affects 10% by age 70. Although more common in men than women, the male predominance is slight (Fig. 3). At any age the prevalence of cardiac enlargement on X-ray was about double that for ECG-LVH (Fig. 4). Either these two procedures measure different phenomena or the ECG finding is a less sensitive measure of the cardiac enlargement. Alternatively, X-ray cardiac enlargement may be less a specific indicator of cardiomegaly. Only 35%—50% of those with ECG-LVH, depending on age and sex, had coexisting cardiac enlargement on X-ray [1]. Because ECG findings are less common and are associated with higher blood pressures than X-ray abnormality,

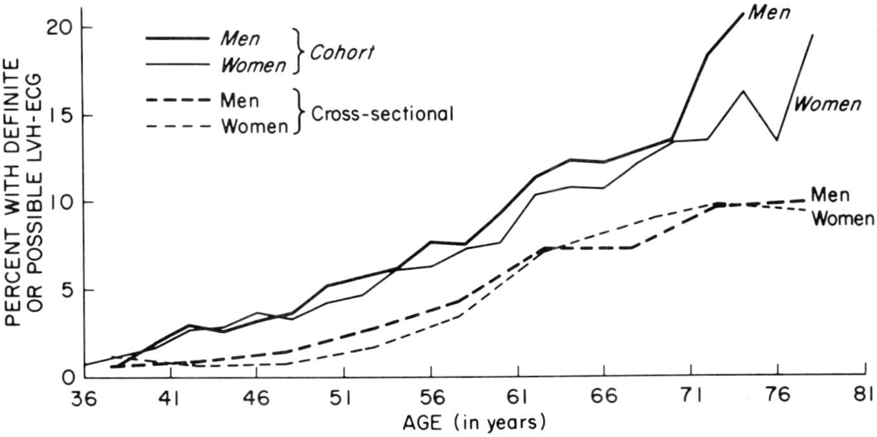

Fig. 3. Average age trends in the prevalence of left ventricular hypertrophy by electrocardiogram, definite or possible, from cross-sectional and cohort data: Framingham Study, Exams 3—10

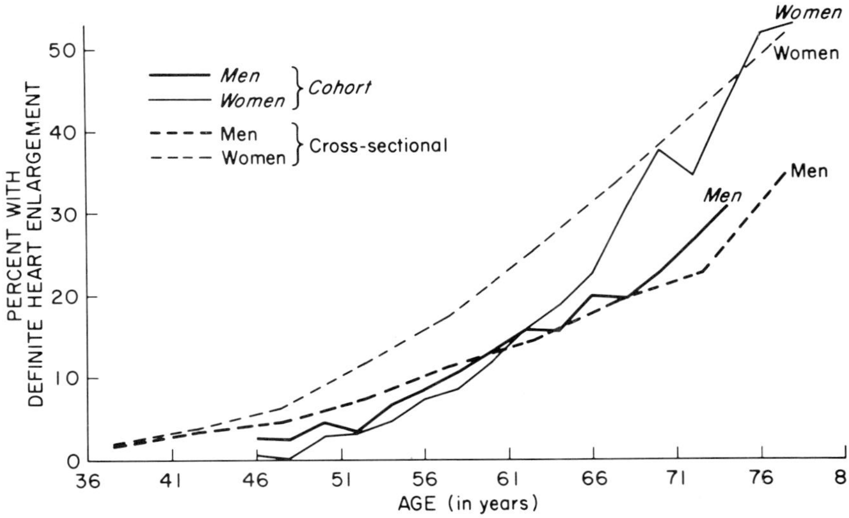

Fig. 4. Average age trends in the prevalence of definite heart enlargement by X-ray for cross-sectional and cohort data: Framingham Study, exams 3—10

there is a clinical tendency to regard X—ray enlargement as an earlier manifestation of hypertrophy than the ECG. Only 16% with X-ray evidence of LVH went on to develop ECG-LVH in the following 12 years. However, this compares with 6% of the general population. Persons with ECG-LVH including S-T and T abnormalities have larger hearts than those with voltage criteria alone [1]. Prevalence estimates based on longitudinal cohort data indicate a higher prevalence with the same slight male predominance (Fig. 3). By contrast, X-ray cardiac enlargement is more prevalent in women (Fig. 4).

Incidence

New development of ECG-LVH occurs at a greater rate than the prevalence data would suggest because persons with the abnormality are removed at a high rate from the population by death and the finding does not necessarily persist. About 3% of the cohort who had not manifested definite ECG-LVH on the initial examination developed it on at least one of the six successive biennial examinations [1]. Another 4.5% developed ECG-LVH characterized by voltage criteria alone (Fig. 5). Thus, one in ten was found to have or develop some manifestation of ECG-LVH during the first 12 years of follow-up when there was little treatment for hypertension. The probability of definite ECG-LVH was distinctly greater for those with the "possible" or borderline LVH finding than for those with a normal tracing [1].

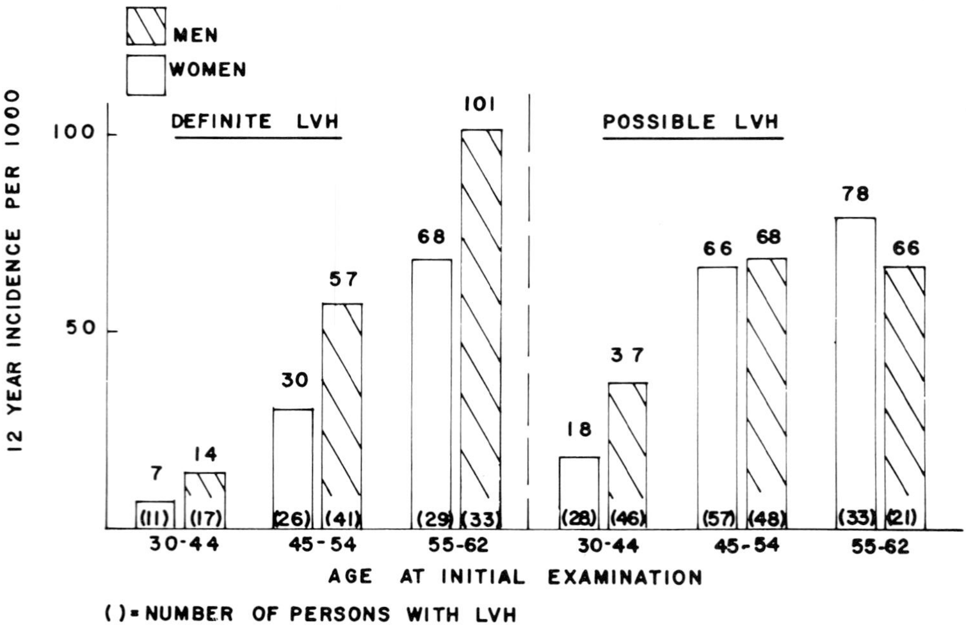

Fig. 5. 12-year incidence of ECG-LVH by age and sex, men and women 30—62 at entry; Framingham Heart Study

Secular Trends

The prevalence of ECG-LVH appears to be less common lately in the cohort than formerly (Table 2). This is especially true for women. The deline must be interpreted while keeping in mind possbile subtle differences in ECG reading practices over the years. It appears to coincide with a decline in the prevalence of hypertension in the cohort, which is also greater for women than men. Hy-

Table 2. Prevalence of definite or possible ECG-LVH at specified ages. Framingham Study — 14 years apart

	Percent with ECG-LVH			
	Men		Women	
Age at exam	exam 3	exam 10	exam 3	exam 10
50—54	5.0	3.0	2.4	2.0
55—59	5.4	3.2	7.1	2.1
60—64	10.9	7.2	8.0	3.9

pertension appears to be the chief determinant of ECG-LVH in the general population.

Relation to Blood Pressure

The higher the pressure the more likely was ECG-LVH to occur (Table 3). The association was no closer for diastolic than systolic pressure [1]. At pressures beyond 180 mm Hg (systolic) some manifestation of ECG-LVH (including possible LVH) appeared on at least one of the first seven biennial examinations in 50% [1]. However, at these pressures the majority exhibit S-T and T-wave changes (definite LVH). Furthermore, abnormalities in repolarization were more common at higher than lower pressures throughout the range of blood pressure [1].

Cardiovascular Hazards

Mortality

The ECG finding of LVH is an extremely lethal risk attribute. About 30% of all deaths within 14 years in the Framingham cohort were preceded by a finding of ECG-LVH. Some 45% of cardiovascular deaths were preceded by the finding [1]. Definite ECG-LVH was associated with an eight fold increased risk of cardiovascular mortality in general and a six fold increased CHD mortality in particular (Table 4). Sudden death risk was also increased six fold. Mortality risks were half as great for ECG-LVH based solely on voltage criteria. The relative odds of death associated with definite ECG-LVH was double that for definite hypertension (Table 5). Within 5 years of its appearance 35% of the men and 20% of the women with the finding were dead (Table 5). Multivariate analysis revealed a significant net effect of ECG-LVH, taking blood pressure and other risk factors into account (Table 5). The relative risk of death associated with ECG-LVH is comparable to that associated with overt CHD (Table 6).

Table 3. Prevalence of definite ECG-LVH any time between exam 1 and 7 by age and sex according to blood pressure. Framingham Study

Systolic pressure Exam 1	Men						Women					
		Age 30–44		Age 45–54		Age 55–62		Age 30–44		Age 45–54		Age 55–62
	(n)	%	(n)	%	(n)	%	(n)	%	(n)	%	(n)	%
< 120	(3)	1.3	(2)	1.8	(2)	5.9	(0)	—	(1)	1.1	(0)	—
120–139	(4)	0.6	(10)	3.4	(7)	5.8	(4)	0.6	(6)	1.9	(2)	1.9
140–159	(12)	3.9	(15)	7.4	(17)	15.2	(5)	2.1	(5)	2.0	(5)	3.9
160–179	(5)	6.2	(13)	15.3	(15)	30.6	(3)	4.4	(8)	5.9	(11)	12.4
180–199	(1)	7.7	(11)	37.9	(4)	25.0	(1)	9.1	(10)	17.2	(7)	15.2
200 +	(2)	33.3	(6)	42.9	(8)	47.1	(2)	33.3	(12)	31.6	(14)	37.8
Total		2.1		7.8		15.2		1.0		4.8		8.9

Table 4. Relative probability of cardiovascular morality in 2 years by ECG-LVH status. Men 45—74. Framingham Study 20-year follow-up

	Smoothed and age-adjusted relative risks		
	Sudden Death	CHD Death	C-V Death
Def. ECG-LVH/No ECG-LVH	5.8	5.9	8.5
Pos. ECG-LVH/No ECG-LVH	2.4	2.4	3.0

Table 5. Overall mortality according to ECG-LVH and hypertensive status. 20 year follow-up. Framingham Study. Persons 45—74. Other Variables: cholesterol, smoking, glucose

	Age-adjusted annual mortality (per 1000)			
	Hypertension		ECG-LVH	
	Men	Women	Men	Women
None	12.1	7.1	13.8	7.8
Borderline	16.7	8.9	31.8	17.6
Definite	23.0	11.1	69.7	38.9
Risk Ratio def/none	1.9	1.6	5.1	5.0
Multivariate regression Coefficient	.194	.102	.835	.716
T-test	3.15	1.39	10.81	7.46

Table 6. Relative risk of mortality following ECG-LVH versus that following coronary desease

	Angina Pectoris		ECG-LVH		Myocardial infarct	
	Observed/ expected	Mortality ratio	Observed/ expected	Mortality ratio	Observed/ expected	Mortality ratio
Men	34/16.3	2.09	70/23.0	3.95	40/15.9	2.52
Women	17/8.3	2.05	32/8.1	3.91	9/2.4	3.75
Total	51/24.6	2.1	102/31.1	3.3	49/18.3	2.7

In persons with already manifest overt heart disease, ECG-LVH is an indicator of the seriousness of this disease, and in persons still free of such disease it forbodes a symptomatic cardiovascular attack.

Definite ECG-LVH carries more than double the risk of a cardiovascular event of that associated with definite hypertension as each is commonly defined (Table 7). Within 5 years 36% of men and 28% of women with ECG-LVH developed a major cardiovascular event.

Table 7. Risk of cardiovascular disease according to hypertensive and ECG-LVH status. Framingham Study 20 year follow-up. Persons 45—74

	Average annual incidence per 1000/year			
	Hypertension		ECG-LVH	
Status	Men	Women	Men	Women
Normal	12.9	5.9	18.7	10.0
Borderline	21.6	11.0	37.7	24.1
Definite	35.7	20.6	72.6	55.6
Age-adjusted regression coefficient:	0.542	0.661	0.763	0.926
T-value	9.95	9.89	8.51	9.38

Table 8. Risk of cardiovascular disease according to ECG-LVH versus X-ray cardiac enlargement. Framingham Study 20 year follow-up. Persons 45—74

	Av. annual incidence per 1000			
	ECG-LVH		X-ray enlargement	
	Men	Women	Men	Women
None	18.7	10.0	18.2	8.5
Borderline	37.7	24.1	23.1	12.6
Definite	72.6	55.6	29.1	18.7
	Probability ratios			
	Men	Women	Men	Women
T-values[a]	8.29	9.19	4.34	6.92
For regression[b]	4.56	4.50	2.20	4.07

[a] Bivariate coefficients (i.e. taking age into account)

[b] Multivariate coefficients (i.e. also taking blood pressure and other cardiovascular risk factors into account)

Definite ECG-LVH carries a greater risk than definite X-ray cardiac enlargement in both sexes (Table 8). Here, too, for cardiovascular morbidity the contributions of each are independent of blood pressure. Also, in subjects with cardiac enlargement there is an increased risk, even taking associated ECG into account.

Although at any age women with ECG-LVH have a lower risk of cardiovascular disease than men, this only reflects their general immunity to cardiovascular disease compared to men. Their *relative risk*, comparing those the same age with and without ECG-LVH in the respective sexes, reveals, if anything, larger coefficients for the regression of cardiovascular disease incidence on LVH in women than men (Table 9). Although the finding of ECG-LVH increases with advancing age, there is no clear evidence of a waning impact of the finding with advancing age in eigher sex. Both the absolute and relative risk associated with ECG-LVH in the elderly is high.

The association of ECG-LVH with the incidence of cardiovascular disease is not accounted for by age, by blood pressure, or by other associated cardiovascular risk factors (Table 10). Multivariate regression coefficients remain sizeable and highly significant in both sexes.

A combination of ECG-LVH with even as closely correlated a risk factor as hypertension further escalates the risk of cardiovascular disease in general and CHD in particular (Table 11). ECG-LVH is also a significant contributor to a multi-

Table 9. Risk of cardiovascular disease according to ECG-LVH status by age and sex. Persons 45—74. Framingham Study 20 year follow-up

ECG-LVH	Men 45—54	55—64	65—74	All ages 45—74[a]
None	12	25	28	19
Borderline	34	29	55	38
Definite	58	110	90	73
Regression coeff.[b]	.887	.748	.671	.750
ECG-LVH	**Women 45—54**	**55—64**	**65—74**	**45—74[a]**
None	5	12	21	10
Borderline	11	35	46	24
Definite	30	77	87	56
Regression coeff.[b]	.960	1.015	.791	.916

[a] Age-adjusted
[b] Regression coefficients for the logistic statistical model. All coefficients statistically significant at P<$^{0}_{1}$.01

Table 10. Net effect of ECG-LVH on incidence of cardiovascular disease. Framingham Study 20 year follow-up

	Regression coefficient Men	Women	T-value Men	Women
Univariate	0.839	1.098	9.41	11.29
Bivariate[a]	0.750	0.916	8.29	9.19
Multivariate[b]	0.467	0.517	4.56	4.50

[a] Bivariate: ECG-LVH and age (men and women 45—74)

[b] Multivariate: ECG-LVH and age, plus: systolic blood pressure, cigarettes/day, S-colesterol, and glucose tolerance

factorial cardiovascular risk profile. Handbooks have been devised by the American Heart Association and the National Heart, Lung and Blood Institute which indicate the probability of an event in relation to the number of risk factors, including ECG-LVH, with risk defined over an extremely wide range (Tabel 11). However, in judging the efficiency of cardiovascular risk profiles with this ECG finding versus without it, it is not clear that ECG-LVH greatly improves the identification of susceptibles in a population. It does, however, identify those with a poor cardiovascular risk profile, who very likely have progressed to the point where they now have a compromised coronary circulation and a myocardium in jeopardy.

Risk of Various Atherosclerotic Cardiovascular Events

In addition to reflecting the severity and duration of exposure to hypertension it appears that ECG-LVH reflects an advancing atherosclerotic process. Risk of each of the major atherosclerotic diseases is substantially increased in those with ECG-LVH, including stroke, CHD, occlusive peripheral arterial disease, and cardiac failure (Table 12). In addition, risk of every clinical manifestation of coronary heart disease is increased in those with ECG-LVH. Risks associated with ECG-LVH are greatest for cardiac failure and brain infarction and least for coronary heart disease, which nevertheless is the commonest sequela of ECG-LVH.

Myocardial Damage

Once ECG-LVH appears there is much to suggest that the myocardium is damaged and in jeopardy. Risk of cardiac failure is high and three times higher than that associated with hypertension in general (Table 13). This risk of failure is comparable to that of a patient with angina.

Table 11. Probability (per 100) of developing coronoary artery disease in six years according to specified characteristics for 45-year old men [a]

	No left ventricular hypertrophy (ECG)								With left ventricular hypertrophy (ECG)							
	Does not smoke cigarettes				Smokes cigarettes				Does not smoke cigarettes				Smokes cigarettes			
	SBP	105	150	195	SBP	105	150	195	SBP	105	150	195	SBP	105	150	195
	Chol				Chol				Chol				Chol			
Glucose	185	1.5	2.5	4.4	185	2.3	3.9	6.7	185	3.0	5.2	8.8	185	4.7	7.9	13.1
Intolerance	260	3.0	5.2	8.7	260	4.7	7.9	13.0	260	6.2	10.3	16.8	260	9.3	15.3	24.0
Absent	335	6.2	10.3	16.7	335	9.3	15.2	23.9	335	12.1	19.4	29.7	335	17.7	27.4	39.8
	SBP	105	150	195	SBP	105	150	195	SBP	105	150	195	SBP	105	150	195
	Chol				Chol				Chol				Chol			
Glucose	185	1.9	3.3	5.6	185	3.0	5.1	8.5	185	3.9	6.7	11.1	185	6.0	10.1	16.4
Intolerance	260	3.9	6.7	11.1	260	6.0	10.0	16.4	260	7.9	13.0	20.8	260	11.8	19.0	29.1
Present	335	7.9	13.0	20.8	335	11.8	19.0	29.1	335	15.2	23.9	35.5	335	21.9	33.0	46.3

[a] Source: American Heart Association with Gordon, T. and Kannel, W.B.: Coronary Risk Handbook — Estimating Risk of Coronary Heart Disease in Daily Practice. 1973. Derived from: Gordon, T., Sorlie, P., and Kannel, W.B.: Coronary Heart Disease, Artherothrombotic Brain Infarction, Intermittent Claudication — A Multivariate Analysis of Some Factors Related to Their Incidence: Framingham Study, 16-year Follow-Up. U.S. Dept. of Health, Education and Welfare, National Institutes of Health, Sect. 27, 1971. SBP, systolic blood pressure (mm Hg); Chol, cholesterol (mg/dl)

Table 12. Risk of atherosclerotic cardiovascular diseases associated with ECG-LVH. Framingham Study 20 year follow-up. Persons 45—74 [a]

	Av. annual incidence per 1000 (age-adjusted)							
ECG-LVH	CHD		ABI		OPAD		CHF	
status	M	F	M	F	M	F	M	F
None	14.3	6.9	1.8	1.6	3.5	1.4	3.1	2.1
Possible	26.1	12.4	3.8	4.6	5.3	3.6	8.6	6.3
Definite	46.3	22.1	8.1	13.2	7.9	9.0	23.3	18.3
Risk ratio[b]	3.2	3.2	4.6	8.4	2.3	6.5	7.6	8.6
T-Value	6.78	5.11	4.09	6.96	2.27	5.30	8.36	8.01

[a] CHD, coronary heart disease; ABI, atherothrombotic brain infarction; OPAD, occlusive peripheral arterial disease; CHF, congestive heart failure

[b] Risk of disease in those with def. ECG-LVH relative to those free of ECG-LVH

Table 13. Risk of cardiac failure by hypertension and ECG-LVH status. Framigham Study 20 year follow-up. Persons 45—74

	Hypertension Rate per 1000/year[a]		ECG-LVH Rate per 1000/year[a]	
Status	Men	Women	Men	Women
Normal	1.7	1.3	3.1	2.1
Borderline	3.8	2.5	8.6	6.3
Definite	8.4	4.7	23.3	18.3

[a] Age-adjusted

Prognosis After Onset of CHD

Once either heart enlargement on X-ray or ECG-LVH is noted after the onset of overt CHD, the mortality is further increased compared to those without these abnormalities. For those with myocardial infarction definite ECG-LVH escalates the risk to four times that of those without the findings. X-ray enlargement doubles the risk (Table 14). For angina, X-ray and ECG-LVH raise the risk an equivalent four-fold amount.

Table 14. Five year mortality following onset of CHD according to evidence of cardiac impairment after event. Framingham Study. Men 30—80. Age-adjusted. Trends all signif. at P = < .05 level

	Risk for myocardial infarction (recognized)					
	Heart enlargement X-ray			ECG-left ventricular (hypertrophy)		
Abnormality	Obs.	Exp.	Obs/exp.	Obs.	Exp.	Obs/exp.
None	12	18.5	0.65	25	29.6	0.85
Possible	6	5.5	1.09	1	0.8	1.33
Definite	14	8.0	1.76	6	1.7	3.57
	Risk for angina pectoris (uncomplicated)					
	Heart enlargement X-ray			ECG-left ventricular (hypertrophy)		
Abnormality	Obs.	Exp.	Obs/exp.	Obs.	Exp.	Obs/exp.
None	10	14.4	0.70	15	17.8	0.85
Possible	1	2.9	0.35	1	1.1	0.93
Definite	9	2.8	3.25	4	1.2	3.42

Type of ECG-LVH

ECG-LVH based on voltage criteria alone carries a risk for cardiovascular events which is only half that noted when S-T and T-wave abnormalities are also included in the criteria (Table 15). Nonspecific abnormality of S-T and T alone carries a risk as low or lower than voltage ECG-LVH, even without excluding from the population at risk those with possible ECG-LVH.

Table 15. Factor of increased risk of cardiovascular events for various criteria for LVH. Framingham Study 20 year follow-up. Persons 45—74

ECG components of ECG-LVH	Probability ratios[a] Cardiovascular disease		CHD	
	Men	Women	Men	Women
Voltage — LVH	2.02	2.42	1.81	1.80
NSA — S-T & T (alone)[a]	1.64	1.60	1.66	1.92
Defin. LVH (Voltage & S-T & T)	3.89	5.58	3.23	3.22

[a] Includes some subjects in population at risk who have voltage-LVH

Voltage-only ECG-LVH (possible or borderline) seems to reflect chiefly the severity and duration of the associated hypertension. When an adjustment is made for coexisting hypertension, the excess risk associated with ECG-LVH without associated repolarization abnormality is virtually obliterated [2]. That risk associated with definite ECG-LVH, including S-T and T, continued to show a substantial residual effect after taking blood pressure into account.

Discussion

ECG-LVH has been reported previously to be associated with an increased risk of CHD and death [2—5]. Not all studies, however, have indicated an *independent* contribution of ECG-LVH to development of cardiovascular disease. This very likely stems from the use of only voltage criteria [6].

The prognostic significance of ECG-LVH *after* myocardial infarction is uncertain. Examination of 3-year mortality in association with ECG-LVH in the Coronary Drug Project placebo group of post-myocardial infarction subjects revealed a mortality double that of those without ECG abnormality. Elevated R-wave amplitude alone, however, had no *independent* prognostic value when other risk factors were taken into account. When combined with S-T and T-wave abnormality, risk was augmented and independently related to prognosis [7]. These findings are in concert with those in Framingham, which stress the importance of accompanying S-T and T-wave abnormality.

A variety of ECG abnormalities occur commonly in association with overt CHD. These include those of myocardial infarction, intraventricular conduction disturbances, atrio-ventricular dissociation, nonspecific abnormality, left ventricular hypertrophy, and all types of premature beats [8, 9]. Aside from the pathognomonic findings of myocardial infarction, the others may be coincidental, nonspecific manifestations of myocardial damage, the result of therapy, or cardiac manifestations of coexisting hypertension.

The ECG pattern is commonly found in association with CHD. In the Framingham cohort a substantial proportion of CHD events were preceded or followed by ECG-LVH. Coronary artery atherosclerosis is at least moderately advanced in the American population by age 20 and it is not unreasonable to assume that a silent asymptomatic phase of ischemic myocardial involvement is also part of the clinical spectrum of CHD. This may be reflected by an ECG pattern of left ventricular hypertrophy when accompanied by abnormalities of repolarization. Lack of symptoms is not incompatible with this hypothesis since one in five actual myocardial infarctions in the Framingham cohort were found to be silent [10].

Since the ECG pattern of left ventricular hypertrophy, when accompanied by S-T and T-wave abnormality, is associated with a striking increase in the risk of every clinical manifestation of CHD and carries the same risk of mortality as angina, it is tempting to hypothesize that it is often an occult manifestation of presymptomatic CHD. The voltage criteria alone may well reflect only the associated hypertensive hypertrophy, since the excess risk of CHD associated with this pattern is eliminated when adjustment is made for accompanying hypertension [2].

Whether or not CHD in the absence of hypertension can produce anatomical cardiac hypertrophy is in dispute [9]. Also, it is not certain whether CHD in the absence of hypertension can produce an ECG pattern of left ventricular hypertrophy. An association of the pathological correlates of pattern of ECG-LVH is confounded by the frequent coexistence of hypertension which predisposes to both anatomical hypertrophy and accelerated coronary atherogenesis.

The pathological and anatomical meaning of the pattern of ECG-LVH is currently unclear. Romhilt et al. in an evaluation of 33 different sets of ECG criteria for LVH against individual chamber dissections of hearts at autopsy found the correlations to be poor [11]. They concluded that new criteria using more information than just voltage were needed. The relation between ECG voltage and left ventricular muscle mass has also been studied in the living by echocardiogram and angiography [12, 13]. Also, using more sophisticated ECG techniques, such as multiple dipole electrocardiography, it would appear that the standard ECG and criteria based on it do not provide a very accurate assessment of left ventricular muscle mass as estimated from angiographic findings [14].

However, although far from perfect, necropsy, X-ray and, more recently, echocardiographic and ventriculographic studies have shown that the ECG pattern of LVH does to some degree reflect anatomical hypertrophy of the left ventricle. The correlation of the components of voltage and repolarization abnormality (S-T and T) is, however, in doubt. Thiry et al. on theoretical grounds, using mathematical models of cardiac electrical activity, indicate that the computer-generated 12-lead ECG for an increase in cardiac cell size is characterized by both an increased QRS amplitude and ventricular activation time and a flattened or inverted T-wave [15].

Cosby et al. concluded from their studies that the increased voltage reflected primarily pure work hypertrophy, whereas that associated with prominent S-T and T-wave abnormality was related to coronary insufficiency [16].

Increased R-wave amplitude and coronary atherosclerosis should be found together because both are related to hypertension. S-T and T-wave repolarization abnormalities may be related to ventricular hypertrophy, hemodynamic overload, or to myocardial ischemia and injury. Although it is clear that ECG-LVH is often associated with impaired cardiac function, the mechanism is not clear. Hypertrophy has been shown to alter coupling of excitation—contraction, energy utilization, and contractile proteins [17]. This may be a result of accompanying myocardial ischemia.

The relation between hypertrophy, relative ischemia, and failure remains unclear. While moderate hypertrophy is probably beneficial, the limit of useful hypertrophy has not been defined [18]. The older view that hypertrophied muscle outgrows its capillary blood supply has been challenged by the suggestion that the main coronary arteries become too narrow. Biochemical evidence of ischemia in hypertrophied muscle is not yet decisive [19, 20].

In general, the adaptation of muscle to increased work is by hypertrophy. In skeletal muscles, which do not change in length, hypertrophy appears as an increase in thickness. Cardiac muscle is able to enlarge either in thickness, or length or both. Increase in length produces a larger cardiac cavity (eccentric hypertrophy) while increase in thickness produces a concentric hypertrophy. The former is alleged to be the response to a volume load and the latter to a pressure load. Hypertrophy, the ventricular adaptation to chronic overload, is abolished if growth hormone is absent [21].

The precise mechanisms involved for different types of hypertrophy remain uncertain. The older view that myocardial cells do not multiply has been challenged. However, it is clear that cardiac hypertrophy involves an increase in cardiac muscle mass largely as a result of individual muscle fiber enlargement and that concentric hypertrophy is the response to increased afterload and eccentric hypertrophy to increased preload [22].

The failure to find a high correlation between ECG findings of LVH and autopsy or other measures of cardiac hypertrophy may stem from the fact that the ECG aberrations are a product of ischemic myocardial damage as much as hypertrophy. Attempts to improve ECG criteria for left ventricular "hypertrophy" should take this into account.

Coronary candidates with a poor CHD risk profile (Table 13) who develop ECG-LVH with changes in repolarization appear to require management equivalent to that prescribed for asymptomatic persons with established overt CHD. This is justified because of ECG finding may well be a hallmark of a compromised coronary circulation (when unexplained by valvular deformity or congenital anomalies). In any event, the appearance of this ECG finding must be regarded as a grave prognostic sign in the course of hypertension or CHD, of stroke, cardiac failure, and premature death. If not an asymptomatic manifestation of CHD, it is clearly a powerful intrinsic risk factor for its development.

References

1. Kannel WB, Gordon T, Offit D (1969) Left ventricular hypertrophy by electrocardiogram. Prevalence, incidence and mortality in the Framingham study. Ann Intern Med 71 : 89
2. Kannel WB, Gordon T, Castelli WP, Margolis JR (1970) ECG left ventricular hypertrophy and risk of CHD. The Framingham study. Ann Intern Med 72 : 813

3. Gordon T, Sorlie P, Kannel WB (1971) Section 27: CHD, atherothrombotic brain infarction, intermittent claudication — A multivariate analysis of some factors ralted to their incidence. Framingham study. 16 year follow-up.
4. Ungerleider HE (1960) The prognostic implications of the electrocardiogram. Am J Cardiol 6 : 35
5. Blackburn H, Parker RW (1960) Antecedents of disease. Insurance mortality experience. Ann NY Acad Sci 134 : 965
6. Blackburn H, Taylor HL, Keys A (1970) The ECG in prediction of 5 year CHD incidence among men aged 45—59. Circulation [Suppl I] 41/42
7. The Coronary Drug Project Research Group (1974) Left ventricular hypertrophy and prognosis. Experience postinfarction in the coronary drug project Circulation 49 : 862—869
8. Graybiel A, White RD, Wheeler L (1954) Electrocardiography in practice, 3rd edn. Saunders, Philadelphia, London, pp 263—298
9. Friedberg CK (1956) Diseases of the heart, 2nd edn. Saunders, Philadelphia, London
10. Kannel WB, McNamara PM, Feinleib M (1970) The unrecognized myocardial infarction: 14 year follow-up. Experience in the Framingham study. Geriatrics 25 : 75—87
11. Romhilt DW, Bove KE, Norris RJ (1969) A critical appraisal of the ECG criteria for the diagnosis of left ventricular hypertrophy. Circulation 40 : 185—195
12. Bennett DH, Evans DW (1974) Correlation of left ventricular mass determined by echocardiography with vectorcardiographic and electrocardiographic voltage measurements. Br Heart J 36 : 981
13. Baxley WA, Dodge HT, Sandler H (1968) A quantitative angiocardiographic study of left ventricular hypertrophy and the electrocardiogram. Circulation 37 : 509
14. Holt JH Jr, Barnard ACL, Kramer JO (1978) Multiple dipole ECG. A comparison of electrically and angiographically determined left ventricular masses. Circulation 57 : 1129—1133
15. Thiry PS, Rosenberg RM, Abbot JA (1975) A mechanism for the electrocardiogram response to left ventricular hypertrophy and acute ischemia. Circ Res 36 : 92—104
16. Cosby RS, Herman LM, Mayo M (1962) Sequential changes in the development of the electrocardiographic pattern of left ventricular hypertrophy in hypertensive heart disease. Am Heart J 63 : 180—187
17. Meersen FZ (1962) Compensatory hyperfunction of the heart and cardiac insufficiency. Circ Res 10 : 250—258
18. Grant C, Greene DG, Bunnell IL (1965) Left ventricular enlargement and hypertrophy. Am J Med 39 : 895—904
19. Olsen RE (1962) Physiology of cardiac muscle. In: Hamilton WF (ed) Handbook of physiology, sect 2, vol 1. American Physological Society, Washington, pp. 226
20. Elliot WC, Cohen LS, Klein LS (1964) Selective cinearteriography study of angina pectoris in valvular heart disease. Circulation 30 : III-73

21. Beznak M (1964) Hormonal influences in regulation of cardiac performance. Circ Res 15 : II–141
22. Schlant RC (1974) Altered cardiovascular function of rheumatic heart disease and other acquired diseases. In: Hurst JW, Logue RB, Schlant RC, Wenger NK (eds) The Heart, arteries and veins, 3rd edn, McGraw-Hill, New York, pp 811–813

Structural Adaptation of the Heart in Hypertension and the Physical Consequences

A.J. LINZBACH

The pathological structural adaptation of the heart in cases of hypertension, valvular disease, myocarditis and coronary disease is characterized by increasing weight of the myocardium and alterations in the shape of the heart.

In the course of pathological structural adaptation the human heart can exceed the maximal heart weight of athletic hearts of 500 g, which corresponds to the *critical heart weight* and increasing frequency of chronic heart failure. When

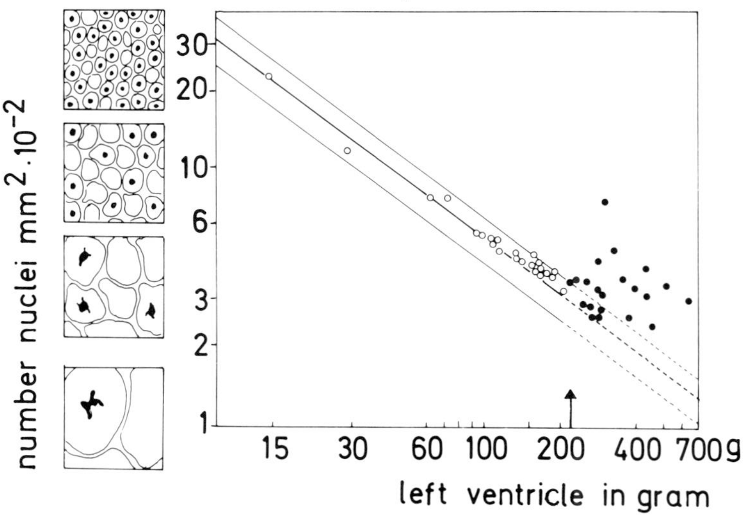

Fig. 1. Number of cardiac muscle cell nuclei per unit area in cross sections of left anterior papillary muscle in relation to weight of the isolated left ventricle with the left part of the septum. Below the critical ventricular weight of 220 g (○) which corresponds to a total critical heart weight of 500 g. Enlargement occurs by growth of the cardiac muscle cells. The number of cells remains constant. Hypertrophy. Above the critical weight (●), the number of cardiac muscle cell nuclei is greater than would be expected if the number of cells were constant. The cross sections of the cardiac muscle cells are too small and therefore the number of nuclei too great to explain the high ventricular weight. Hyperplasia

the cardiac weight exceeds the critical value of 500 g, it can be demonstrated that the adaptive growth of the heart muscle cells is not only performed by an increase in size as in athletic hearts (hypertrophy) but also in number (hyperplasia). Nevertheless we call it hypertrophy. (Fig. 1)

This hyperplasia is managed by splitting in length of the heart muscle cells and their nuclei and a corresponding augmentation of the myocardial capillaries. Therefore, in hyperplasia the relation of one capillary to one muscle fibre is the same as in the normal heart (Fig. 2).

In cases of hypertension we distinguish two phases of adaptive growth:

1. *The concentric pressure hypertrophy* (Fig 3b), and

2. *The excentric pressure hypertrophy* (see Fig. 3c, d)

In comparison to the normal heart *concentric pressure hypertrophy* is macroscopically shown by a marked to an extreme thickening of the left ventricular

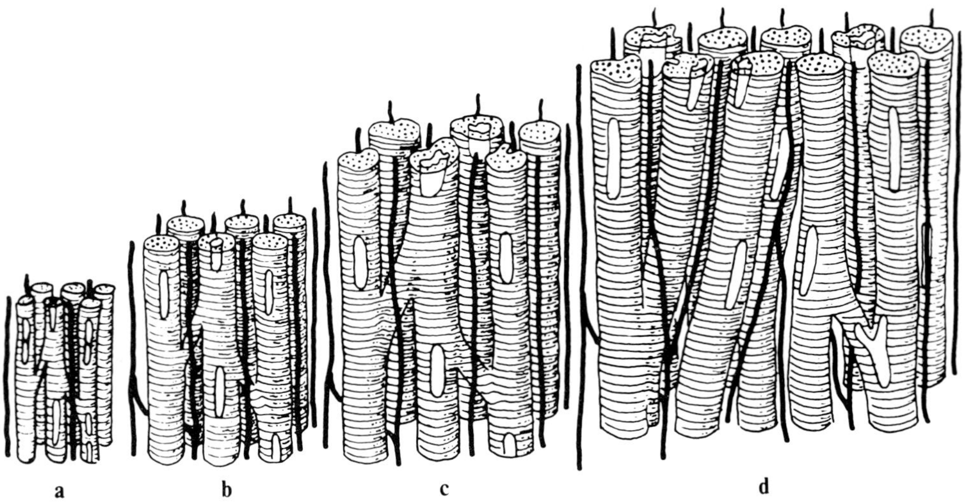

Fig. 2a—d. Growth of six muscle fibres and their capillaries. (a) Infant. Left ventricular weight 10 g. One capillary supplies four muscle fibres. (b) Adult. Left ventricular weight 150 g. One capillary per muscle fibre. Harmonious growth of cardiac muscle fibres with a constant number of cells and nuclei. Compared with the infant heart the number of capillaries has increased fourfold, (c) Athletic heart. Left ventricular weight 220 g. Weight of the heart 500 g. One capillary per muscle fibre. Growth has occurred, but the number of cells and nuclei has remained constant. (d) Concentric pressure hypertrophy. Left ventricular weight more than 400 g. Number of muscle fibres and cardiac muscle cell nuclei increased from 6 to 10. Longitudinal cleavage (splitting) of the muscle fibres and their nuclei, beginning at the branching angels. Hypertrophy and hyperplasia. From Linzbach [2]

wall and a characteristic elongation of the ventricle (Fig. 3b). The residual capacity in rigor mortis and also the systolic residual capacity of the left ventricle during life may be smaller than in the norm.

Microscopically the thickening of the ventricular wall is caused by a corresponding thickening of the heart muscle cells in the sense of hypertrophy. The number of muscle layers in the compact part of the left ventricle is approximately the same as in the norm and amounts to a mean value of 520. In contrast to the thickening of the wall the elongation of the ventricle is performed by a hyperplasia of the heart muscle cells (Figs. 2d, 3b).

A heart with concentric pressure hypertrophy is an effective pressure pump which works with normal or diminished stroke volume and with normal or diminished systolic residual blood volume. These hearts appear to be compensated, but in many cases the right ventricles develop small hypertrophy. This indicates the beginning left ventricular failure caused by increasing rigidity of the thick left ventricle wall with impaired diastolic filling the sense of diastolic insufficiency (Fig. 3b).

In the further course of events in hypertrophy coronary insufficiency is developing, caused by retardation of the growth of the great coronary vessels in relation to the growing muscle mass and additive coronary disease of the great epicardial and small intramural coronary vessels. Due to this coronary insufficiency with impairment of the myocardium the concentric hypertrophy changes to *excentric pressure hypertrophy* with progressive tendency in the development of chronic dilatation and heart failure (Fig. 3 c, d).

The small focal necroses and scars in the myocardium in consequence of the coronary insufficiency impair the quality of the heart muscle and the conductive system, but they are not the direct cause of heart failure.

In contrast to acute cardiac dilatation chronic dilatation is not associated with stretching or overstretching of heart muscle cells. The medium distance of Z-bands (length of sarcomeres) in chronic dilatation is the same as in normal hearts, even when the capacity of the left ventricle post mortem amounts to more than 300 ml (Fig. 4). Starling's law is not applicable for an explanation of heart failure in these chronic cases.

Chronic dilatation is a *structural dilatation* which arises from sliding displacement (slippage) and rearrangement of the heart muscle cells in the myocardium, which leads to a decrease in the number of muscle layers in the compact part of the left ventricular wall from 520 to 350 (Fig 5 and Fig 3c, d). In comparison to a normal ventricle the structural dilatation without corresponding stretching of the muscle cells severely impairs the working conditions, the efficiency and the effectiveness of the heart muscle.

The force developed by a ventricle during a cardiac cycle is proportional to the intraventricular pressure times the inner surface area. This is valid not only for the whole ventricle but also for the tension times unit cross section of heart muscle cells.

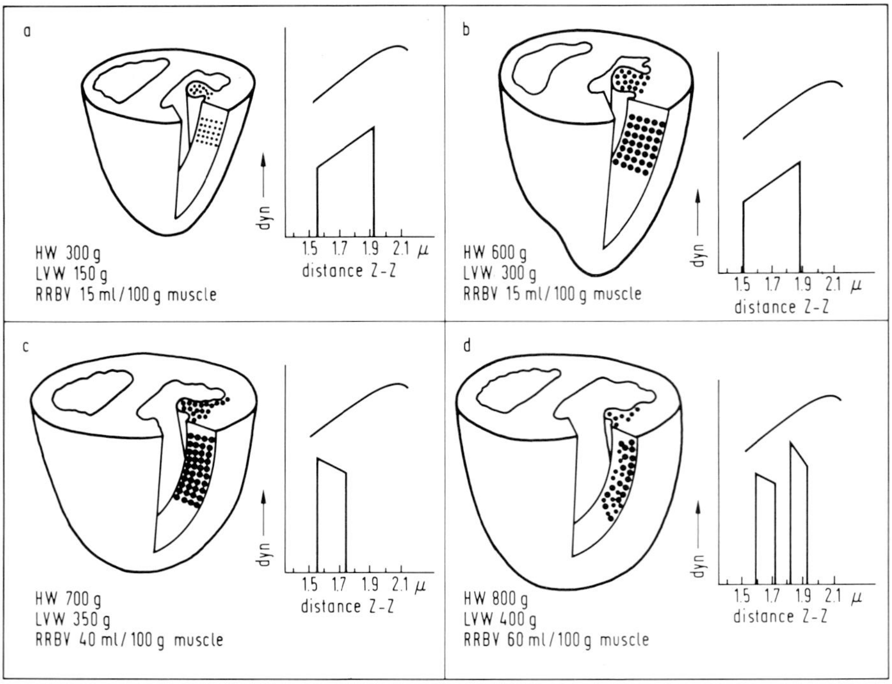

Fig. 3a–d. *HW* = total heart weight; *LVW* = left ventricular weight; *RRBV* = relative residual blood volume (capacity) of the left ventricle in rigor mortis in ml per 100 g muscle; *Z–Z* = length of sarcomeres. All schemata true to scale. The *dots* represent the number and layers of heart muscle cells and if multiplied by one hundred, approximate the actual values. On the *right side* of the hearts constructed work diagrams. (a) Normal heart. (b) Concentric pressure hypertrophy. Hypertrophy and hyperplasia of heart muscle cells. The number of circular muscle layers in the wall of the left ventricle is the same as in a. The elongation of the left ventricle is performed by hyperplasia of muscle cells. Minor diastolic failure is indicated by slight hypertrophy of the right ventricle and probably by a small reduction of the diastolic and systolic length of the sarcomeres. (c) Pressure hypertrophy with structural dilatation. Beginning left heart failure, indicated by hypertrophy of the right ventricle. Hypertrophy, hyperplasia and reduction of the number of muscle layers (to 400) due to slippage of the muscle cells in the wall of the left ventricle. In spite of the good adaptive growth of the heart muscle mass, the amount of work per unit cross section of heart muscle is smaller than in the norm (a) or in cases of concentric pressure hypertrophy (b), because the lift or the distance between diastolic and systolic length of the sarcomeres is reduced. In contrast to a and b the force increases in the ejection phase. To perform the same amount of work the muscle mass of the left ventricle must be greater as in *a* or *b*. This state may be reversible. (d) Final state of pressure hypertrophy with irreversible structural dilatation and scars, especially in the inner layers of the wall of the left ventricle, following coronary insufficiency. Irregular hypertrophy and hyperplasia of muscle cells

A healthy ventricle of normal proportions develops its highest force in the isometric phase when the inner diastolic surface is great and the diastolic aortic pressure must be compensated for by generating a corresponding tension. During the ejection phase the force decreases because the inner surface of the ventricle diminishes more rapidly than the intraventricular pressure rises to the value of the systolic aortic pressure (Fig. 3a, work diagram).

The normal cardiac cycle is performed by a special and highly efficient afterload contraction of the heart muscle cells in which the developed force decreases when the muscle contracts and generates increasing intraventricular pressure. The same is valid for the concentric pressure hypertrophy (Fig 3b, work diagram). In cases of structural dilatation the number of muscle layers in the ventricular wall is diminished (Fig. 3c, d). The inner surface of the ventricles is much greater than normal and therefore the developed forces during the cardiac cycle must be greater than in normal ventricles (Fig. 3d, work diagram). In addition to this the force does not decrease but increases during the ejection because the shortening of muscle cells and the reduction of the inner surface are smaller than the increase of the pressure.

This alteration of the muscle mechanics results in a remarkable reduction of work performed by unit cross section of muscle in cases of structural dilatation. The more a structural dilatation is expanded, the shorter the distance or lift and the smaller the amount of work performed by unit cross section of heart muscle has to be (Fig. 3c, d)

A compensation for the impaired mechanical working conditions is not possible by an additional stretching of muscle cells in accordance with the Starling law, because even minor additional stretching of muscle cells would cause an excessive enlargement of the diastolic volume with its deadly consequences (Fig. 3d; compare the left and right work diagrams).

In structural dilatation adaptation is only possible by additional growth of muscle mass which has the effect of reducing the force developed by unit cross section of muscle. This is only possible as long as coronary supply is sufficient. But in the final states of structural dilatation the reduced shortening of muscle cells and the reduced work per unit cross section of muscle are irreversible, leav-

---

with decreasing number of muscle layers in the wall of the left ventricle to 350. Chronic left heart failure. With increasing structural dilatation, the lift and the distance between diastolic and systolic length of the sarcomeres and the amount of work per unit cross section of muscle decreases more and more. Coronary insufficiency impairs adaptive growth of the muscle. Additional stretching of muscle cells (*right diagram*) is associated with increasing force and further reduction of lift and amount of work per unit cross section

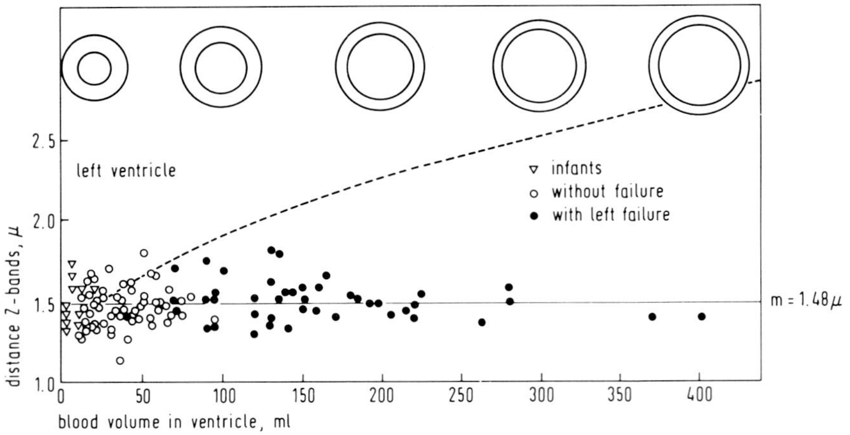

Fig. 4. Mean distance between Z-bands, i.e. length of sarcomeres in μm in relation to absolute residual blood volume in the left ventricle in rigor mortis. (An average number of 600 sarcomeres was measured for every single case). *Broken-line curve* indicates length of sarcomeres if dilatation were due to stretching of the muscle fibres. The areas of the concentric circles (*above*) are a true to scale illustration, taking into account the mean ventricular weights in five groups of increasing structural dilatation

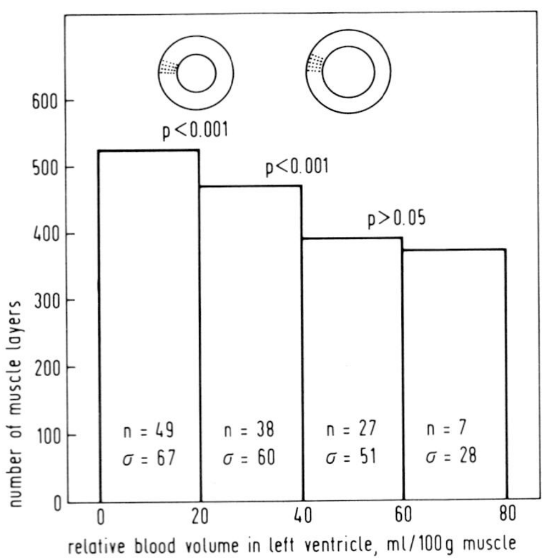

Fig. 5. Number of muscle layers in the compact part of the left ventricle in relation to the relative capacity of the left ventricle. The areas of the concentric circles (*above*) show true to scale the degree of dilatation for a ventricular capacity of 20 ml and 50 ml per 100 g muscle. On the average about 3000 muscle fibres were counted per ventricle

ing out surgical interaction (compare work diagrams in Fig. 3c and the right diagram in Fig. 3d).

The reduced lift or distance of the length of sarcomeres during contraction is more important for the comprehension and understanding of chronic heart failure in cases of structural dilatation than the rise of force or tension in accordance with the Laplace law. The rise of force can be normalized by adapture growth of muscle mass. The reduced distance is irreversible in the final state.

In structural dilatation a much greater muscle mass is necessary to perform the same amount of work in comparison to a normal ventricle, even when the dilated ventricle has performed adaptive growth of heart muscle mass (Fig. 3c, d work diagrams).

With increasing structural dilatation and progressive coronary insufficieny the weight of the ventricular muscle mass is in the end too small to perform the work which is necessary to drive out a sufficient stroke volume. Therefore, I think it is important to discuss not only metabolic but also physical changes of the heart to explain the mechanisms of chronic heart failure in cases of hypertension.

References

1. Linzbach AJ (1960) Heart failure from the point of view of quantitative anatomy. Am J Cardiol 5 : 370–382
2. Linzbach AJ (1966) Die pathologische Anatomie der Herzinsuffizienz. In: Springer, Berlin Heidelberg New York, Handbuch der inneren Medizin, vol 9/1, pp 706–800
3. Linzbach AJ (1976) Hypertrophy, hyperplasia and structural dilatation of the human heart. Adv Cardiol 18 : 1–14

Performance, Wall Dynamics and Coronary Function of the Left Ventricle in Hypertensive Heart Disease[1]

B.E. Strauer

Introduction

Arterial hypertension is the most frequent of left ventricular pressure load in man [1—4]. Its cardiac consequences closely depend on the degree of myocardial hypertrophy and on the progression of coronary artery disease [3, 4]. There have been relatively few reports [5, 6] on cardiac performance in human hypertension, in part because the disease in often asymptomatic and not thought to justify left ventricular catheterization. This study was, therefore, undertaken to investigate the cardiac manifestations of essential hypertension with special reference to left ventricular (LV) function, wall geometry, coronary hemodynamics, and myocardial energy demand. Moreover, the role of ventricular mass, volume, mass-to-volume ratio, and wall stress on the oxygen demand of the human LV myocardium has been studied in various clinical conditions of the chronic hypertrophic heart. The results indicate that systolic wall stress, as a consequence of the degree of ventricular hypertrophy, plays the predominant role in ventricular function and overall myocardial energy demand in chronic hypertrophic heart disease.

Methods

Study Patients. The results reported are based on a total of 251 patients, 114 of whom were hypertensive. The latter all had essential hypertension (World Health Organization classifications I—III). Left ventriculography and coronary angiography were performed during otherwise indicated invasive procedures (cardiac catheterization or renal arteriography). On the basis of these tests, the first 88 patients were classified into four subgroups as follows (Fig. 1):

Group I. Fifteen patients with compensated essential hypertension New York Heart Association (NYHA) class O/I [7], without coronary artery disease (mean age 44 years);

---

1 Supported by the Deutsche Forschungsgemeinschaft

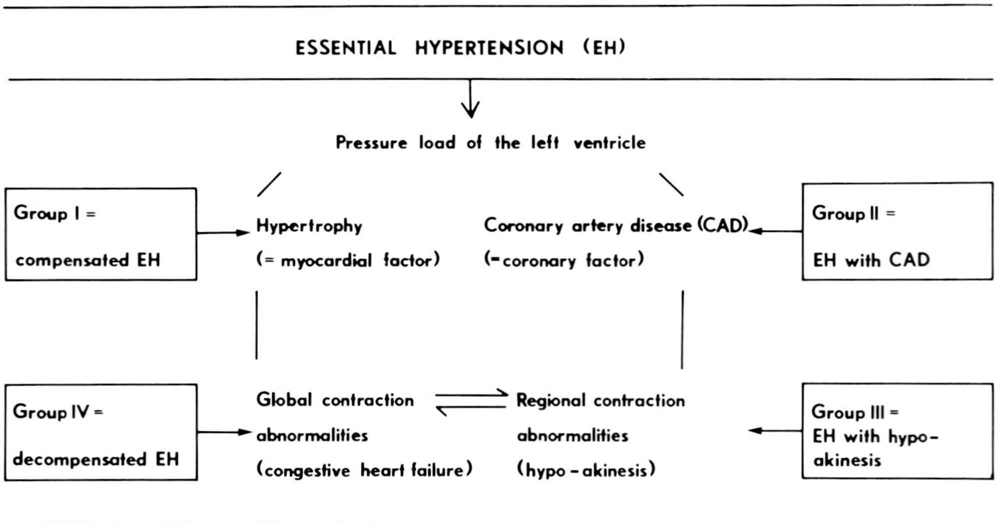

Fig. 1. Schematic representation of the four patient groups investigated. *CAD*, coronary artery disease; *EH*, essential hypertension

Group II: Thirty-two patients with compensated essential hypertension (NYHA class O/I) with 75% or greater stenosis of the left anterior descending coronary artery and without regional wall contraction abnormalities (mean age 41 years);

Group III: Twenty-nine patients with essential hypertension and regional wall motion abnormalities (hypokinesis and akinesis) due to coronary artery disease (mean age 39 years); and

Group IV: Twelve patients with decompensated essential hypertension (NYHA class IV) on the basis of global wall contraction abnormalities (mean age 49 years).

Coronary hemodynamics were specifically investigated in an additional group of 26 hypertensive patients (mean age 42.5 years). Of the 114 hypertensive patients, the majority (78) were untreated ; in the remaining 36, all drugs were discontinued 8–14 days before examination. Treatment in the latter had consisted mainly of diuretic drugs, clonidine, or reserpine; six had been taking propranolol. No significant differences in hemodynamic, coronary, or, ventricular responses could be detected between untreated subjects and those who discontinued therapy.

The results in hypertensive patients were compared with findings in the following groups of subjects: (1) 12 patients with no evidence of cardiovascular disease (normal subjects); (2) 36 normotensive patients with coronary artery disease; (3) 12 patients with hypertrophic obstructive cardiomyopathy; (4) 15 patients with aortic stenosis (six with NYHA class I/II disease, nine with class III/IV disease); and (5) 12 patients with aortic incompetence (NYHA class III/IV).

Cardiac Catheterization and Angiography. Left ventricular and aortic pressures were measured through catheters (pigtail, Cordis) that were directly connected to pressure transducers (Statham F23 Gb). The catheter system had a natural frequency above 20 Hz and a phase lag which was linear with frequency in this frequency range.

Left ventriculograms were obtained with multiple-hole catheters using power injections (Contrac) and 40—60 ml 76% meglumine sodium diatrizoate. The projection was 30° in the right anterior oblique view. Left ventricular volumes were calculated with the methods of Greene et al. [8, 9], i.e., $V = \pi LM^2/6$ (V = volume; L = longest measured chamber axis; and M = internal transverse diameter at the midpoint of L). L was taken directly from the ventriculogram and M was derived from the area (F) of the left ventricle ($M = 4.F/\pi L$). In each patient the correction factor was determined considering magnification and distortion. Volume measurements were performed for end-diastole as well as for each frame during systole until the peak value of systolic circumferential wall stress was obtained [8—16].

Peak systolic wall stress was determined from intraventricular pressure, radius, and wall thickness with use of the Laplace equation ($T_{syst} = P.r/2d$, where P = peak systolic developed pressure, r = internal left ventricular radius, and d = wall thickness). The LV internal radius has been derived from volume measureements ($r = \sqrt[3]{3.V/4 \cdot \pi}$). Wall thickness (d) was taken frame by frame as the averaged thickness of a 4-cm segment of the free wall on the anterior projection one-third of the distance from the apex. Each value for (1) intraventricular pressure, (2) ventricular radius, and (3) ventricular wall thickness was taken for the instantaneous wall stress calculation until the peak value of systolic circumferential wall stress was obtained. The stress calculated by this procedure represents mean values across the thickness of the wall. This mean value underestimates maximal stress, which occurs at the endocardium, and it overestimates minimal stress at the outer layers (epicardium); however, application of the mean value does not lessen the validity of this stress value because it deviates from thin-walled calculations by approximately 10—15%.

Determinations of LV mass were made from end-diastolic chamber dimensions, that is, from end-diastolic measurements of wall thickness and volume. These calculations were based on the determinations of shell volume created by adding lateral wall thickness to calculated ellipsoidal chamber dimensions and subtracting adjusted chamber volume. Shell volume was converted to mass by multiplying by the specific gravity of heart muscle: left ventricular muscle mass (LVMM) = LVTV — EDV (LVTV = left ventricular total volume; EDV = end-diastolic volume), where $LVTV = 4/3 \cdot \pi (L/2 + d)(M/2 + d)^2$ and $LVMM = 4/3 \cdot \pi (L/2 + d)(M/2 + d)^2 - EDV$. Left ventricular mass-to-volume ratio was obtained by dividing LV mass by the end-diastolic volume.

Coronary Blood Flow. A Goodale-Lubin catheter (CH. 7) was inserted through the left antecubital vein and introduced into the coronary sinus for coronary sinus blood sampling and determination of coronary blood flow. Coronary blood flow was measured after right and left heart catheterization and before left ventriculography by means of the argon method with gas chromatographic analysis of argon in arterial and coronary venous blood. Details as well as a record of the accuracy of this method, which allows measurements for coronary blood flow up to 400—500 ml/min per 100 g, have previously been published [17—22]. The linearity of this method over the whole range of physiologically existing coronary blood flow was proved by comparisons with flowmeter and coronary sinus sampling techniques [17, 18]. Argon blood concentrations were determined after extraction through a specially designed extraction chamber with use of gas chromatography (trace gas analyzer 1533 B, Varian, Darmstadt, Federal Republic of Germany). Measurements of coronary blood flow were carried out under resting conditions and during maximal coronary vasodilation. The latter was achieved by the intravenous injection of a potent coronary vasodilator (dipyridamole, 0.5 mg/kg body wt.), which was given to each patient in fractions that would exert no significant effects on aortic pressure or heart rate [18—22]. Coronary vascular restisance (mm Hg/ml per min per 100 g) was determined as the ratio of coronary perfusion pressure to coronary flow; the former was calculated as mean diastolic aortic pressure minus mean LV diastolic pressure. Coronary vascular reserve, or coronary reserve, was defined as the ratio between coronary vascular resistance in the resting state and the resistance during maximal coronary vasodilation [21]. Left ventricular oxygen consumption (ml/min per 100 g) was determined as the product of coronary blood flow (ml/min per 100 g) and the arterial-coronary venous oxygen difference (vol percent). Arterial and coronary venous oxygen saturation levels were measured with carbon monoxide oximetry.

Results

Central Hemodynamics and Left Ventricular Function

Mean arterial pressure was increased in hypertension by approximately 50% without significant differences among the four hypertensive subgroups I to IV (Table 1, Fig. 2). In contrast, LV muscle mass, which is a consequence of chronic pressure overload, progressively increased from group I to group IV. Accordingly, the LV mass to pressure load ratio was markedly elevated in the groups III and IV with advanced hypertension. It would be reasonable to assume that this progression of cardiac hypertrophy was related to the duration and severity of hypertensive heart disease.

End-diastolic pressure and end-diastolic volume were considerably increased in the hypertensive groups III and IV (Table 1, Fig. 3). In contrast, end-diastolic volume was nearly normal in clinically compensated essential hypertension, whether or not it was associated with coronary artery disease (groups I and II), and end-diastolic pressure was only moderately elevated in these patients. The

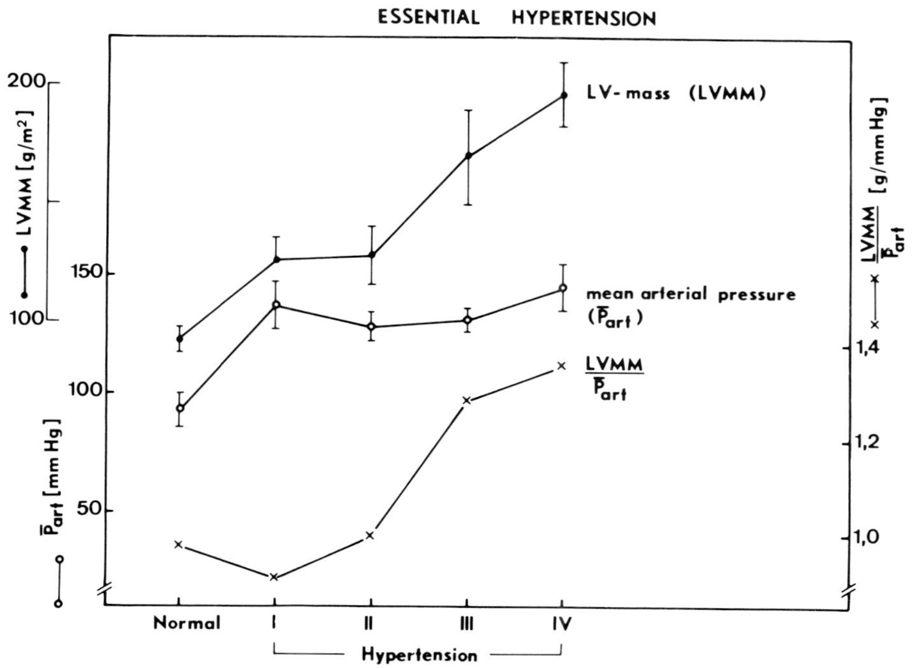

Fig. 2. Left ventricular (*LV*) mass, mean arterial pressure ($\overline{P}_{art}$), and mass to pressure ratio ($LVMM/\overline{P}_{art}$) in the four hypertensive groups

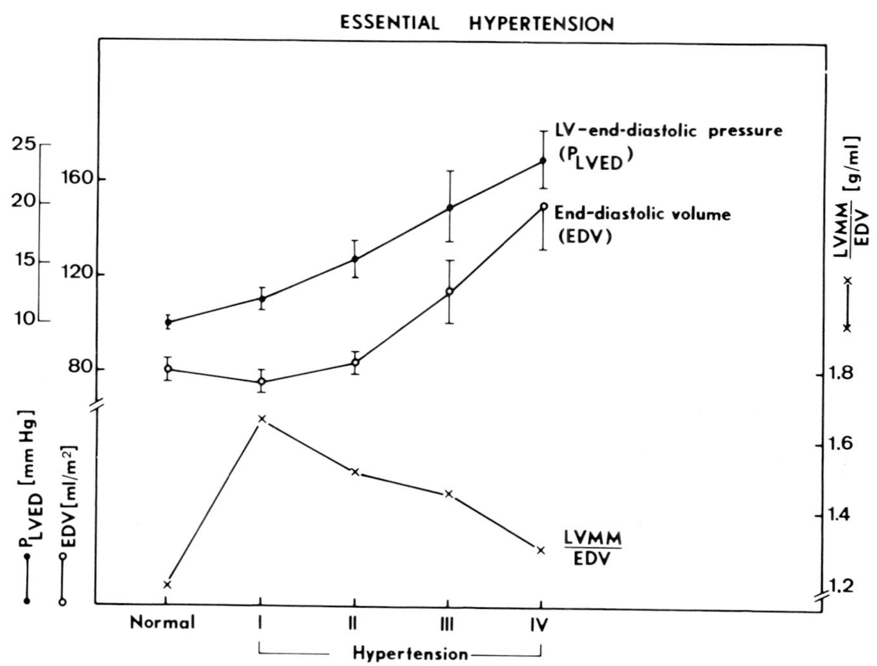

Fig. 3. Left ventricular end-diastolic pressure (P_{LVED}), end-diastolic volume (*EDV*), and mass to volume ratio. *LVMM* = LV mass

Table 1. Haemodynamics and ventricular function values in 12 normal subjects and in the four subgroups of essential hypertension (EH)[a]

	$\bar{P}_{art}$ [mm Hg]	LVMM [gm/m²]	LVMM/$\bar{P}_{art}$ [gm/m²·mmHg]	P_{LVED} [mm Hg]	EDV [ml/m²]	LVMM/EDV [g/ml]
Normals	91 ± 9	92 ± 6	1.01	10 ± 1	81 ± 6	1.14
EH I	136 ± 9[b]	122 ± 11[d]	0.90	12 ± 2	74 ± 6	1.65
II	128 ± 6[b]	129 ± 14[e]	1.01	15 ± 4	80 ± 5	1.61
III	131 ± 3[b]	168 ± 16[b]	1.28	19 ± 7[c]	112 ± 16	1.50
IV	146 ± 4[b]	192 ± 15[b]	1.32	23 ± 6[d]	147 ± 17[d]	1.31

	CI [l/min·m²]	EF [%]	dp/dt_{max} [mm Hg/s]	V_{CF} [circ/s]	T_{syst} [10^3 dyn/cm²]	MVO_2 [ml/min·100 g]
Normals	3.82 ± 0.09	72 ± 2	1690 ± 90	1.62 ± 0.13	220 ± 9	7.98 ± 0.52
EH I	3.95 ± 0.08	78 ± 5	2460 ± 110[b]	1.71 ± 0.12	232 ± 8	8.21 ± 0.31
II	3.93 ± 0.09	69 ± 5	2400 ± 94[b]	1.36 ± 0.11	208 ± 19	7.13 ± 0.19
III	3.22 ± 0.10[b]	61 ± 6[c]	2310 ± 88[e]	0.74 ± 0.14[e]	256 ± 18	9.62 ± 0.34[d]
IV	3.24 ± 0.11[b]	40 ± 8[d]	2190 ± 102[d]	0.44 ± 0.14[e]	369 ± 26[b]	12.8 ± 0.61[e]

[a] Statistical analysis was performed by means of the *t*-test (mean ± standard error of the mean). *P* values listed in table are given for comparison of normal subjects and groups with essential hypertension. *P* values within subgroups with essential hypertension (I to IV) are as follows: $\overline{P}_{art}$ (II vs. IV, $P < 0.005$); LVMM (I vs. III, $P < 0.025$; I vs. IV, $P < 0.001$; II vs. IV, $P < 0.005$); P_{LVED} (I vs. IV, $P < 0.05$); EDV (I vs. IV, II vs. IV $P < 0.001$); CI (I vs. III, I vs. IV, II vs. III, II vs. IV, $P < 0.001$); EF (I vs. IV $P < 0.001$, II vs. IV, $P < 0.005$); V_{CF} (I vs. III, I vs. IV, II vs. III, II vs. IV, $P < 0.001$); T_{syst} (I vs. IV, II vs. IV, III vs IV, $P < 0.001$); MVO_2 (I vs. II, I vs. III, $P < 0.005$; I vs. IV, II vs. III, II vs. IV, III vs. IV, $P < 0.001$). Significance for LVMM/$\overline{P}_{art}$ (tested against normal subjects) was $P < 0.001$ for groups III and IV; for LVMM/EDV, *P* values were $P < 0.001$ (groups I and II) and $P < 0.05$ (group III). CI = cardiac index; circ = circumference; dP/dt_{max} = maximal rate of left ventricular pressure development; EDV = end-diastolic volume; EF = ejection fraction; LVMM = left ventricular muscle mass; MVO_2 = left ventricular oxygen consumption; $\overline{P}_{art}$ = mean arterial pressure; P_{LVED} = left ventricular end-diastolic pressure; T_{syst} = peak circumferential systolic wall stress; Vcf = mean circumferential fiber shortening

[b] $P < 0.001$

[c] $P < 0.05$

[d] $P < 0.01$

[e] $P < 0.005$

mass-to-volume ratio was greatly increased in compensated hypertension because of a considerable mass increase per volume, whereas the mass-to-volume ratio tended toward normalization in decompensated hypertension (group IV). The latter finding was attributable to a progressive increase in volume despite further augmentation of LV mass. Cardiac index, stroke volume index, and ejection phase indexes were normal in groups I and II, but they were depressed in hypertensive patients with wall motion abnormalities and with cardiac decompensation (groups III and IV) (Table 1). The maximal rate of LV pressure development (dP/dt_{max}) was increased in all groups; however, the ratio of dP/dt_{max} to its corresponding isovolumic pressure was normal in groups I (38 ± 4 s) and II (42 ± 5 s), and it was depressed in groups III (29 ± 4 s) and IV (22 ± 3 s).

Ventricular Size and Function

Left ventricular size as determined by the end-diastolic volume showed an inverse relationship with LV function as evidenced by the LV ejection fraction (Fig. 4). Similar relationships were present between the end-diastolic volume and time or velocity-related auxotonic ejection phase parameters (MNSER: mean normalized systolic ejection rate, V_{CF} : mean circumferential fiber shortening). With increases in end-diastolic volume the ejection fraction decreased for all groups. However, steepness of this characteristic was quite different: lowest decrease in LV function with increase in end-diastolic volume was present for volume-overloaded aortic incompetence, whereas the largest decrease was found for chronic pressure overload due to aortic stenosis and essential hypertension as well as for coronary artery disease. This means that considerable decrease in LV function occurs at an only small LV enlargement in chronic pressure overload and in coronary artery disease, whereas in chronic volume overload even a large increase in LV size may have normal LV function.

The different course of these characteristics most probably may be related to different contractile state and/or to different loading conditions of the left ventricle. At an equal end-diastolic volume an increase in contractility increases shortening and, hence, the LV ejection fraction. Likewise, therapeutic reduction of afterload may enhance LV function. The opposite effects should be expected with negatively inotropic interventions, with an increase in afterload, and with abnormal increase or decrease in LV preload. Thus, it seems probable that the different course of this relationship in chronic volume and pressure overload reflects different LV performance. From the diagnostic point of view, these relationships may help to evaluate LV function from the heart size in chest X-ray, provided the reason for LV hypertrophy is known (e.g., pressure overload, volume overload, or coronary artery disease).

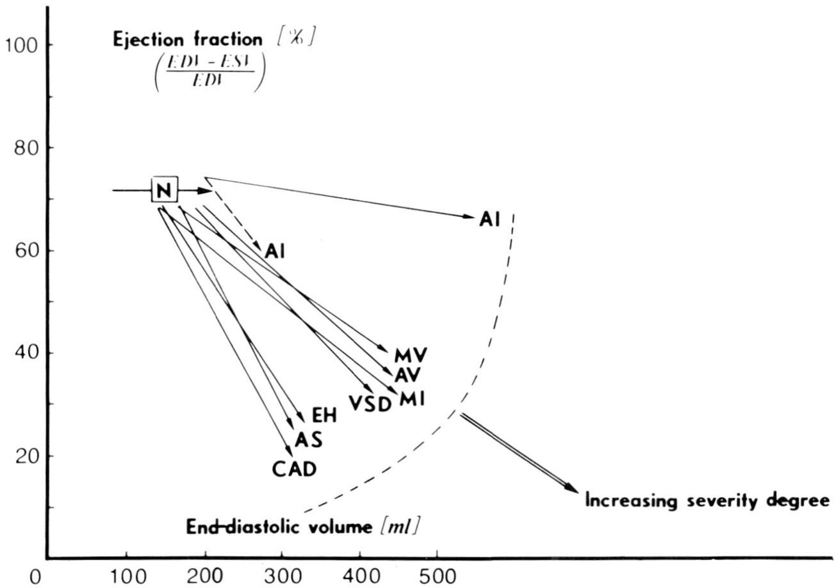

N	Normals	y = 71.5 − 0.00479 x
AI	Aortic incompetence	y = 78.5 − 0,022 x
CMV	Comb. mitral valve lesions	y = 84.7 − 0,11 x
CAV	Comb. aortic valve lesions	y = 110.0 − 0,17 x
MI	Mitral incompetence	y = 85.9 − 0,12 x
VSD	Ventricular septal defect	y = 98.2 − 0,16 x
AS	Aortic stenosis	y = 117.7 − 0,29 x
CAD	Coronary artery disease	y = 114.9 − 0.33 x
EH	Essential hypertension	y = 106.5 − 0,24 x

Fig. 4. Relationship between the end-diastolic volume of the left ventricle and the ejection fraction. Note the inverse relationship between both variables. Note further that coronary artery disease as well as pressure overload (aortic stenosis, essential hypertension) have marked reduction in the LV ejection fraction with increase in end-diastolic volume

Left Ventricular Wall Dynamics

Peak circumferential systolic wall stress was normal in the groups I and II (essential hypertension), whereas it was considerably increased in groups III and IV (Table 2). An inverse relation was present between mass to volume ratio and peak systolic wall stress, indicating a characteristic decrease in peak systolic wall

Table 2. Dynamical and energetical measures in normals, in coronary artery disease and in chronic pressure and volume overload

	N =	Ejection fraction [%]	LV mass [gm/m^2]	LV mass to volume ratio [gm/ml]	T_{syst} [10^3 dyn/cm^2]	MVO_2 [ml/min·100 g]	LVO_2 [ml/min]
Normals	12	72 ± 2	92 ± 6	1.21 ± 0.12	220 ± 9	7.98 ± 0.52	13.3 ± 2.1
CAD	36	52 ± 11	145 ± 22[d]	1.12 ± 0.16	236 ± 18	7.9 ± 0.39	20.6 ± 3.2
SVD	8	69 ± 8	84 ± 14	1.18 ± 0.21	206 ± 22	6.4 ± 0.6 [d]	9.7 ± 0.91[d]
AS[b]	6	74 ± 4	145 ± 10[e]	2.1 ± 0.31	192 ± 23	8.1 ± 0.8	21.1 ± 2.3 [e]
AS[c]	9	46 ± 11	190 ± 17[f]	1.01 ± 0.11	396 ± 95[e]	14.9 ± 1.6 [f]	51.0 ± 6.9 [f]
AI	12	58 ± 7	174 ± 22[f]	1.12 ± 0.13	329 ± 36[d]	14.2 ± 1.4 [f]	45.4 ± 4.7 [f]
HOC	12	78 ± 6	~228	~3.78	142 ± 52	8.6 ± 1.21	35.3 ± 3.6
EH	92	62 ± 6	152 ± 12[f]	1.52 ± 0.33	266 ± 18[e]	10.7 ± 0.38[f]	29.3 ± 4.1 [f]
MI	20	63 ± 9	132 ± 11[d]	1.19 ± 0.09	267 ± 11[d]	9.82 ± 0.21[e]	21.6 ± 0.92
MV	44	62 ± 12	149 ± 9[e]	1.20 ± 0.10	248 ± 32[d]	9.22 ± 0.99[d]	24.9 ± 2.9 [d]

a AI = aortic incompetence; AS = aortic stenosis; CAD = coronary artery disease; EH = essential hypertension; HOC = hypertrophic obstructive cardiomyopathy; LVMM = left ventricular muscle mass (g/m^2); LVMM/EDV = left ventricular muscle mass to volume ratio (g/ml); LVO_2 = total left ventricular oxygen consumption (ml/min); MVO_2 = myocardial oxygen consumption per weight unit (ml/min x 100 g); SVD = small vessel disease; T_{syst} = peak circumferential systolic wall stress (10^3 $dynes/cm^2$)

b Clinically compensated (NYHA I°/II°), concentric hypertrophy

c Clinically decompensated (NYHA III°/IV°), LV dilatation

d $P < 0.05$

e $P < 0.01$

f $P < 0.001$

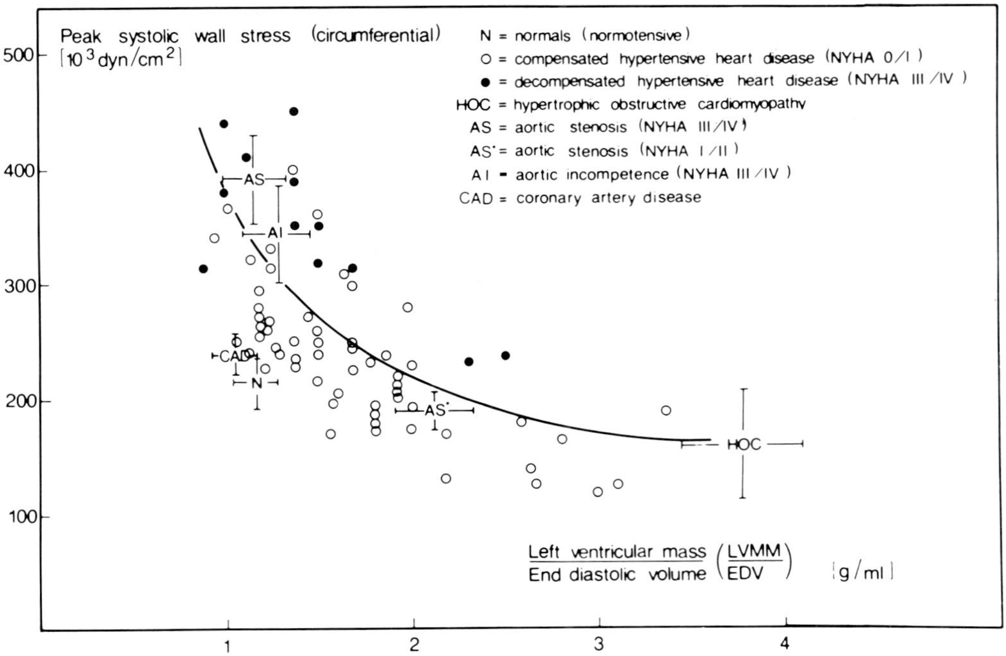

Fig. 5. Relation between LV mass to volume ratio (LVMM/EDV) and peak systolic wall stress. A decrease in wall stress with an increase in mass to volume ratio is demonstrated. The *curve* (isobar for all patients with essential hypertensio) was calculated by polynome fitting (Y = 31.2 + 371.2 x 1/X, where Y = wall stress, X = mass to volume ratio). Note the following points: (1) normotensive normal subjects (*N*) and normotensive subjects with coronary artery disease have shifts to lower wall stress at comparable mass to volume ratio (= lower isobar); (2) the appropriateness of LV hypertrophy in essential hypertension may be derived from the course of this curve. At a normal mass to volume ratio, an increased wall stress is present for decompensated hypertensive disease (class III or IV, high stress hypertrophy), whereas an appropriate increase in mass to volume ratio, despite an enhanced systolic pressure load, may maintain normal systolic wall stress (normal stress hyprtrophy). In contrast, excess augmentation of LV mass out of proportion to volume may lead to a decrease in systolic wall stress (low stress hypertrophy); (3) hypertrophic heart disease (AS, AI, HOC) may be situated within the isobaric characteristics of hypertensive heart disease if systolic pressure is increased at comparable mass to volume ratio; and (4) LV hypertrophy due to aortic stenosis may have increased wall stress (AS; III or IV; high stress hypertrophy) or normal wall stress (AS′, I or II; normal stress hypertrophy), and wall stress my be even reduced, despite increased intraventricular systolic pressure load in hypertrophic obstructive cardiomyopathy (low stress hypertrophy), *NYHA*, New York Heart Association

stress with increase in the mass to volume ratio (Fig. 5). The largest mass-to-volume ratio was found in the patients with hypertrophic obstructive cardiomayopathy and the lowest values were present for decompensated subgroups with pressure and volume overload. Compensated LV hypertrophy due to essential hypertension and aortic stenosis was within this hypertensive correlation, whereas in the normotensive patient groups there was a shift to lower peak systolic wall stress at equal mass to volume ratio or to lower mass to volume ratio at equal peak systolic wall stress.

With a chronic pressure load an increase in the mass to volume ratio would be expected. However, correlation between these two variables, that is, between systolic pressure and the mass to volume ratio, was not present (Fig. 6). When all patients are considered with regard to equal peak systolic wall stress (isostress ranges), a graduated arrangement of all values becomes possible (Fig. 7). At comparable systolic pressure the peak systolic wall stress decreases with an increase in the mass to volume ratio. Conversely, at comparable mass to volume ratios the peak systolic wall stress increases with an increase in systolic pressure.

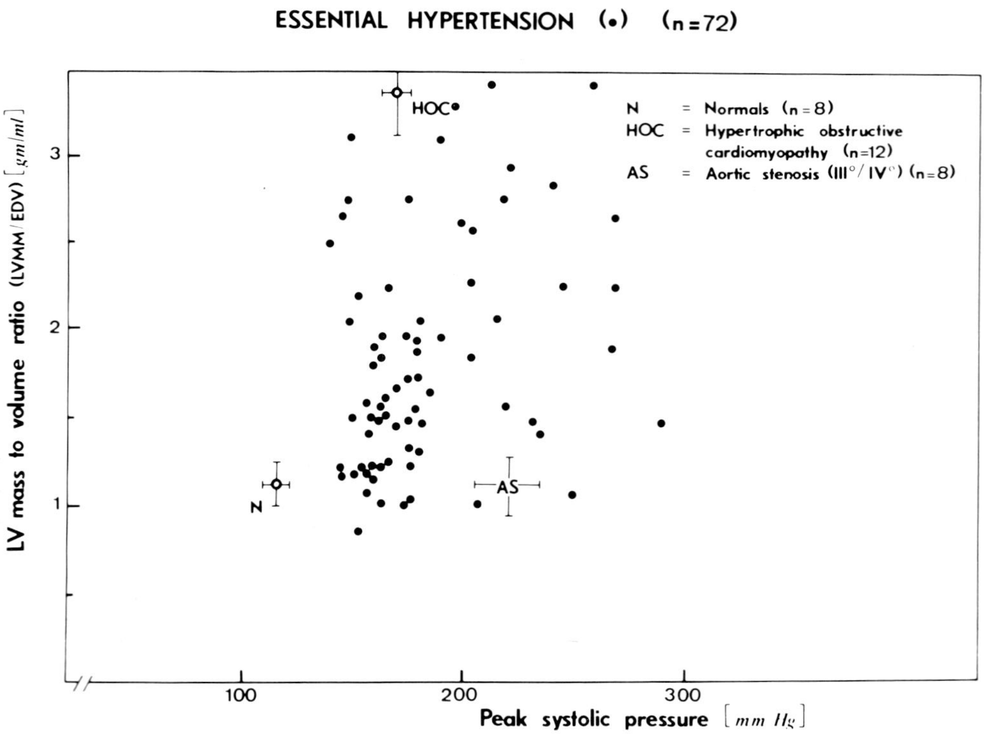

Fig. 6. Relationship between peak systolic pressure and the LV mass to volume ratio. Note the scatter "relationship" without any correlation. Patient groups with normal pressure (*N*), with aortic stenosis (*AS*), and with hypertrophic obstructive cardiomyopathy (*HOC*) have been considered for reasons of comparison

ESSENTIAL HYPERTENSION (•) (n=72)

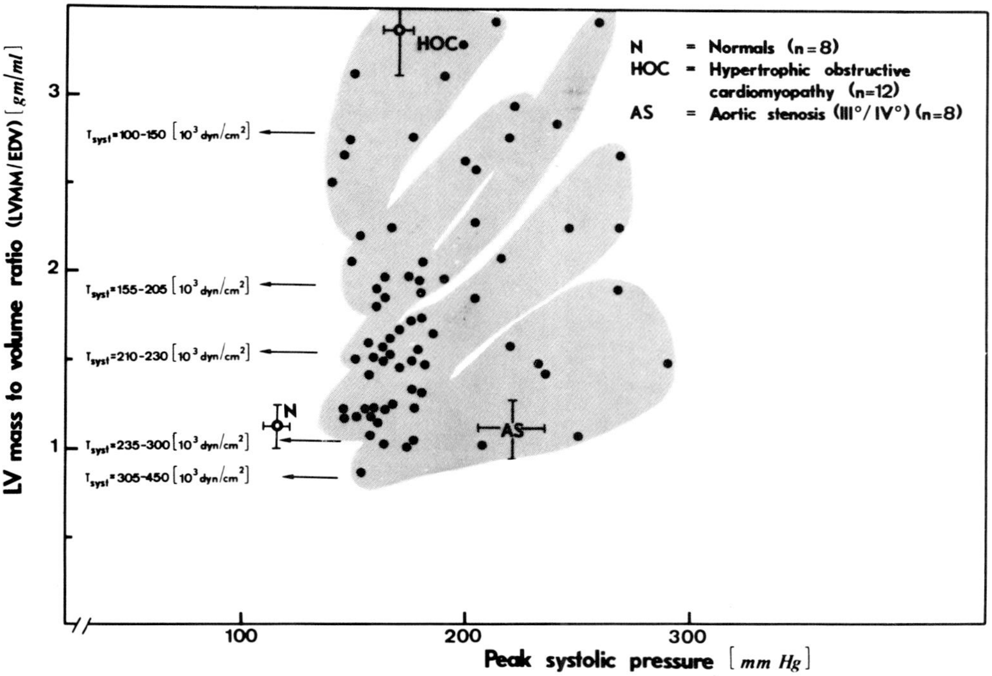

Fig. 7. Relation of peak systolic pressure and LV mass to volume ratio separated on the basis of nonoverlapping isostress ranges with same patients and points as in Fig. 6. At comparable systolic pressure, the peak systolic wall stress (T_{syst}) decreases with increase in mass to volume ratio. At comparable mass to volume ratio the peak systolic wall stress increases with increase in systolic pressure. However, peak systolic wall stress may remain normal even at an extreme increase in pressure, provided that the mass to volume ratio also increases in proportion to pressure load. *Closed circles* indicate patients with essential hypertension. *III°*, *IV°*, New York Heart Association functional classes III and IV

However, within any isostress range the peak systolic wall stress remained unaltered, even at extreme pressure load, provided the mass to volume ratio increased in proportion to systolic pressure load.

Stress and Function

Except for changes in contractility, the altered LV loading conditions may decrease LV function with increase in heart size. At comparable systolic pressure and mass an increase in end-diastolic volume leads to an increase in systolic wall stress. Accordingly, the relationship between wall stress and function has been determined for a large number of hypertensive and normotensive patients (Fig.

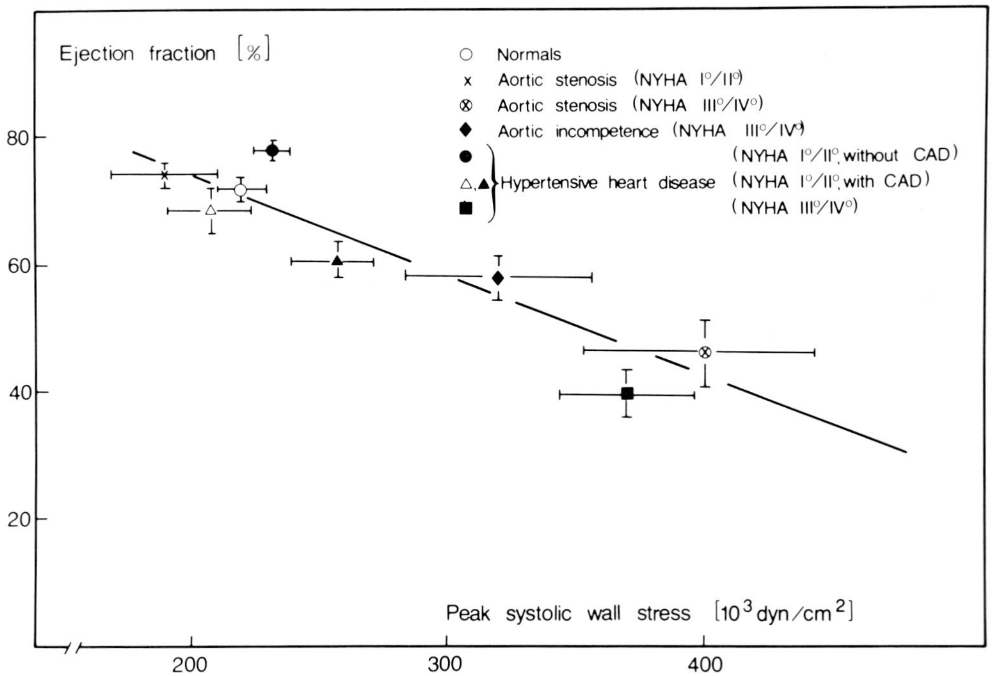

Fig. 8. Relation between peak systolic wall stress (= left ventricular afterload) and ejection fraction. Note the decrease in ejection fraction with an increase in stress

8). With an increase in systolic wall stress the ejection fraction markedly decreased. Doubling of stress led to reduction in the LV ejection fraction by approximately 50%. Since systolic wall stress results from systolic pressure and mass to volume ratio, it equals the afterload which is imposed on the left ventricular wall. Therefore, it may be concluded that heart size, i.e., end-diastolic volume, and systolic wall stress are important determinants of LV performance.

Regional Wall Hypertrophy

Regional Degree of Hypertrophy. For quantification of the degree, extent, and regularity of the regional hypertrophy the regional wall thickness values and the end-diastolic/end-systolic wall thickness changes were analyzed in five ventricular segments (Fig. 9). The end-diastolic as well as the end-systolic thickness of the anterior wall of the left ventricle in all patients examined was greatest at the heart basis. The thickness decreased up to the ventricular equator, where it reached its minimum and thereafter again increased towards the apex. The differences in regional wall thickness at the end-diastole or end-systole were smallest in decompensated hypertensives with LV dilatation and they were greatest in compensated hypertensives with concentric hypertrophy and coronary stenoses as determined by coronary angiogrphy (Figs. 10, 11).

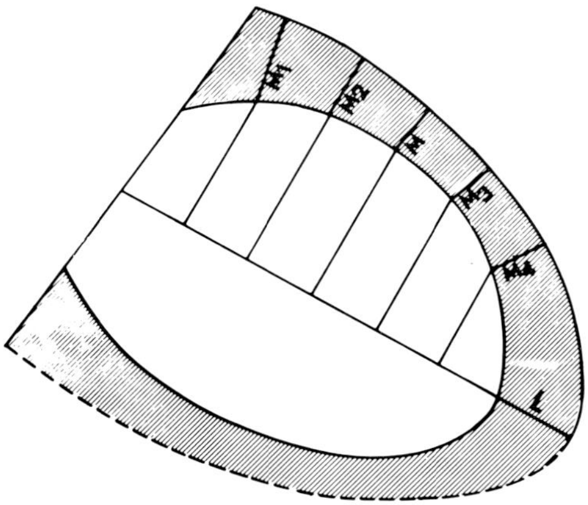

Fig. 9. Model for evaluation ventricular wall thickness in various regions of the LV wall. Projection: 30° RAO. The regional wall thickness was established from the section points of short diameters at the endocardial surface and the connection to the epicardial surface, perpendicular to the tangent of the LV epicardium

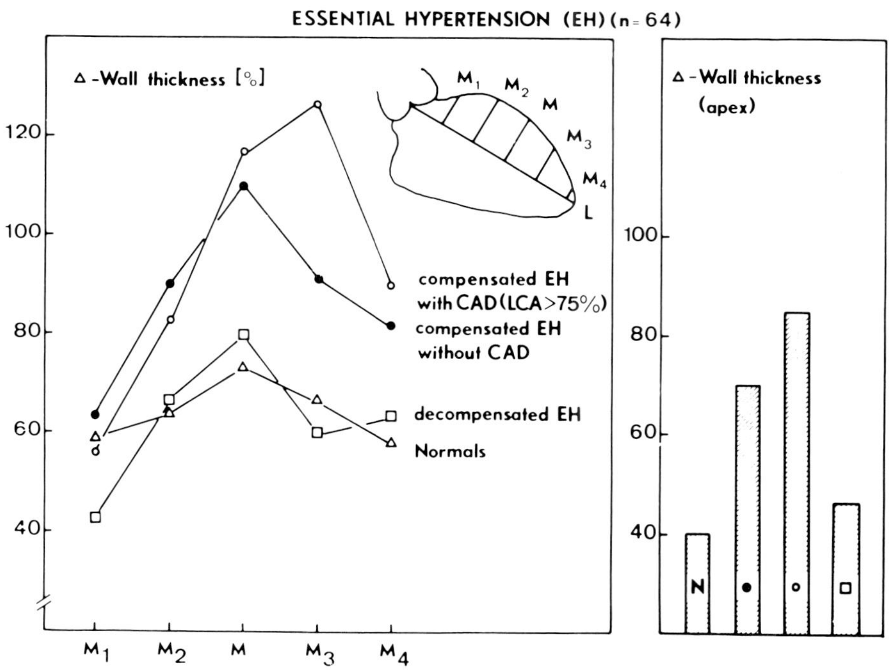

Fig. 10. Percent changes of LV wall thickness (end-diastolic — end-systolic); end-diastolic = 100%; *CAD* = coronary heart disease; *LCA* = left coronary artery; *M* = minor axis; *L* = long axis

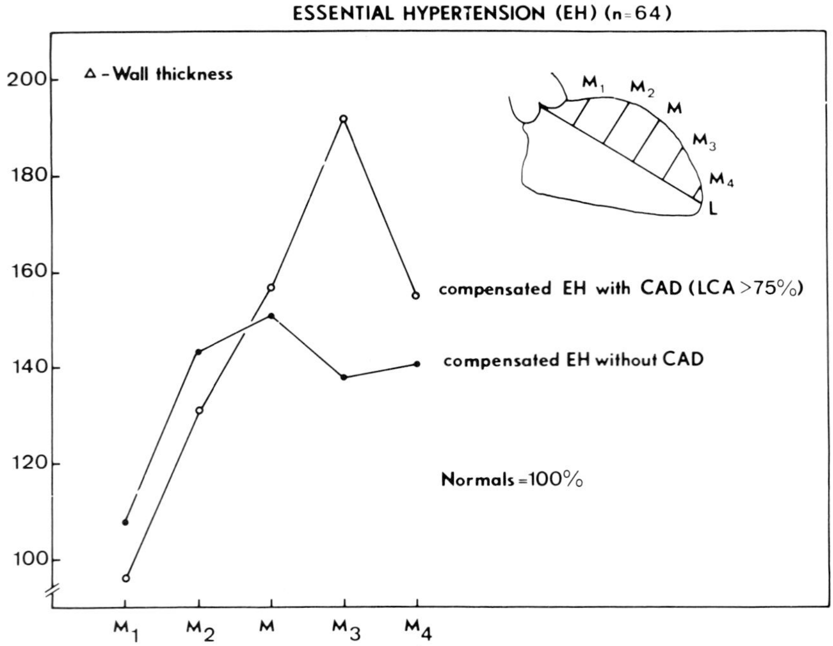

Fig. 11. Percent changes of LV wall thickness (end-diastolic — end-systolic) in patient groups with compensated essential hypertension and with and without coronary artery disease. Note the considerable wall thickness increase during systole in (M, M_3) compensated hypertensive heart disease with coronary artery disease; *CAD*, coronary heart disease; *LCA*, left coronary artery

The maximal thickening of the anterior wall of the left ventricle during the course of a cardiac action, i.e., the end-diastolic/end-systolic change in wall thickness, was greatest in the near of the equator in apical direction (M, M_3) (Figs. 10,11). This means that the ventricular wall region with the greatest end-diastolic/end-systolic change in distance and the greatest hemiaxis shortening also showed the greatest relative increase in the ventricular wall thickness during a cardiac cycle. The wall thickness increase measured in this ventricular wall region in the hypertension groups was greatest in compensated hypertensives with coronary heart disease proven by coronary angiography. This means that this group revealed the greatest relative differences in the regional end-diastolic/end-systolic wall thickness changes and that it is in these cases where the highest degree of asymmetry or irregularity of the ventricular wall hypertrophy, particularly in the middle of the ventricle, is to be expected.

Coronary Haemodynamics

Left ventricular coronary blood flow was increased in essential hypertension by a mean of 18% ($P < 0.005$), whereas coronary perfusion pressure (that is, mean diastolic aortic pressure minus mean diastolic LV pressure) was increased by 56% (Table 3). In consequence, coronary vascular resistance was significantly ($P < 0.001$) increased by 38%. Arterial-coronary venous oxygen difference in hypertensive patients was not different from normal values. Coronary reserve, which averaged 4.8 in normal subjects, was significantly ($P < 0.01$) reduced in those with essential hypertension (Fig. 12). In hypertensive patients with concomitant coronary artery disease (group II), the coronary reserve was quantitatively similar to that found among normotensive patients with coronary artery disease. However, even in the absence of evident coronary artery disease, patients with essential hypertension (group I) had a significant reduction in coronary reserve; this averaged 34% below normal ($P < 0.01$).

Myocardial Oxygen Consumption

Myocardial oxygen consumption per LV weight unit (MVO_2) was lowest in the normotensive patients with small vessel disease and largest in those with aortic valve disease with a dilated heart (Table 2, Fig. 13). There was no correlation between MVO_2 and ventricular function (as manifested by cardiac index, stroke work index, external cardiac work, pressure-time index, isovolumic contractility indexes, ejection phase indexes, systolic pressure, and other measures).

Table 3. Coronary perfusion pressure, arterial-coronary venous oxygen difference, coronary blood flow of left ventricle, and coronary resistance in normal subjects, in patients with essential hypertension and in normotensive coronary artery disease. Note the increase of both coronary perfusion pressure and coronary resistance in essential hypertension. Arterial-coronary venous oxygen difference and, hence, coronary oxygen extraction were unchanged in the three groups[a]

		P_{cor} [mm Hg]	$avDO_2$ [Vol %]	V_{cor} [ml/min·100 g]	R_{cor} [mm Hg·min ·100 g·ml^{-1}]
Normals	(n = 12)	82 ± 2	12.2 ± 0.1	71 ± 3	1.15 ± 0.04
EH	(n = 63)	129 ± 8[b]	12.9 ± 0.2	83 ± 2[c]	1.57 ± 0.06[b]
CAD	(n = 38)	87 ± 5	12.8 ± 0.6	64 ± 3[d]	1.36 ± 0.09

[a] $avDO_2$ = arterial-coronary venous oxygen difference; CAD = (normotensive) coronary artery disease; EH = essential hypertension; P_{cor} = coronary perfusion pressure; R_{cor} = coronary resistance; V_{cor} = coronary blood flow of left ventricle
[b] $P < 0.02$
[c] $P < 0.005$
[d] $P < 0.001$

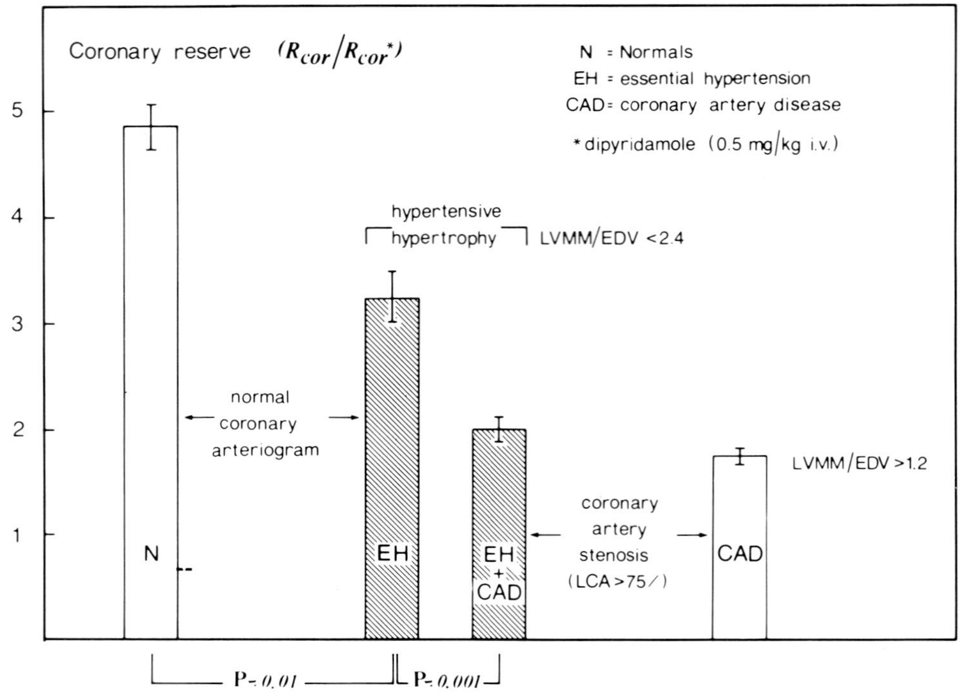

Fig. 12. Coronary reserve, defined as the ratio of coronary resistance (R_{cor}) under control conditions and coronary resistance under maximal coronary dilatation (R_{cor}), in normal subjects (*N*), in those with essential hypertension (*EH*) with a normal coronary arteriogram, in those with essential hypertension with coronary arterial stenosis, and in normotensive patients with coronary artery disease (*CAD*). Note the decreased coronary reserve even in hypertensive hypertrophy with normal coronary arteriogram. *LCA*, left coronary artery; *LVMM/EDV*, left ventricular mass to volume ratio; P = probability

Total LV oxygen consumption was linearly correlated with total LV muscle mass in normal subjects and in hypertensive patients with normal stress hypertrophy (Fig. 14). At comparable LV mass, increased oxygen consumption occured in patients with high stress hypertrophy due to decompensated aortic stenosis and aortic incompetence (functional classes III and IV), whereas decreased oxygen consumption was found in those with coronary artery disease, aneurysm, or small vessel disease.

The mass to volume ratio was inversely related to MVO_2 (Table 2, Fig. 15). At isobaric conditions, the largest mass to volume ratio and lowest MVO_2 was found in patients with hypertrophic obstructive cardiomyopathy, whereas in those with decompensated aortic stenosis and aortic incompetence the lowest mass to volume ratio was associated with the largest MVO_2. Normotensive patients with normal LV function or with coronary artery disease had a lower MVO_2 at a comparable mass to volume ratio.

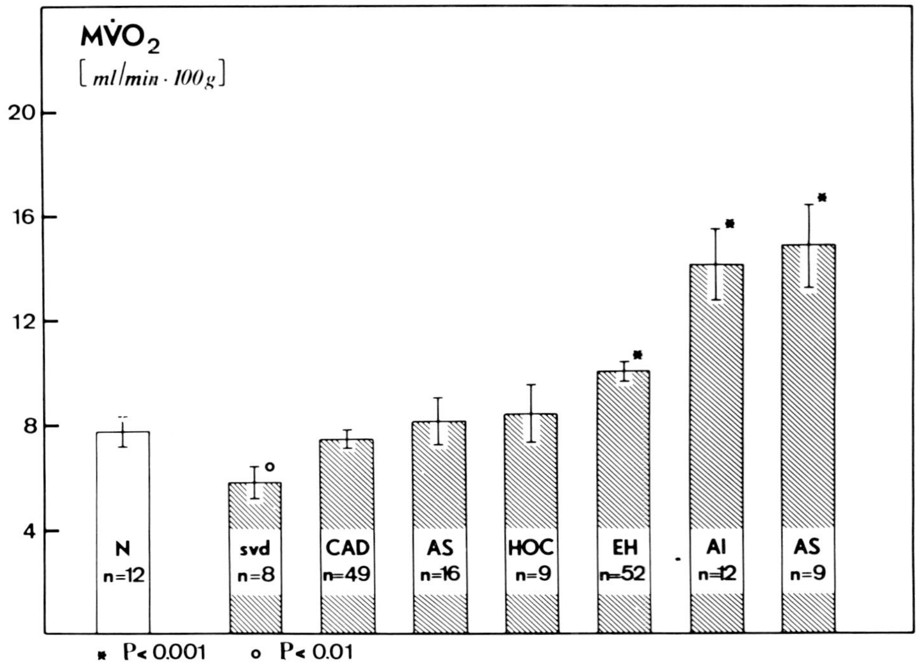

Fig. 13. Myocardial oxygen consumption (ml/min x 100 m) in hypertrophic heart disease in man. *N*, normals; *svd*, small vessel disease; *CAD*, coronary artery disease; *AS*, aortic stenosis (compensated); *HOC* hypertrophic obstructive cardiomyopathy; *EH*, hypertensive heart disease (essential hypertension); *AI*, aortic incompetence; and *AS*, aortic stenosis (decompensated)

Because the mass to volume ratio at equal systolic pressure represents the major determinant of peak systolic wall stress, correlation was performed between peak systolic wall stress and the MVO_2. A significant relation was found between both variables (Fig. 16). Patients with decompensated aortic stenosis and aortic incompetence were within the upper range, and the normotensive normal subjects were within the lower range of this relation. Extrapolation to zero stress resulted in an intercept of 3.28 ml/min x 100 g. This value, althoug somewhat increased, corresponds quite well with the oxygen consumption of the empty beating heart. Steepness of this regression indicates an increase in MVO_2 by 2.8 ml/min x 100 g for an increase in peak systolic wall stress by 100 (10^3 dynes/cm^2) for normal subjects as well as for those with coronary artery disease and hypertrophic heart disease.

Systolic Stress Reserve

The lowest peak systolic wall stress, which was found in patients with chronic hypertensive hypertrophy, was ~100±12 (10^3 dynes/cm^2) and the largest peak systolic wall stress was ~450±46 (Table 4, Fig. 17). In comparison with the nor-

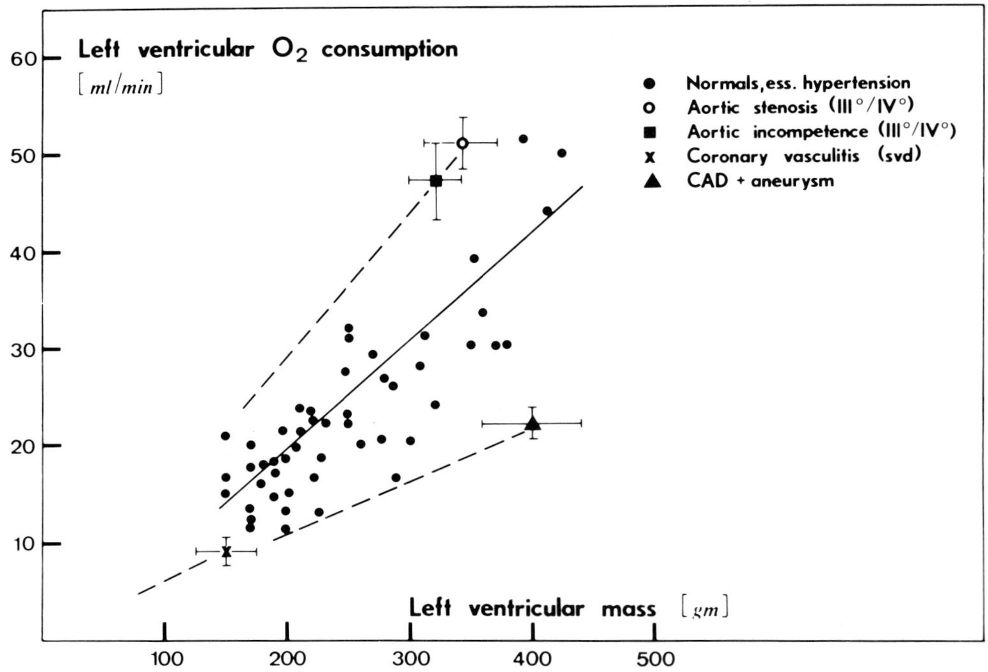

Fig. 14. Left ventricular mass and total LV oxygen consumption

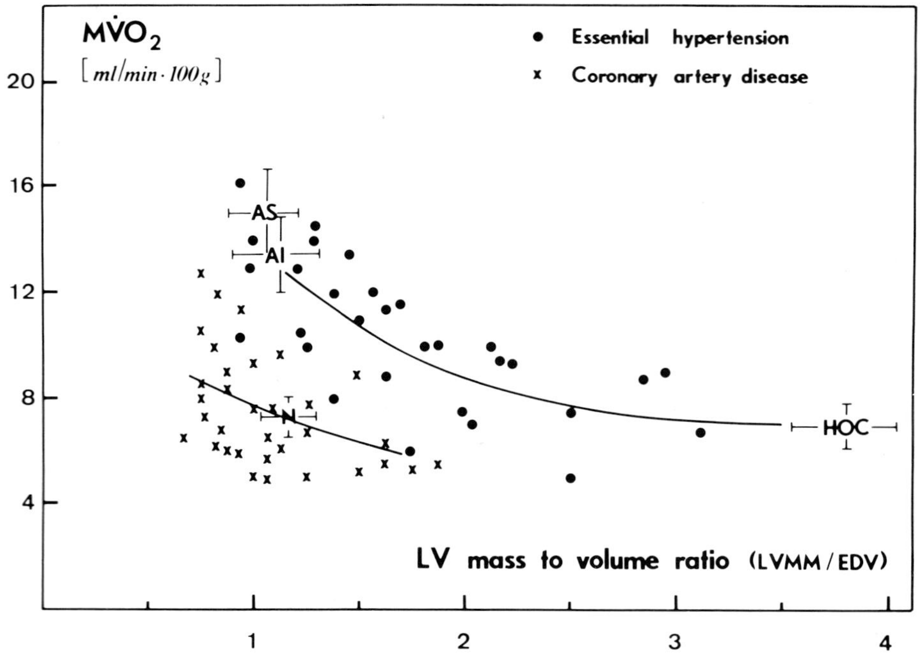

Fig. 15. Relation between LV mass to volume ratio (*LVMM/EDV*) and LV oxygen consumption per weight unit (MVO_2). *AI*, aortic incompetence; *HOC*, hypertrophic obstructive cardiomyopathy; *EDV*, end-diastolic volume; *AS*, aortic stenosis

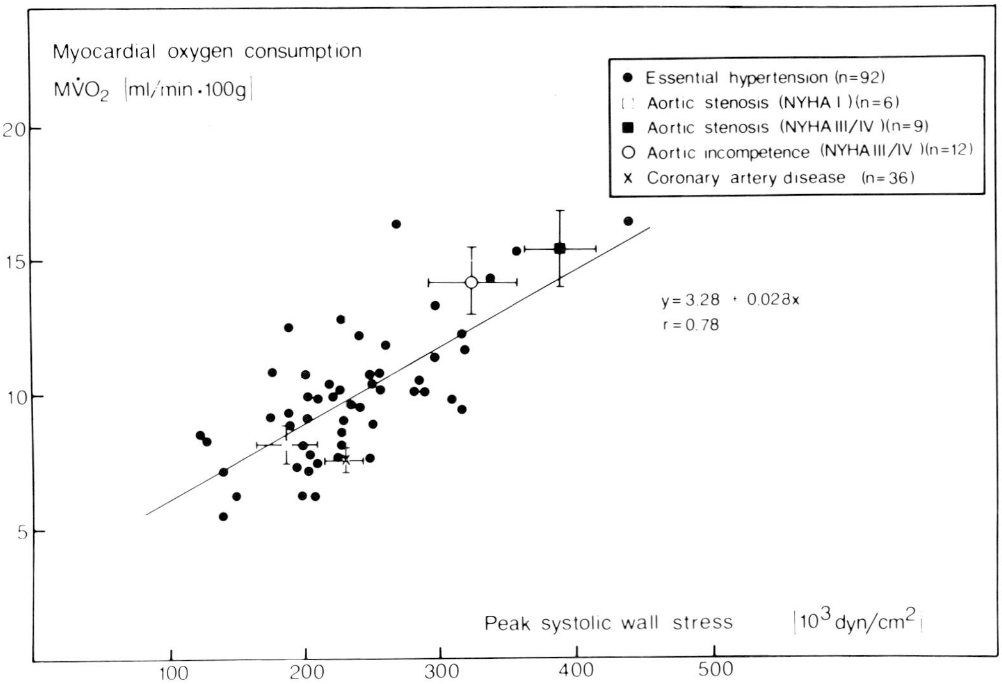

Fig. 16. Relation between peak systolic wall stress per cross-sectional area unit (abscissa) and the myocardial oxygen consumption per 100 g of LV weight unit (MVO_2, *ordinate)*. Note the following: (1) MVO_2 in essential hypertension may be normal, increased or even decreased, the amount of myocardial energy demand being closely related to systolic wall stress, and hence to both systolic pressure load and to the appropriateness of left ventricular hypertrophy. (2) Extrapolation of regression to zero stress results in an intercept of 3.28 ml/min x 100 g. This value, although somewhat higher, corresponds quite well with the oxygen consumption of the empty beating heart. *n*, number of subjects; *NYHA*, New York Heart Association; and *r*, correlation coefficient

mal subjects (peak systolic wall stress = 220 ± 9 x 10^3 dynes/cm^2), patients with chronic hypertrophy may have a decreased, normal, or increased peak systolic wall stress. Thus, both low and high stress hypertrophy may occur, with the ratio between maximal and minimal stress averaging 4.5 (Table 4).

Discussion

Left Ventricular Function. This study has shown that LV function in hypertensive heart disease may remain normal in the presence of marked LV hypertrophy (group I), even when associated with coronary arterial stenosis (group II). Thus, an increase in LV mass due to chronic pressure overload need not necessarily be associated with impaired LV function [3, 4]. The data on hypertensive

Table 4. Reserve capacities of the human heart

		Minimum	Maximum	Maximum / Minimum	
T_{syst}	$[10^3 dyn/cm^2]$[a]	100 ± 12	450 ± 46	4.5	= Stress reserve
$M\dot{V}O_2$	[ml/min·100 g][b]	5.2 ± 0.3	24 ± 2.9	4.6	= Metabolic reserve
V_{cor}	[ml/min·100 g][c]	79 ± 12	392 ± 26	4.9	= Coronary reserve

[a] Essential hypertension
[b] Chronic valvular and hypertensive pressure overload
[c] Normals (before and after dipyridamole: 0.5 mg/kg)

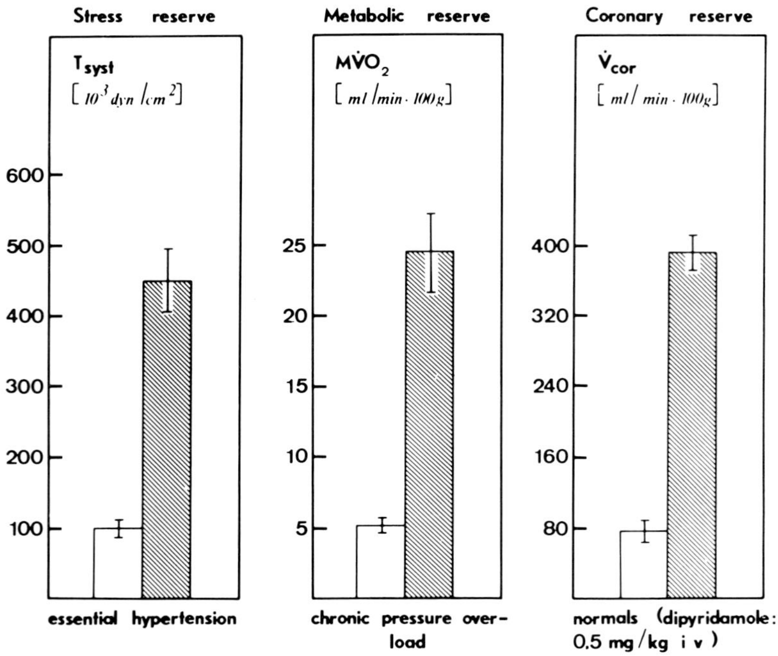

Fig. 17. Stress reserve, metabolic reserve, and coronary reserve

hypertrophy in our patients appeared to diverge in this respect from data reported in other types of pressure-induced left ventricular hypertrophy (such as aortic stenosis or coarctation of aorta); in the latter conditions, studies by others [24–26] indicated that depression of ventricular function was the rule, as evidenced by decreases of both isovolumic and ejection phase indexes. Normal contractile behavior of hypertrophied myocardium was also reported in rats with spontaneous hypertension [27–29]. It may be reasonable to assume that the specific circumstances of the hypertensive disease as well as the type of chronic pressure overload play an important role in the ventricular performance in hypertensive hypertrophy.

Stress and Function. Left ventricular function in hypertensive heart disease depended closely on heart size and, with comparable systolic pressure, on the systolic stress that is imposed at the LV wall [23]. Peak systolic wall stress and LV function were inversely related (Fig. 8). Systolic wall stress may be considered the fundamental correlate of the LV afterload. Therefore, the characteristic inverse relation between stress and function underlines the important influence of systolic wall stress or afterload on LV performance in hypertrophic heart disease. Since other factors, such as contractility and heart rate, may influence LV performance, the steepness of regression between stress and function may presumably be modified at various contractile states and heart rates.

Appropriateness of Left Ventricular Hypertrophy. Systolic wall stress is the consequence of changes in mass, ventricular volume, and systolic pressure. In acute pressure overload, systolic stress increases in parallel with an increase in pressure, because the mass to volume ratio (or wall thickness to radius ratio) remains nearly unaltered. In chronic pressure and volume overload, systolic stress is altered in accordance with chronically altered LV geometry (mass to volume ratio). In either condition, systolic stress reflects the response in ventricular hypertrophy to the acute or chronic LV overload. Therefore, LV hypertrophy may be appropriate or inappropriate with regard to the systolic stress changes that depend on the mass or volume changes relative to load [20—22]. This concept implies that systolic stress represents the afterload imposed on the LV wall [3, 4, 30].

The degree or appropriateness of left ventricular hypertrophy may be described by: (1) the relation between the mass to volume ratio and peak circumferential systolic wall stress (Fig. 5) or (2) the relation among systolic pressure, mass to volume ratio, and peak systolic wall stress when considering instantaneous systolic pressure (Fig. 7). With regard to this relation at least three types of LV hypertrophy may be separated in chronic hypertrophic heart disease [3, 4, 30] (Fig. 18): (1) appropriate hypertrophy, which keeps peak systolic stress normal, even at an extreme pressure load, as a result of an appropriate increase in mass to volume ratio parallel with pressure load; (2) inappropriate excess hypertrophy (low stress hypertrophy), which is associated with marked increase in LV mass out of proportion to intraventricular volume; and (3) inappropriate low hypertrophy (high stress hypertrophy), which is characterized by excess ventricular dilatation out of proportion to ventricular mass development. Thus, at least two forms of inappropriate hypertrophy may occur in chronic hypertrophic heart disease.

Appropriateness of Left Ventricular Hypertrophy, Ventricular Function, and MVO_2. The degreee of appropriateness of LV hypertrophy profoundly influenced both LV function and myocardial oxygen consumption (Fig. 8, 16):

1. Hypertrophy with an increase in wall stress associated with normal or decreased mass to volume ratio was regularly associated with increased MVO_2.

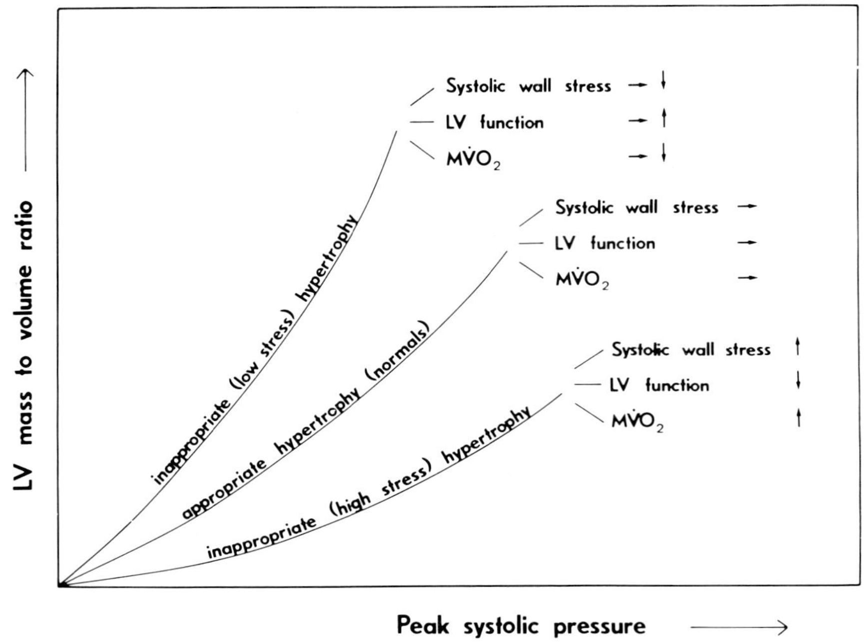

Fig. 18. Classification of hypertrophic heart disease with regard to the degree or appropriateness of LV hypertrophy (see Fig. 2, 7). MVO_2, myocardial oxygen consumption

Ventricular performance was depressed under these conditions, and LV hypertrophy was inappropriate and out of proportion to the pressure and volume demand of the left ventricle.

2. Hypertrophy associated with normal wall stress and normal LV function and MVO_2 or LV hypertrophy was appropriate with regard to the pressure and volume demand.

3. In hypertrophy associated with low peak systolic wall stress and large mass to volume ratio there was normal or increased LV function and normal or decreased MVO_2. Left ventricular hypertrophy was inappropriate, that is, out of proportion to the pressure and volume demand of the left ventricle.

The existence of both low and high stress hypertrophy in chronic heart disease may help to explain the difference in oxygen demand as well as the variable results that have been reported for LV oxygen consumption in patients with a chronically hypertrophied heart. For example, in aortic stenosis a 4.14-fold variation in MVO_2 has been reported (from 5.8 to 24 ml/min x 100 g). In essential hypertension the range of MVO_2 extends from approximately 5.2 to 16 ml/min x 100 g (3.1-fold) [8, 22, 31, 32]. These variations seem controversial and may be due in part to variations in heart rate, cardiac work, or contractility.

It appears somewhat surprising that a large MVO_2 was found in patients with the lowest values for LV function and contractility and that the lowest MVO_2 was present in patients with normal LV function and contractility, particularly in those with essential hypertension, who had significant increases in the maximal rate of pressure development (dP/dt_{max}) (Tables 1 and 2). This result may be the consequence of a minor influence of contractility on overall MVO_2 in chronic heart disease or the result of a disproportionate interplay between the contractile state and systolic wall stress in favor of a dominant influence of peak systolic wall stress on cardiac oxygen demand. There is little question that contractile state influences myocardial oxygen consumption, especially also valid for chronic hypertrophic heart disease in relation to acute inotropic interventions [33, 34]. However, in chronic hypertensive heart disease, the oxygen consumption of the heart is mainly governed quantitatively by alterations in wall stress. This phenomenon obviously reflects a mismatch between stress and contractility in favor of a predominant influence of stress on myocardial energy demand in chronic hypertrophic heart disease.

In a quantitative sense, systolic wall stress, as demonstrated by our study, may play the major role and may predominantly influence MVO_2. Thus, a depressed contractile state may be associated with an increase in MVO_2 when peak systolic wall stress is increased (essential hypertension group IV, aortic stenosis, and aortic incompetence in functional classes III and IV), and decreased MVO_2 may be present during normal contractility when peak systolic wall stress is decreased (essential hypertension group I, aortic stenosis, and aortic incompetence in functional classes I and II).

Pressure-Induced Stress Alterations and MVO_2. An increase (hypertensive crisis) or decrease (antihypertensive treatment) in systolic pressure is associated with alterations in systolic wall stress and, hence, in MVO_2. However, pressure-induced stress alterations depend on the individual isobaric conditions as well as on the initial mass to volume ratio (Fig. 19). An equal rise in pressure (for example, from 120 to 200 mm Hg). ($A' \rightarrow B'$), at a mass to volume ratio of 4 g/ml leads to a stress increase of only 80×10^3 dynes/cm^2, whereas the same rise in pressure ($A \rightarrow B$) at a mass to volume ratio of 1.2 is followed by a considerable increase in stress of 180×10^3 dynes/cm^2. The same calculations and consequences as to systolic stress and, hence, MVO_2 are valid for therapeutically induced pressure reductions. This means that from a diagnostic and prognostic point of view, a rise in systolic pressure in a dilated hypertensive heart causes a greater increase in peak systolic wall stress and in MVO_2 than the same pressure increase in a nondilated, hypertensive heart. Because both stress and metabolic reserve are limited in man, the left ventricular stress capacity is increasingly reduced with: (1) an increase in initial systolic stress, (2) a decrease in mass to volume ratio, and (3) an increase in systolic pressure. However, a therapeutic reduction in systolic pressure will lead to greater reduction in both

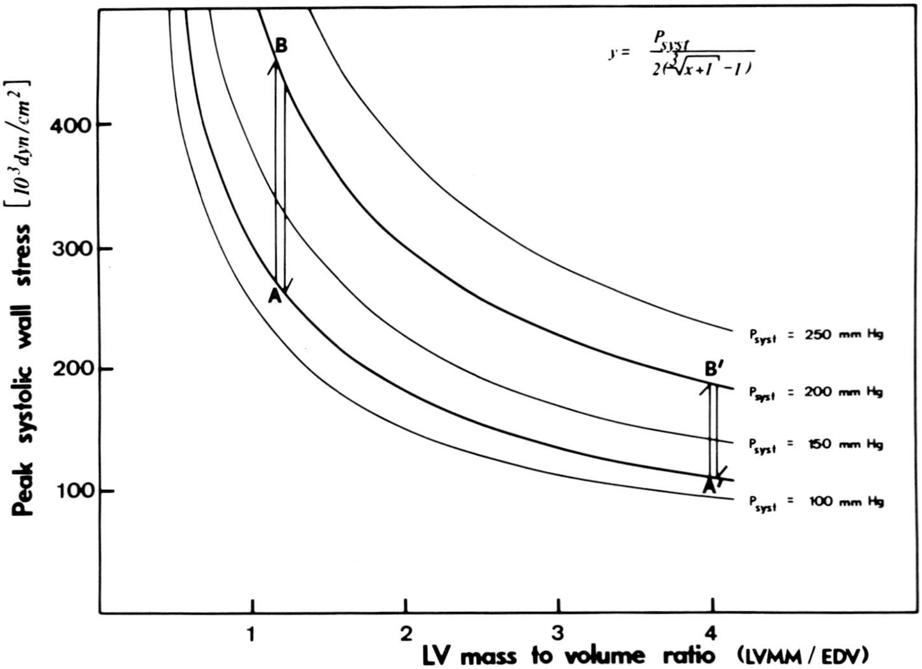

Fig. 19. Representation of concept of the relation between mass to volume ratio (*abscissa*) and peak systolic wall stress (*ordinate*) for different isobaric conditions (for original data, see Table 1). Calculation of isobars was performed with use of the Laplace equation. The lack of parallelism and curvature of these isobaric relations implies that systolic pressure (P_{syst}) changes occurring at points with a high mass to volume ratio lead to fewer stress changes than the same systolic pressure variations at a low mass to volume ratio. An equal increase in systolic pressure, for example, from 120 to 200 mm Hg (that is, from B to A), at a mass to volume ratio of 3.5 leads to a stress increase of only 80 units (10^3 dynes/cm^2). However, with the same increase in pressure (that is, from B′ to A′) at a mass to volume ratio of 1.5, systolic wall stress is considerably increased (by 160 units). The same consequences are valid for therapeutically induced pressure reductions (from A′ to B′ and from A to B, respectively). This means that the increase in systolic wall stress at a given rise in systolic pressure in hypertensive heart disease is greater in the dilated than in the nondilated heart. Conversely, systolic and metabolic unloading of the left ventricle at equal pressure reduction is greater or more effective in a dilated than in a nondilated heart. This relation between mass to volume ratio and stress emphasizes the importance of heart size and systolic wall stress on changes in stress and, hence, in ventricular function and myocardial energy demand

stress and oxygen consumption in patients with LV dilatation than in patients with concentric hypertrophy. Thus, the relation between mass to volume ratio and peak systolic wall stress elucidates the importance of pressure-dependent changes in systolic stress and, hence, in myocardial stress and metabolic reserve.

Coronary Reserve. The increase in coronary resistance under resting conditions (Table 3) can presumably be related to increased tone of the coronary vascular bed in essential hypertension. However, there may be at least three possible reasons for the reduced coronary reserve: (1) In theory, the responsiveness to dipyridamole, which was used as the test agent, could be altered; however, no alteration in coronary sensitivity to dipyridamole-induced coronary dilatation has been documented to date. (2) The hypertrophied ventricular wall could restrict coronary dilatation. However, in aortic stenosis as well as in hypertrophic obstructive cardiomyopathy normal coronary reserve has been found with a normal coronary arteriogram [35, 36]. (3) Increased coronary vascular tone could limit complete coronary dilatation. Because the coronary resistance is already increased in essential hypertension at rest, the minimal coronary resistance after maximal coronary dilatation would be increased, even with normal coronary reserve. Thus, a functional increase in the tone of coronary resistance vessels could limit coronary reserve.

Coronary Reserve, Systolic Wall Stress and MVO_2. The decrease in coronary reserve with the increase in peak systolic wall stress may be related to the increase in MVO_2 in parallel with augmentation of peak systolic wall stress (Fig. 16). Because a rise in MVO_2 is accomplished by a rise in coronary flow, the lattter is already increased at resting conditions. Consequently, the dipyridamole-estimated coronary reserve becomes progressively decreased with an increase in MVO_2, with a decrease in the mass to volume ratio, and with an increase in systolic wall stress (Fig. 20). The coronary reserve would be influenced by myocardial contraction abnormalities as well as by coronary arterial lesions, primarily as a result of coronary stenosis [31, 37]. In patients with coronary artery disease a marked decrease in coronary reserve (mean 2.01 ± 0.12) was found. This is most obviously due to coronary atherosclerosis and, hence, to the impaired dilating capacity of the coronary vascular bed. In vasculitis, lupus erythematosus, and scleroderma heart disease a considerable reduction in coronary reserve may occur even with normal coronary arteries and normal heart size [4, 19, 21]. This has been referred to as vasculitic involvement of the small coronary arteries, which in a great percentage of cases are histologically affected [3].

Independent from coronary lesions the coronary reserve may even be greatly reduced in LV enlargement associated with high end-diastolic pressure. In these diseases (congestive heart failure and congestive cardiomyopathy, for example) an increased myocardial, that is, extravascular, component will be responsible for the decrease in coronary reserve. This may be attributed to enhancement of the extraordinary tissue resistance, reduction in the driving coronary perfusion pressure, impaired course of contraction and relaxation and, hence impaired coronary perfusion.

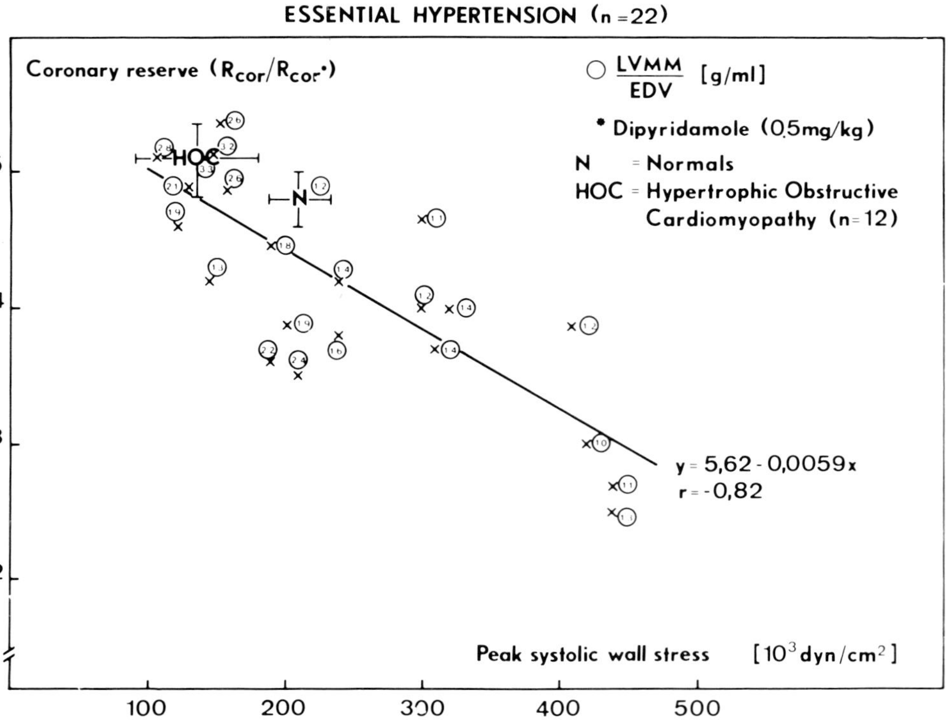

Fig. 20. Relation between peak systolic wall stress and coronary reserve in the normal subjects and in patients with hypertrophic obstructive cardiomyopathy (*HOC*) and essential hypertension (*crosses*). *Encircles numbers* represent the mass to volume ratio (*LVMM/EDV*), *r*, correlation coefficient; R_{cor}, coronary resistance; $R_{cor}*$, coronary resistance under maximal conditions

Finally, clinical diseases with an increased resting MVO_2 (high stress hypertrophy, for example, in decompensated hypertrophic heart disease) may limit coronary reserve. Thus, the coronary reserve depends on coronary and extracoronary (that is, myocardial) factors. In a quantitative sense, the coronary lesions may affect or reduce the coronary reserve more than extravascular and myocardial abnormalities [38—40].

Fig. 22. Relationship between LV mass to volume ratio and systolic wall stress. ▶ The *hatched region* indicates maximum stress that can be developed and obtained from human myocardium. Data have been derived from experiments on the isolated human ventricular myocardium [31]. The *vertical arrows* indicate ranges of stress that can be developed. At large initial mass to volume ratio (i.e., at low initial systolic wall stress) large stress can be additionally developed until the maximum stress value is reached. However, at initially low mass to volume ratio (i.e., at initially large systolic wall stress) the additional systolic stress is reduced; hence, the systolic stress reserve is diminished in the high stress hypertrophies. *LVMM*, left ventricular mass; *EDV*, end-diastolic volume

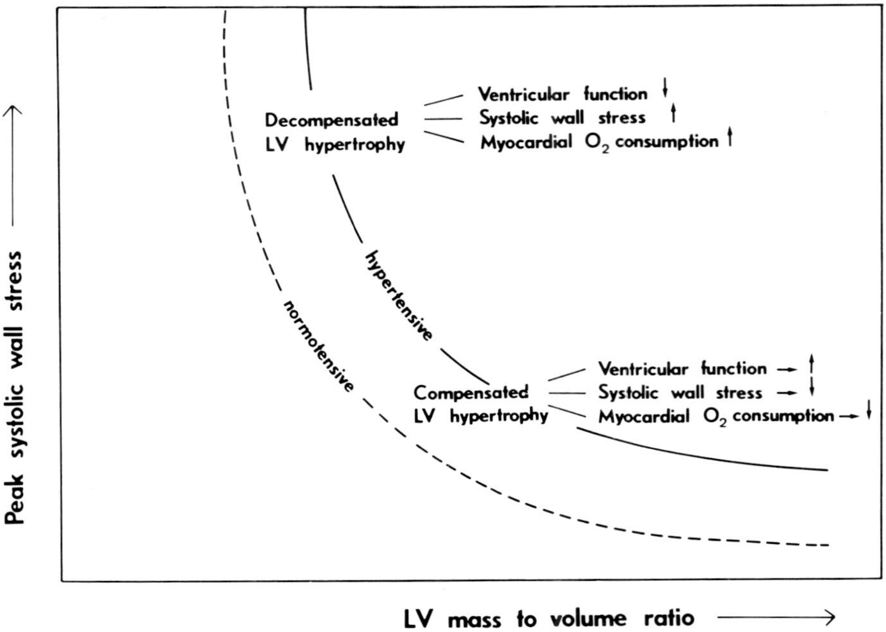

Fig. 21. Representations of the appropriateness of LV hypertrophy as derived from the inverse relationship between LV mass to volume ratio and systolic wall stress

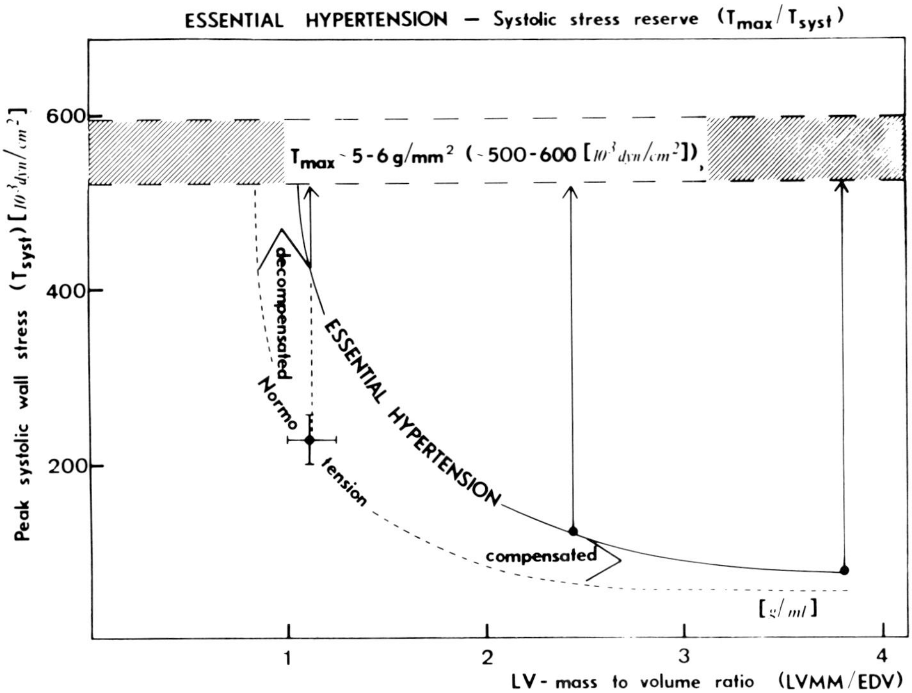

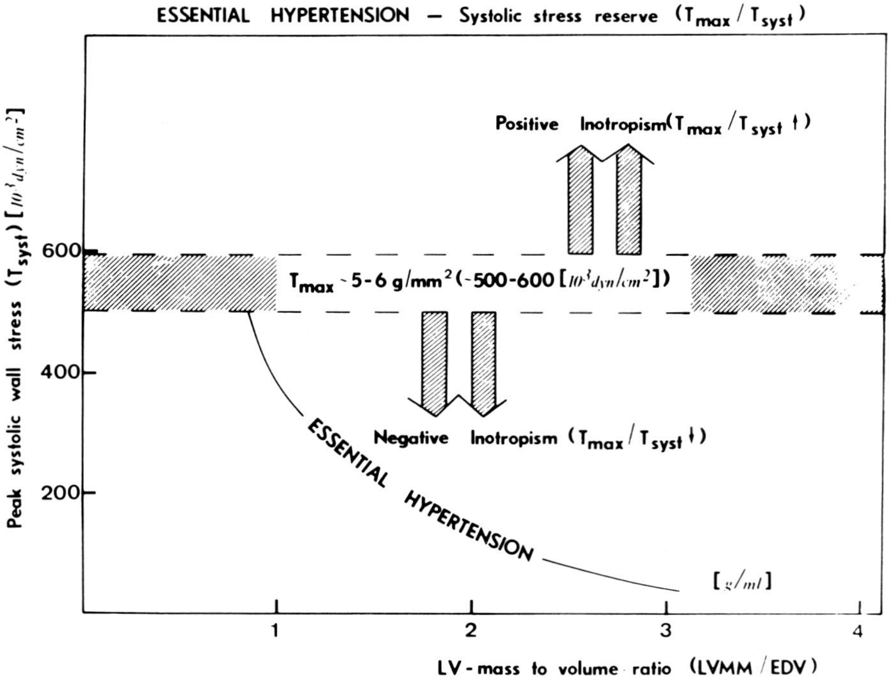

Fig. 23. Variation of systolic stress reserve by inotropic interventions

Relations Among Coronary, Metabolic, and Systolic Stress Reserves. A close relation seems to be present among the coronary, metabolic and systolic stress reserves (Table 4, Figs. 21—23) of the LV. This obviously helps to explain the limited LV function or reserve capacity, or both, in disorders associated with coronary (for example, in coronary artery disease), metabolic (for example, in hyperthyroidism) and systolic wall stress abnormalities (for example, in decompensated LV pressure overload). Because the human heart works almost exclusively aerobically, an increase in left ventricular function may be accomplished preferably by an increase in myocardial oxygen supply. In coronary artery disease, the coronary reserve is limited because of coronary stenosis. Accordingly, the coronary factor is the limiting link that diminishes the oxygen availability to the myocardium, thereby restricting both the metabolic and systolic stress reserves. In hyperthyroid heart disease an increased MVO_2 occurs due to excess increase in heart rate, cardiac output, and contractility [41—43], thus narrowing both the coronary and systolic stress reserves. Here the increased metabolism seems to play the limiting role. In decompensated LV pressure overload, as has been shown previously, both the coronary and metabolic reserves are reduced because the stress level is already elevated at rest. Thus, increased LV loading conditions at rest may skim off maximal stress capacity.

It can be concluded from these results that systolic wall stress reflects the major determinant of the degree of LV hypertrophy and plays a predominant role in both LV function and myocardial energy balance. The coronary, metabolic, and systolic stress reserves of the human heart seem to be closely correlated with each other, and it is reasonable to assume that determination of coronary reserve gives important insight into the LV metabolic and working capacity reserves.

Summary

Left ventricular function, wall geometry, and coronary hemodynamics were analyzed in 114 patients with essential hypertension during diagnostic left heart catheterization, left ventriculography, and coronary arteriography. The findings were compared with data from patients with normotensive and hypertensive, hypertrophic heart disease.

1. Left ventricular function (as assessed from the cardiac index, stroke volume index, ejection fraction, mean velocity of circumferential fiber shortening, mean normalized systolic ejection rate, and isovolumic indexes) was normal in patients with hypertensive hypertrophy, even with a large increase in muscle mass and even in the presence of concomitant coronary artery disease. Left ventricular function was impaired when regional contraction abnormalities or ventricular dilatation, or both, occurred and was inversely related to both cardiac size and systolic wall stress.

2. Coronary blood flow (+ 18%), coronary resistance (+ 38%), and MVO_2 (+ 21%) were increased in essential hypertension. Coronary reserve was reduced even in hypertensive hypertrophy without evidence of coronary artery disease. MVO_2 per mass unit was directly correlated with systolic wall stress per cross-sectional area of LV wall.

3. The appropriateness of LV hypertrophy may be defined by the relation between pressure, mass to volume ratio, and systolic wall stress. In hypertensive heart disease at least two types of inappropriate LV hypertrophy occur: (1) low stress hypertrophy, with an increased mass to volume ratio, with normal LV function, and with normal or reduced MVO_2 ; and (2) high stress hypertrophy, with normal or low mass to volume ratio, impaired LV function, and increased MVO_2.

4. The range of systolic wall stress was 100—450 x 10^3 dynes/cm^2 and reflects the stress that could be altered by inotropic interventions and changes in systolic pressure. A similar reserve capacity is present for both the metabolic and the coronary reserves. Total LV oxygen consumption is related to total LV mass. This relation is influenced by the degree of viability of LV mass, by the mass to volume ratio, and by inotropic interventions. Left ventricular oxygen consumption per viable mass unit (MVO_2) is significantly correlated with the systolic force per unit corss-sectional area of the LV wall, that is, with LV systolic wall stress.

It can be concluded that the appropriateness of LV hypertrophy, as a result of mass to volume ratio and stress, is a major determinant of LV performance and of myocardial oxygen consumption and that the individual history of LV pressure load may specifically influence LV function.

References

1. World Health Organisation (1959) Hypertension and coronary heart disease: Classification and criteria for epidemiological studies. First report of the expert committee on cardiovascular diseases and hypertension. WHO Tech Rep Ser 168
2. World Health Organisation (1962) Arterial hypertension and ischemic heart disease, preventive aspects. Report of an expert committee. WHO Tech Rep Ser 231
3. Strauer BE (1977) Ventrikelfunktion und koronare Hämodynamik bei der essentiellen Hypertonie. Verh Dtsch Ges Kreislaufforsch 43 : 41—55
4. Strauer BE (1979) Das Hochdurckherz. Springer, Berlin Heidelberg New York
5. Lund-Johansen P (1970) Physiological symptoms and signs of incipient cardiac insufficiency in arterial hypertension: Changes in the physiological data announcing failure. In: Symposium on incipient cardiac insufficiency, European Society of Cardiology. Locarno, Sandoz pp 119—125
6. Frohlich ED, Tarazi RC, Dustan HP (1971) Clinical-physiological correlations in the development of hypertensive heart disease. Ciruculation 44 : 446—455
7. Criteria Committee of the New York Heart Association (1973) Nomenclature and criteria for the diagnosis of diseases of the heart and great vessels, 7th edn. Little Brown, Boston p 286
8. Strauer BE, Beer K, Heitlinger K, Höfling B (1977) Left ventricular systolic wall stress as a primary determinant of myocardial oxygen consumption: Comparative studies in patients with normal left ventricular function, with pressure and volume overload and with coronary heart disease. Basic Res Cardiol 72 : 306—313
9. Greene DG, Carlisle B, Grant C, Bunnell I (1967) Estimation of left ventricular volume by one-plane cineangiography. Circulation 35 : 61—69
10. Hood WP (1971) Dynamics of hypertrophy in left ventricular wall of man. In: Alpert NR (ed) Cardiac hypertrophy. Academic Press, New York 445—452
11. Rackley CE, Dodge HT, Coble YD, Hay RE (1964) Method of determining left ventricular mass in man. Circulation 29 : 666—671
12. Hood WP, Rackley CE, Rolett EL (1968) Wall stress in the normal and hypertrophied human left ventricle. Am J Cardiol 22 : 550—558
13. Sandler H, Dodge HT (1963) Left ventricular tension and stress in man. Circ Res 13 : 91—104
14. Sandler H, Dodge HT (1968) The use of single plane angiocardiogram for the calculation of left ventricular volume in man. Am Heart J 55 : 325—334

15. Hugenholtz PG, Kaplan E, Bull E (1969) Determination of left ventricular wall thickness by angiocardiography. Am Heart J 78 : 513—522
16. Gaasch WH, Battle WE, Oboler HH, Banas JS, Levine HJ (1972) Left ventricular stress and compliance in man. Circulation 45 : 746—762
17. Bretschneider HJ, Cott L, Hilgert G, Probst R, Rau G (1966) Gaschromatische Trennung und Analyse von Argon als Basis einer neuen Fremdgasmethode zur Durchblutungsmessung von Organen. Verh Dtsch Ges Kreislaufforsch 32 : 267—273
18. Tauchert M (1973) Koronarreserve und maximaler Sauerstoffverbrauch des menschlichen Herzens. Basic Res Cardiol 68 : 1—83
19. Strauer BE, Brune I, Schenk H, Knoll D, Perings E (1976) Lupus cardiomyopathy: Cardiac mechanics, hemodynamics, and coronary blood flow in uncomplicated systemic lupus erythematosus. Am Heart J 92 : 715—722
20. Strauer BE, Scherpe A (1976) Ventricular function and coronary hemodynamics after intravenous nitroglycerin in coronary artery disease. Am Heart J 95 : 210—219
21. Strauer BE (1977) Die quantitative Bestimmung der Koronarreserve in der Diagnostik koronarer Durchblutungsstörungen. Internist (Berlin) 18 : 579—587
22. Strauer BE, Tauchert M, Cott L, Kochsiek K, Bretschneider HJ (1970) Simultane Bestimmung des Sauerstoffverbrauches und der Coronardurchblutung des linken Ventrikels bei Mitral- und Aortenklappenfehlern mit einem neuen hämodynamischen Parameter und der Argon-Fremdgasmethode. Verh Dtsch Ges Inn Med 76 : 217—220
23. Strauer BE, Bürger SB (1977) Dynamic geometry of the left ventricle in essential hypertension (abstr). Circulation [Suppl III] 56 : 118
24. Meerson FS (1969) Hyperfunktion, Hypertrophie und Insuffizienz des Herzens. Volk & Gesundheit, Berlin
25. Simon H, Krayenbühl HP, Rutishauser W, Preter B (1970) The contractile state of the hypertrophied left ventricular myocardium in aortic stensosis. Am Heart J 79 : 587—602
26. Spann JF, Buccino RA, Sonnenblick EH, Braunwald E (1967) Contractile state of cardiac muscle obtained from cats with experimentally produced ventricular hypertrophy and heart failure. Circ Res 21 : 341—354
27. Bürger SB, Strauer BE (1977) Dynamics of left ventricular hypertrophy and contraction in spontaneously hypertensive rats (abstr). Circulation [Suppl III] 56 : 234
28. Bürger SB, Strauer BE (1978) Left ventricular geometry and wall stress in various stages of hypertrophy due to spontaneous essential hypertension (abstr). Circulation [Suppl II] 57/58 : 158
29. Bürger SB, Meinardus A, Strauer BE (1978) Hypertrophiegrad und Dynamik des linken Ventrikels bei der spontanen essentiellen Hypertonie der Ratte. Klin Wochenschr 57 : 207—209
30. Weber KT, Janicki JS (1977) Instantaneous force-velocity-length relations: Experimental findings and clinical correlations. Am J Cardiol 40 : 740—747
31. Strauer BE (1975) Dynamik, Koronardurchblutung und Sauerstoffverbrauch des normalen und kranken Herzens. Karger, Basel, pp 72—81

32. Johnson LL, Sciacca RR, Ellis K, Weiss MB, Cannon PJ (1978) Reduced left ventricular myocardial blood flow per unit mass in aortic stenosis. Circulation 57 : 582—590
33. Braunwald E (1971) Control of myocardial oxygen consumption. Physiological and clinical considerations. Am J Cardiol 27 : 416—432
34. Bretschneider HJ (1967) Aktuelle Probleme der Koronardurchblutung und des Myokardstoffwechsels. Regensburger Aerztl Fortbild 1 : 11
35. Kochsiek K, Heiss HW, Tauchert M, Strauer BE (1971) Koronarreserve und Sauerstoffverbrauch bei hypertrophischer obstruktiver Cardiomyopathie. Verh Dtsch Ges Inn Med 27 : 880—883
36. Kochsiek K, Tauchert M, Cott L, Neubaur J (1970) Die Koronarreserve bei Patienten mit Aortenvitien. Ver Dtsch Ges Inn Med 76 : 214—218
37. Kathke N (1955) Die Veränderungen der Koronararterienzweige des Myokards bei Hypertonie. Beitr Pathol Anat 115 : 405
37a. James TN (1977) Small arteries of the heart. Circulation 56 : II—114
38. Strauer BE, Heitlinger KH, Bürger SB (1977) Coronary hemodynamics and myocardial oxygen consumption in essential hypertension (abstr). Circulation [Suppl II] 56 : III—818
39. Strauer BE (1979) Myocardial oxygen consumption in chronic heart disease: Role of wall stress, hypertrophy and coronary reserve. Am J Cardiol 44 : 730—740
40. Strauer BE (1980) Hypertensive heart disease. Springer, Berlin Heidelberg New York
41. Bretschneider HJ (1967) Aktuelle Probleme der Koronardurchblutung und des Myokardstoffwechsels. Regensburg Aerztl Fortbild 15 : 1—27
42. Strauer BE, Scherpe A (1975) Myocardial mechanics and oxygen consumption in experimental hyperthyroidism. In: Roy PE, Harris P (ed) The cardiac sarcoplasm. University Park Press, Baltimore, pp 495—502
43. Strauer BE, Scherpe A (1975) Experimental hyperthyroidism IV. Myocardial muscle mechanics and oxygen consumption in eu- and hyperthyroidism. Basic Res Cardiol 70 : 246—255

Part II: Afterload Changes and Ventricular Function

The Pressure-Overloaded Heart: Physiological and Clinical Correlates[1]

K.T. WEBER, N. REICHEK, S. JANICKI AND S. SHROFF

The view of the heart as a mechanical pump has emerged from the classic experiments of Otto Frank and Ernest Starling. According to this concept cardiac performance is expressed in terms of the displacement of blood from its ventricles. The relationship between stroke volume, cardiac output or stroke work, and the diastolic volume of the ventricle has been termed the ventricular function curve. Alterations in the functional state of the ventricle are described by a "family" of such function curves.

In more recent years it has become apparent that the heart is not simply a mechanical pump. The development of pressure and the generation of flow are functions of the muscular fibers which comprise the myocardium surrounding each ventricular chamber. The interrelationship between the force which these fibers must sustain during contraction, their length during contraction, and the contractile state will determine the extent (and rate) of their shortening and consequently the extent of wall shortening and chamber volume displacement. Consequently, the heart may be more logically thought of as a muscular pump [5, 39, 45, 48].

An inverse relation exists between the extent of fiber shortening and the force which these muscular fibers must sustain during their contraction. This represents an important property of the muscular pump. The pressure-overloaded left ventricle (e.g., aortic stenosis, coarctation, or systemic hypertension) is required to generate and maintain an augmented force in order to provide an adequate cardiac output. Through the process of hypertrophy this elevated force is distributed over a larger cross-sectional area of myocardium, thereby maintaining a normal wall stress (i.e., force per unit area of muscle) and pump performance. Eventually, however, and for reasons which are not clearly understood, the pressure-overloaded ventricle fails. In this review we wish to describe the contractile behavior of this mucular pump, the role of hypertrophy in the

1 This work was supported by National Heart, Lung and Blood Institute Grants HL-17441 and HL-18749 and Program Project Grant HL-08805. Drs. Weber and Janicki are the recipients of National Heart, Lung and Blood Institute Research Career Development Awards HL-00187 and HL-00411, respectively

diseased heart, and the results of several clinical studies which utilize these physiological principles to describe cardiac function and the results of therapy in the pressure-overloaded heart.

The Heart as a Muscular Pump

The Concept of Wall Force and Fiber Length

A simple, global description of the muscular pump may be formulated which does not require the precise correlation of force and length at the individual fiber level. Instead, the concept of wall force and a representative fiber length may be used to describe the summated contraction of all fibers [51].

Let us begin by taking an imaginary plane to divide the heart in half as shown in Fig 1. The plane includes a cross-sectional area of each ventricle and the surrounding myocardium. A force is created on either side of the plane which tends to pull the ventricle apart. The magnitude of this force is a function of the pressure inside the chamber and the area of the chamber subtended by the plane. This force, according to Newton's theorem, must be counterbalanced by an equal and opposite force which exists within the rim of myocardium and holds the halves of the ventricle together. In calculating force in this manner we are not dependent on the shape, area, or thickness of the subtended myocardium, the orientation of fibers, or the distribution of forces generated by individual fibers or between fibers. Hence, a net *wall force*, in grams, may be calculated as the product of chamber pressure and the subtended cross-sectional area of the chamber [51]. This concept has been experimentally validated [20].

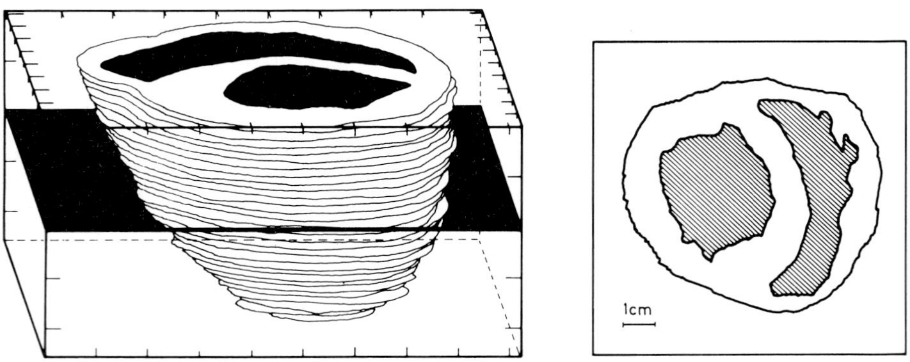

Fig. 1. A computer reconstruction of a sectioned canine heart divided by an imaginary plane. The plane subtends a cross-sectional area of the myocardium, and each ventricle as indicated on the *right*. The net wall force existing in either the right or left ventricular myocardium may be calculated from the produced chamber pressure and the cross-sectional area of the chamber included in the plane

If the ventricle were a perfect thick-walled sphere, then wall force and stress would be equally distributed throughout. The ventricles, however, have irregular shapes and, consequently, the magnitude of force along any given plane will vary according to the dimension of the chamber included in that plane. For the left ventricle, which resembles a truncated ellipsoid of revolution, the force along the minor axis (i.e., meridional force) will be less than that existing along the major axis (i.e., circumferential force), and this difference will be related to the difference in the minor and major axes, respectively.

A representative *length* of muscle fiber may be derived on the basis of the data available on the orientation and distribution of fibers within the myocardium. Streeter et al. [41] have shown that in the left ventricular myocardium of the dog the orientation of fibers may be described as a continuum; discrete muscle bundles are not present. Moreover, the majority of fibers, excluding those within the subendocardium or subepicardium, have a circumferential direction [41] with fibers joined to one another by acute angular branchings. Pearlman and co-workers [30] have recently reported similar observations for the normal human heart. Thus, a circumferential length, calculated for the midwall of the left ventricle, may be used as a reasonable approximation of fiber length.

Properties of the Muscular Pump

The Maximum Force-Length Relation. The contractile behavior of the muscular pump may be described using the concepts of wall force and fiber length. As with any muscle, whether cardiac or skeletal, the relationship between developed force and muscle length provides a useful means to describe its behavior. The maximum force which the muscular wall of the ventricle can develop for any given stretch of its wall is observed in the isovolumetrically beating heart [39, 45, 48, 49, 51, 52]. An isovolumetric beat results when the wall contracts around its ventricular chamber without blood being displaced from the chamber. The essentially linear relation between maximum developed pressure and ventricular volume is shown in panel A of Fig 2. The pressure within the chamber is a result of the contracting fibers and the force which they produce within the wall. Recall that this wall force can be approximated as the product of chamber pressure and chamber area. As a consequence of this transformation the relation between calculated wall force and volume at lesser filling volumes (i.e., corresponding to filling pressure < 5 mm Hg) becomes nonlinear. For the remainder of the physiologic range of filling, however, (i.e., pressures of 5—25 mm Hg) the relation can be considered linear [52]. As previously discussed a circumferential length for the midwall of the left ventricle can be calculated (i.e., assuming the ventricle to be a sphere and using chamber volume and myocardial mass) as a reasonable approximation of fiber length [51, 52]. An example of the relation between midwall circumferential length and chamber volume is given in panel C. Even though this relation is nonlinear, the relation between wall force and fiber length (panel D) is not substantially different in form from that of wall force and volume (panel B). From any of the

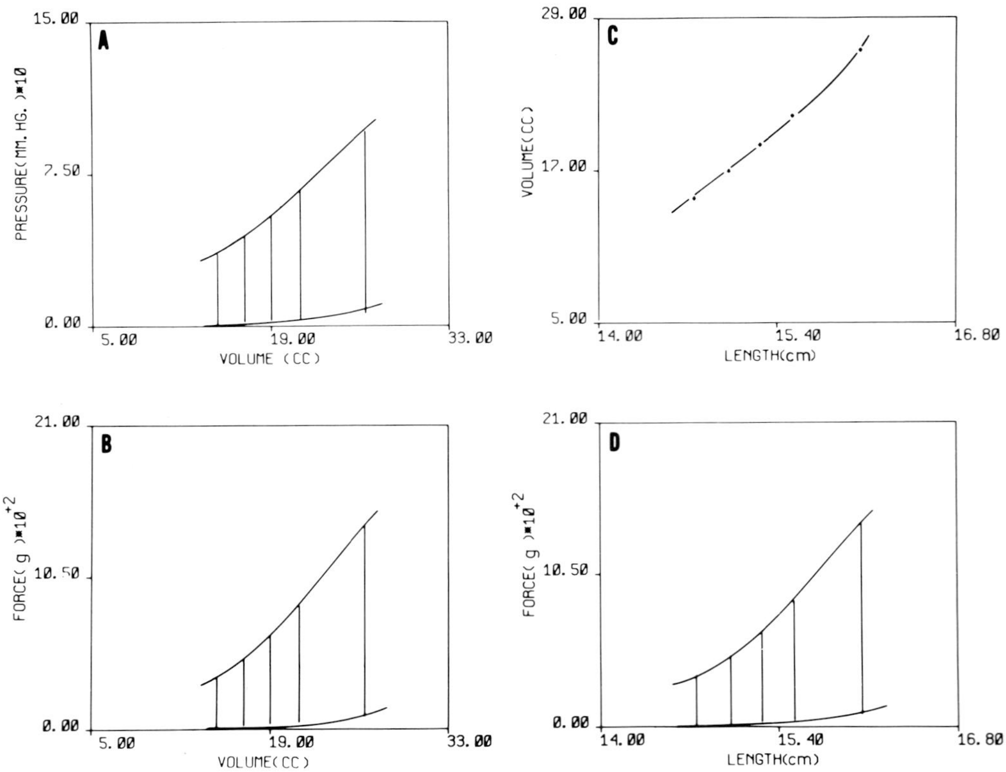

Fig. 2. The interrelationships between peak developed left ventricular pressure and left ventricular volume (A), developed net wall force and filling volume (B), chamber volume and midwall circumferential fiber length (C), and force-length (D) are shown for fiber isovolumetric beats of the intact canine heart. The transformation of pressure and volume to force and fiber length impart a nonlinearitiy to these relations at lower filling volumes

aforementioned relations it is apparent that quite unlike isolated cardiac muscle, a length at which developed force peaks and then subsequently declines has not been observed for the intact ventricle operating within the physiological range of filling pressure. Hence, the intact heart does not demonstrate a maximum length [51, 52].

Pharmacologic or intrinsic alterations in myocardial contractile state produce nonparallel shifts in the developed force-stretch relation [51—53]. As shown in Fig. 3, the sympathomimetic amine, dobutamine, increases the force developed from a given diameter for the minor axis of the left ventricle; negative inotropic agents, such as propranalol, shift the curve downwards and to the right. The extent to which positive inotropic interventions, such as catecholamines or pacing, will augment the force developed for any particular end-diastolic fiber length is determined by the level of 0_2 availability [47, 49]. Once the aerobic capacity of the ventricle has been reached, further increments in contractile

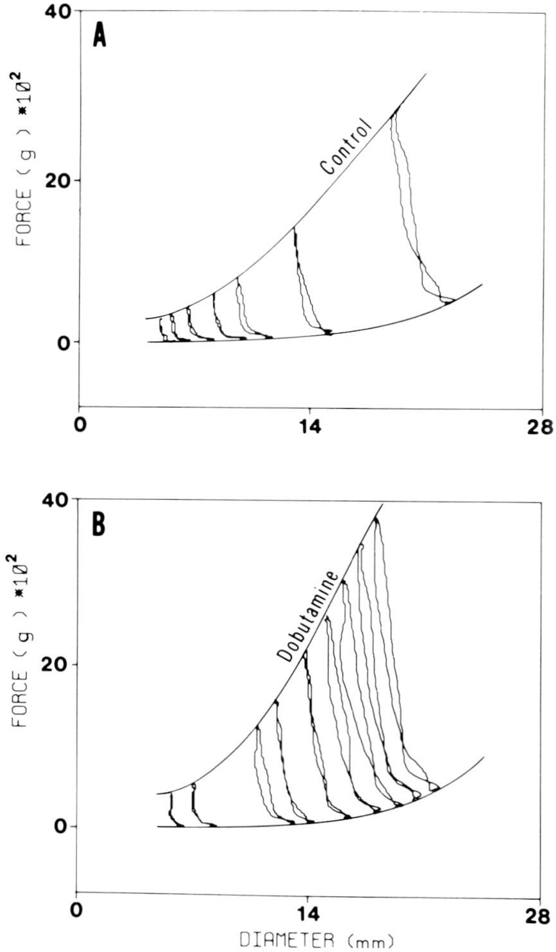

Fig. 3. The augmentation of the left ventricular maximally developed force-minor axis diameter relation following the infusion of the sympathomimetic amine, dobutamine (12 μg/min). Note also that the diameter of the ventricle changes during an isovolumetric contraction and therefore the term isometric (i.e., constant length) does not apply. Reproduced from [50] with permission

state are not possible. In fact, at the aerobic limit, increments in metabolic demand result in the onset of lactate production and the appearance of pulsus alternans [49].

The Limit to Shortening. The maximum developed force-length relation also establishes the limit to which the ejecting ventricle will reduce its size [43, 45, 52] or the length to which contracting muscle will shorten [7]. The force which exists in the wall at end ejection is equal to the maximum force which the given length can sustain. The interrelationship between the isovolumtric

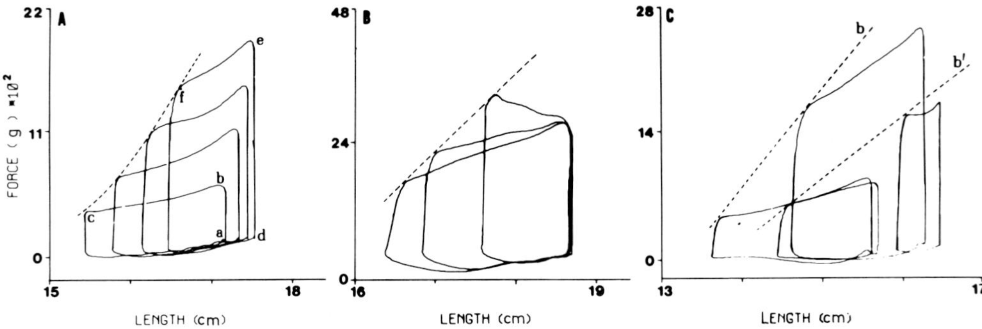

Fig. 4. The interrelationship between the isovolumetric developed force-length relation (*dotted line*) and the end-systolic force-length relation is shown for contractions having different shortening loads (A and B) and following the infusion of propanolol (0.5 mg/min, C). Each panel represents a different heart. See text. Reproduced from [50] with permission

developed force-length and the *end-systolic force-length* relations is shown in Fig. 4 where several force-length loops are given for the ejecting ventricle. From an initial end-diastolic length, given as point *a* in panel A, the ventricle generates force and a corresponding chamber pressure until ejection commences (point *b*). Following its initial rise, force peaks shortly after aortic valve opening and then declines during the remainder of the ejection period. When a force is achieved which is maximal for the given shortening length the muscle fibers are no longer able to shorten and ejection ceases (point *c*). Conceptually, the ventricle has reached its isovolumetric condition. Another contraction, having different loading conditions represented by *def* in Fig. 4 also ceases to shorten when the maximum force-length relation (the dotted line in panel A) is approximated. In panel B of Fig. 4 instantaneous shortening force has been varied from the same onset ejection force. Because these contractions reach the maximal force-length relation differently, three different end-systolic lengths result. Moreover, it is apparent that end-systolic length is independent of the end-diastolic length and onset ejection force which both serve only to establish the starting points of the contraction. The isovolumetric maximum force-length relation also establishes the limit of fiber shortenting following the infusion of catecholamines [43, 52] or negative inotropic interventions [52]. Panel C of Fig. 4 illustrates the interdependence of these relations before (line b) and after beta blockade with propranolol (line b′). As we will discuss subsequently, the derivation of the end-systolic force-length relation may therefore be used to provide an estimate of the contractile state dependent on maximal force-length relation and thereby the contractile state of the myocardium [43, 45, 52].

Determinants of Shortening. From the foregoing discussion, it should be apparent that the shortening of the muscular pump is independent of those conditions of length and force which exist at the onset of shortening (i.e., aortic valve opening). The contracting fibers are responsive to the force which exists at each

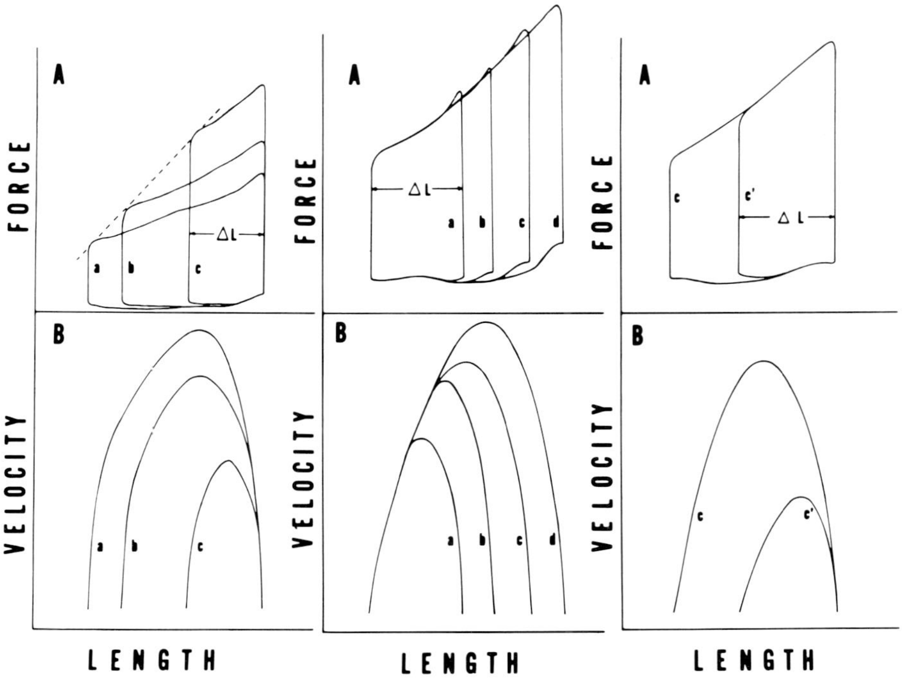

Fig. 5. The extent (ΔL) and rate (velocity) of shortening of the muscle fibers are regulated by instantaneous shortening load (*left hand* A and B), instantaneous shortening length (*middle panels*), and myocardial contractile state (*right hand panels*, before and after beta blockade with propranolol, beats c and c′, respectively). Adapted from [48] with permission

instant of ejection. The influence of *instantaneous shortening load*, or ejection force, on fiber shortening represents an important property of cardiac muscle [4] and the intact heart [45]. The inverse relation between the rate and extent of midwall circumferential fiber shortening and shortening load is demonstrated in the left hand panels of Fig. 5. Because fiber shortening is determined by the instantaneous force opposing that shortening, beat *a*, having the lowest shortening force, has the greatest extent and rate (velocity) of shortening. The response of the muscular wall to instantaneous shortening load is further underscored by the three variably loaded contractions given in panel B of Fig. 4, where that beat, having an ejection force of ever increasing magnitude, has the smallest change in fiber length or shortening. In the enlarged and failing heart the reduction in ventricular dimension is markedly attenuated. As a result the absolute level of ejection force is elevated. Hence, the failing heart has lost the advantage of being able to unload itself and consequently works at a mechanical disadvantage [5, 45, 48].

Instantaneous shortening length is another major determinant of shortening. In the middle panels of Fig. 5, instantaneous shortening load has been held constant while instantaneous shortening length has been raised by increasing the onset (end-diastolic) contraction length. Contraction *d*, having the greatest instantaneous length, shortens to a greater extent (and with greater speed) than the other beats of lesser length. The ventricular function curve of the traditional pump concept may be derived from these shortening-length relations (vide infra) [48, 50].

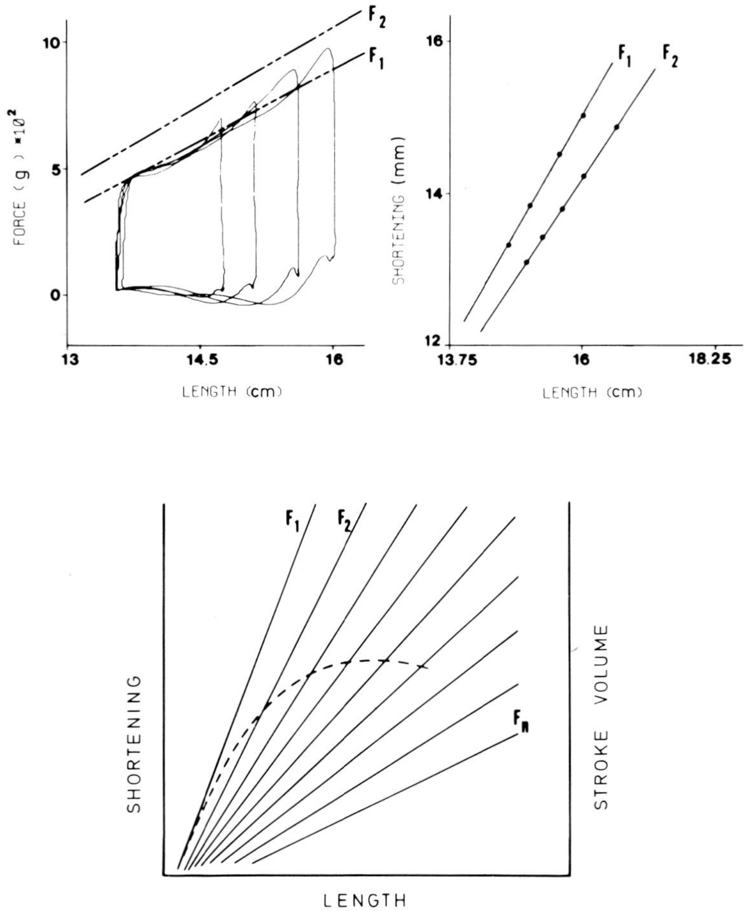

Fig. 6. The ventricular function curve may be derived from the shortening-length relationship of the muscular pump. In the *upper left hand panel*, the extent of shortening is seen to be a function of instantaneous shortening length for a given shortening load trajectory (F_1). As this shortening load is increased to a higher plane (F_2) shortening is less for an equivalent shortening length examined for F_1. Similarly, the shortening end-diastolic length relation is shifted downward and to the right for F_2 *(upper right panel)*. A function curve is derived by determining the response in stroke volume during the expansion of intracardiac and intravascular volume and a result during progressive increments in wall force. Hence, the function curve traverses a series of shortening-length relations. Reproduced from [50] with permission

The other major determinant of shortening relates to the *contractile state* of the myocardium. In the right hand panels of Fig. 5 are shown two contractions having essentially equivalent instantaneous shortening loads and lengths. Contraction c', however, was examined following beta blockade. As a result of the depression in contractile state, the extent and velocity of shortening are reduced. A positive shift in contractility, on the other hand, would increase shortening and consequently stroke volume.

The ventricular function curve may be derived from the shortening-length relations of this muscular pump [48, 50]. As shown in Fig. 6 (upper left panel) the extent of shortening, or change in fiber length, is a function of instantaneous shortening length, provided that the time course of the instantaneous shortening load trajectory is common to each beat. Such a common trajectory is indicated by F_1. For a higher shortening load, F_2, the extent of shortening is less for equivalent shortening lengths examined during F_1. The relation between the extent of shortening and the initial, or end-diastolic, length is given in the upper right panel. The description of pump performance by the function curve consists of the determination of stroke volume for a variety of filling volumes. Volume expansion with dextran, for example, provides a range of diastolic volumes for examination. Intravascular and intracardiac expansion raises arterial pressure and chamber size. Consequently, wall force rises progressively with the result that the ventricle traverses a series of ever increasing force trajectories (i.e., $F_1 < F_2 < ... < F_n$). A reduction in contractile state would reduce the slope of each shortening-length relation. In turn, the function curve would be depressed downward and to the right. As the depressed ventricle enlarges, instantaneous shortening load increases abnormally so that shortening is markedly restricted and a descending limb of the curve results. An increment in contractility raises the slope of each shortening-length relation; consequently, the function curve would be shifted upward and to the left. The derivation of the ventricular function curve during the rapid withdrawal and reinfusion of blood raises the issue of an altered sympathetic response and thereby a variable level of contractile state.

The Pressure Overloaded Heart: Physiological and Theoretical Considerations

Tension, Stress, and Hypertrophy

The concept of net wall force provides a useful means to describe the contractile behavior of the muscular pump. However, when considering the complex geometry of the ventricle and hypertrophy in the diseased heart, it is more appropriate to use the terms wall tension and wall stress. The concept of tension was first applied to the heart in 1892 by Woods [54]. Tension [(T), g/cm] describes the force existing along a unit length of a surface, for example, as a thin-walled structure such as the alveolus. The tension existing anywhere in the alveolus is determined by the pressure inside the alveolus and the principle radii of curvature along the segment in question. Because the ventricle is a thick-walled

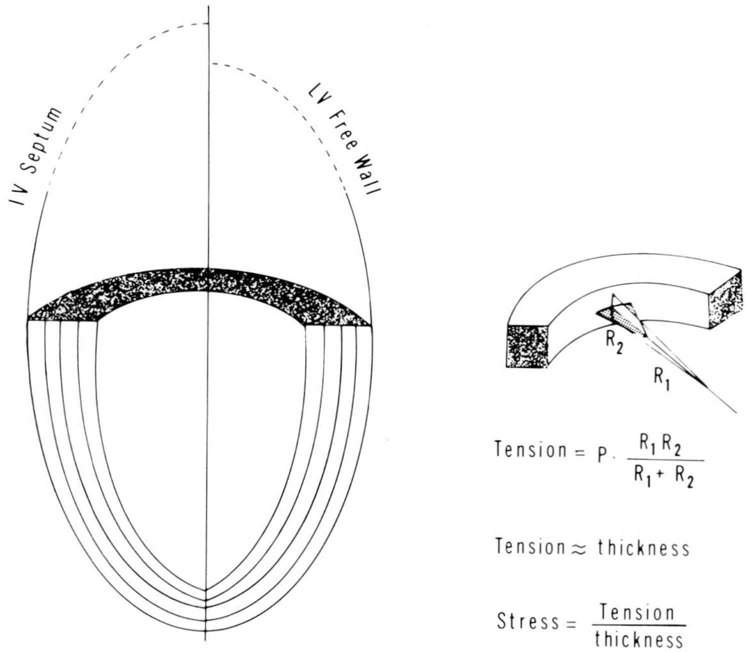

Fig. 7. The concept of tension is best applied to thin-walled structures. If the left ventricle is viewed as consisting of a series of nested shells of finite thickness than the tension existing at any point along the surface of one of these shells is related to the produce of chamber pressure and the two principle radii of curvature (R^1 and R_2). Because the radius of curvature is larger for the septum than the free wall apex of the left ventricle than septal tension and thickness must be greater than the other regions of the ventricle. Stress expresses tension per unit wall thickness

structure, the application of the tension concept is somewhat cumbersome. For this purpose it is helpful to view the ventricle as consisting of a set of nested, concentric shells of finite thickness as shown in Fig. 7. The tension existing at a point along the surface of any given shell is related to the pressure and the principle radii of curvature (R_1 and R_2) at that point. The orientation of muscle fibers within the myocardium may be thought of as a set of these nested shells [41] and the force existing along a unit lenght of fiber or group of fibers as represented by tension.

For any given ventricular pressure, the tension developed within the myocardium is a function of its geometry. Hence, one would expect regional differences in tension based on the complex shape of the ventricle. For example, the tension existing along the interventricular septum, having a large radius of curvature (see Fig. 7), would be greater than that found along the free wall of the left ventricle or at its apex. Woods [54] and Burton [6] have reasoned that the thickness of the ventricular wall at any point is proportional to the systolic tension in the wall. Thus, for any chamber pressure the thickness of the ventricular wall would also be a function of its regional configuration. For example, at the apex of the left ventricle, where the radius of curvature is small compared to that of the septum, the wall is thinner. These variations in wall thickness suggest that *average wall stress*, or tension per unit thickness, is maintained constant throughout the ventricle despite its obviously complex shape. Implicit in this view is the assumption that tension must regulate protein synthesis and therefore muscle mass. The homogeneous distribution of stress permits uniform wall motion and the ordered process of contraction. If such were not the case, pump function would be compromised by abnormal segmental wall motion at regions of high stress. This simplified view of wall stress, however, does not consider that stress, like tension, varies across the wall and is greatest along the subendocardium. Moreover, stress in the cirucumferential direction is greater than meridional stress because of the differences in the length of the major and minor axes of the ventricle. The functional architecture of the heart is well suited to these differences, however, since the majority of muscle fibers are oriented in the circumferential direction [30, 41], thereby supporting the larger circumferential stress. The smaller number of semiventricular fibers, located along the subendo- and subepicardium, are shortening principally in the meriodional direction agianst the meridional stress.

When the ventricle is placed under an excessive hemodynamic load, e.g., the pressure overload of aortic stenosis, coarctation, or systemic hypertension, wall tension is elevated. Compensatory increments in muscle mass, or hypertrophy, follow, thereby attempting to normalize wall stress. Chronic increments in ventricular volume (e.g., aortic or mitral valve incompetence) and the radii of curvature also serve to raise tension and promote wall hypertrophy. In the case of the pressure overloaded heart, hypertrophy occurs without a change in chamber size. Because the growth in muscle mass and increase in wall thickness occurs around the symmetrical axis of the chamber it has been termed *concentric* hypertrophy. In the volume-overloaded ventricle, on the other hand, cardiac muscle increases in length as chamber size increases. Hence, muscle growth presumably does not occur around the same symmetrical axis as that of the chamber, and therefore, the term *eccentric* hypertrophy has been used. Validation of the concentric or eccentric growth of the myocardium, however, requires careful examination. Moreover, such an analysis dicates that the axis of symmetry of the left ventricle must be identified.

Geheb et al. [12], in our laboratory, have recently provided this information by describing the centers of gravity of the myocardium and its two ventricular chambers. Nevertheless, it is tempting at this time to speculate that because of its larger curvature the interventricular septum would hypertrophy in advance of the free wall in the pressure-overloaded heart. The fact that asymmetric septal hypertrophy has been noted in patients with a variety of cardiac diseases, including pressure overload [27], lends support to this notion. Moreover, the assymmetric hypertrophy and subvalvular muscular obstruction, noted postoperatively following valve replacement in some patients with aortic stenosis, may also indicate an accelerated regional hypertrophy of the septum which has now been unmasked. Proof of these differences in regional hypertrophy, however, requires verification.

If indeed hypertrophy is a mechanism whereby average wall stress is maintained constant in various disease states, then wall thickness, chamber geometry, and systolic pressure should be interrelated. The irregular shape of the ventricle makes the determination of the two principle radii of curvature difficult under most circumstances. Hence, simpler expressions relating shape, thickness, and pressure have been sought, including the ratio of wali thickness to chamber radius (h/r) and the ratio of muscle mass to end-diastolic volume (M/V [9]. The first expression, using the minor axis to relate h/r to systolic pressure, assumes that ventricular shape does not change during the disease process. This may be true for the pressure overloaded heart; it is unclear, however, whether this applies to the enlarged, volume-overloaded heart. A cruder approximation, representing the average of the h/r ratios in all dimensions, is the M/V ratio. Because the measurement of mass and end-diastolic volume is complex and requirescine-angiography and several assumptions concerning shape, the h/r ratio obtained directly by echocardiography is a more promising technique for determining the appropriateness of ventricular hypertrophy and for estimating the level of systolic pressure to which the myocardium has chronically adapted (vide infra).

As we have already noted, the foregoing discussion presumes that muscle growth and hypertrophy are related to increased levels of wall tension. The compensatory increment in muscle mass serves to normalize tension, or stress, and to maintain pump function. What is not clear is why this should be so. The energy requirements of the myocardium are also a function of wall force or tension [40, 46]. By increasing myocardial 0_2 utilization and protein synthesis [31], increments in wall tension initiate a series of mechanisms which not only preserve the distribution of force per unit area of muscle but, more importantly, minmize the energy requirements of the myocardium [49]. Thus, the heart appears to carry out its work load under conditions of minimal energy expenditure (i.e., maximal efficiency). However, for reasons which are poorly understood, the heart eventually fails.

Some [17] have suggested that an inappropriate amount of hypertrophy is responsible for elevated wall stress and impaired performance of the muscular pump. From the foregoing discussion, it is obvious that an elevated stress will impair pump function. What is not clear is why hypertrophy should be limited. Others [1, 8, 26, 44, 49] have suggested that the 0_2 requirements of the overloaded heart, e.g., aortic stenosis, eventually exceed its coronary vascular reserve. With the resultant impairment in 0_2 availability, protein synthesis becomes the limiting factor to the further growth of cardiac muscle. Morover, increments in work and 0_2 demand will now exceed 0_2 supply, leading to the onset of anaerobic metabolism and a further progressive deterioration in performance.

Wall Stress

Interest in the role of wall stress in clinical disorders actually preceded the development of methods for determining wall stess in man. In 1960, Linzbach [26] theorized that wall stress was a critical determinant of the extent of hypertrophy in the compensated pressure-overloaded heart. He suggested that hypertrophy occurred to a degress sufficient in keep wall stress within its normal range. This hypothesis could be tested only after the development of quantitative angiography methods for determination of wall stress [14, 22, 37]. In general, these early studies confirmed Linzbach's hypothesis. In the compensated pressure-overloaded left ventricle, angiographic peak circumferential and meridional wall stress were normal. More recent studies by Peterson and co-workers [31], however, indicate that there may actually be a slight elevation in peak stress in this setting, which presumably serves as a continued stimulus to ongoing hypertrophy. In decompensated hearts, on the other hand, all are agreed that peak stress is consistently elevated [22, 37]. Hence, wall stress is normalized as long as the continued growth of the myocardium is unimpeded. Once hypertrophy is limited, stress is increased and the function of this muscular pump declines.

Echocardiography provides quantitative data on left ventricular dimensions and wall thickness that can be substituted for angiographic data in the computation of wall stress. Grossman and co-workers [3, 17], using M mode, or single plane echocardiography have shown that results for meridional wall stress are quite comparable to those obtained from angiographic data in the same subject. They, too, have demonstrated a tendency toward normalization of peak stress. Using the equitation for meridional stress and several simplifying assumptions, we have developed a totally noninvasive echocardiographic method for the estimation of peak and end-systolic wall stress [5]. Estimates of peak stress by this method are quite comparable to those obtained angiographically by Gould and co-workers [14] in normal subjects and patients with cardiomyopathy or aortic regurgitation. In hypertension an elevated peak meridional stress is seen only in the dilated failing ventricle. In aortic regurgitation peak stress is elevated in symptomatic patients with either normal or depressed angiographic ejection fraction. In contrast, asymptomatic patients with severe aortic regurgitation and normal left ventricular function have normal peak stress [17, 53].

The performance of the muscular pump is not merely regulated by peak stress, however, but in point of fact by the time course of wall stress throughout the ejection period. As we have pointed out earlier, the failing, enlarged heart operates at a mechanical disadvantage because stress remains elevated throughout ejection. Others [11, 32] have documented this abnormal stress trajectory in patients with myocardial disease. As a result of the increased stress, instantaneous fiber shortening and, thereby, stroke volume are reduced. As long as ejection fraction remains normal we would not expect the trajectory of instantaneous shortening load to be altered in pressure-overloaded heart, irrespective of the absolute level of systolic pressure. Increments in muscle mass with hypertrophy serve to normalize stress at onset ejection, i.e., peak stress under most circumstances. The increment in wall thickness during ejection, however, will determine whether instantaneous shortening load is normalized. It would appear reasonable to assume that if end-systolic stress is normal, then stress throughout ejection is normalized by wall thickening.

The h/r Ratio and the Prediction of Systolic Pressure

The relation between hypertrophy, chamber size, expressed as the ratio of thickness to chamber radius (h/r), and ventricular pressure has been examined by a number of investigators. Levine et al [25] found that in aortic stenosis the increase in h/r was proportional to the increase in ventricular systolic pressure. In patients with outflow obstruction and normal diastolic volume, Grant and coworkers [15] found h/r to increase twofold, while h/r was unchanged in patients with valvular incompetence and chamber dilation. Similar results were obtained by Grossman et al. [17] in volume-overloaded hearts. Alternatively, in the pressure-overloaded heart h/r was increased in proportion to the rise in ventricular pressure.

The echocardiographic end-systolic ratio of wall thickness to chamber radius (h/r) has been used to predict peak left ventricular pressure in the compensated pressure-overloaded left ventricle of valvular aortic stenosis [2, 13, 23]. When manifestations of cardiac failure are absent and velocity of circumferential fiber shortening is normal, peak pressure is accurately predicted from the simple formula: P=k (PWTs/LVIDs), where P is peak pressure, PWT is end-systolic posterior wall thickness, LVID is end-systolic left ventricular dimension, and the constant k is derived from the meriodional wall strss formula [17]. This analysis implies that in the compensated ventricle stress is normalized by hypertrophy at end-systole as well as at peak stress, which occurs early in systole. Moreover, it is assumed that peak pressure falls late in ejection as is the case in aortic stenosis and cardiac failure. When left ventricular function is more variable, as is generally the case in unselected adult populations with aortic stenosis, this analysis breaks down. Our own data indicate that in such a population end-systolic h/r correlates less well with peak ventricular pressure than does end-diastolic h/r [34].

Table 1. Prediction of left ventricular peak pressure from h/r ratio at end-diastole

h/r Ratio	Pressure range
< 0.45	< 140 mm Hg
0.45—0.50	140—180 mm Hg
> 0.50	> 180 mm Hg

As a practical matter, only a rough categorization of the range of peak pressure is therefore possible in an unscreened adult population (Table 1).

End-Systolic Stress

As mentioned earlier, a normal end-systolic stress implies that instantaneous shortening load is normalized by wall thickening during ejection. We have examined end-systolic echocardiographic wall stress both invasively and noninvasively [35, 53]. The noninvasive approach appears to be valid, since a good correlation exists between cuff and micromanometer end-systolic pressure, and an excellent correlation exists between invasive and noninvasive end-systolic stress in normal, cardiomyopathic and pressure- and volume-overloaded hearts. The noninvasive method breaks down in severe mitral regurgitation and, presumably, in other conditions in which the left ventricle is not truly isovolumetric at end systole. Our data (Table 2) indicate that end-sytolic stress is normal in aortic stenosis with depressed ejection fraction and in failing hearts due to hypertension, cardiomyopathy, or aortic regurgitation, as well as compensated asymptomatic aortic regurgitation.

The end-systolic stress-length relation may be used experimentally to represent the maximally developed stress-length relation and thereby myocardial contractile state. The linearity of the end-systolic pressure-diameter relationship in the intact human circulation has recently been demonstrated by several investigators [28,29, 36]. We have examined the end-systolic meriodional wall stress-length relationship using echocardiographic left ventricular diameter and either

Table 2. Estimated end-systolic meridional stress[a]

Group	**n**	**Mean end-systolic stress** ($\times 10^3$ dynes/cm^2)
Normal	22	65 ± 13
Aortic stenosis, (normal EF)	24	56 ± 24
Aortic stenosis, (decreased EF)	6	97 ± 28[b]
Treated hypertension	14	57 ± 17
Cardiomyopathy	4	157 ± 41[b]

[a] EF, ejection fraction; all values ± 1 s.d.: In aortic stenosis, peak left ventricular pressure at catheterization was used to calculate end-systolic stress. In all other groups, cuff systolic blood pressure was used

[b] Significantly higher than normal ($P < 0.05$)

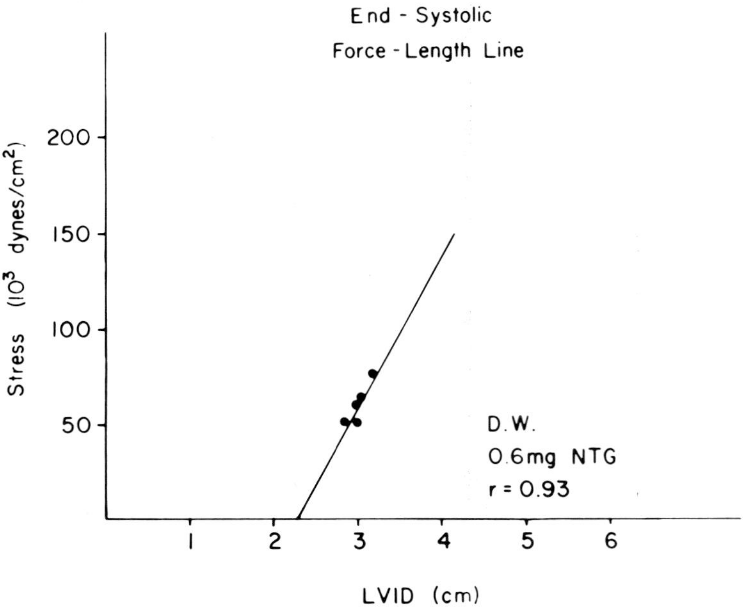

Fig. 8. The end-systolic force-length relationship in a normal subject derived from cuff arterial pressure and echocardiographic wall thickness and ventricular diameter, before and after administration of sublingual nitroglycerin (NTG). A linear relationship between end-systolic stress (*vertical axis*) and left ventricular diameter *(LVID) (LVID, horizontal axis)* is apparent

high fidelity micromanometry or sphygmomanometry to measure left ventricular pressure following load alteration with nitroprusside, neosynephrine, or sublingual nitroglycerin. Our analysis indicates that the end-systolic stress-diameter relationship is essentially linear for a given inotropic state (Fig. 8), provided that end ejection is truly isovolumetric. In severe mitral regurgitation or inhomogeneous segmental ventricular wall function due to ischemic disease where end systole is not isovolumetric, the application of this concept will not hold. A good correlation exists between invasive and noninvasive stress-length analyses in the same patient. In our experience, acute increments in contractile state, noted in the post-potentiated beat following a premature ventricular contraction, increase the slope of the end-systolic stress-length line.

Therapy and the Pressure-Overloaded Heart

Antihypertensive therapy produces an abnormally high end-diastolic h/r ratio in relationship to peak left ventricular pressure [34]. Consequently, noninvasive estimates of peak stress are abnormally low in this setting. In contrast, end-systolic stress in treated hypertension is normal, indicating that these ventricles shorten to a normal end-systolic force-length value. Regression in left ventricular hypertrophy following treatment of hypertension has been described [37a].

However, the persistence of high h/r ratios in retreated hypertensives suggest that such regression may be incomplete or slow in occurrence. Using an echocardiographic quantitation of left ventricular mass, we have documented a substantial regression (i.e., up to 200 g or 40% of total left ventricular mass) of hypertrophy in several hypertensives with severe left ventricular hypertrophy following several months of treatment. Various forms of antihypertensive therapy may differ as to the extent to which they reduce load. Thus, systematic differences in the effects of antihypertensive therapy on mechanics and hypertrophy would be predicted. In particular, the cardiac effects of blood pressure reduction by agents which depress contractility need to be closely scrutinized.

In aortic stenosis, valve replacement leads to abrupt reduction in load. Consequently, h/r ratios are uniformly high relative to left ventricular pressure in the early postoperative period [23]. Thereafter, regression of hypertrophy of considerable degree generally occurs in ventricles that were well compensated preoperatively. In decompensated aortic stenosis, regression of hypertrophy occurs, but may be less complete [24]. Residual hypertrophy and chamber enlargement appear to be important risk factors in both aortic stenosis and hypertensive heart disease [21, 38].

Although existing data on the effects of therapy on the mechanics and myocardial mass of the pressure overloaded human heart are intriguing, it is clear that major gaps exist with respect to our understanding of the optimal design and timing of therapeutic interventions.

References

1. Badeer HS (1964) Biological significance of cardiac hypertrophy. Am J Cardiol 14 : 133–138
2. Bennett DH, Evans DW, Raj MVJ (1975) Echocardiographic left ventricular dimensions in pressure and volume overload. Their use in assessing aortic stenosis. Br Heart J 37 : 971–977
3. Brodie BR, Grossman W, McLaurin LP (1975) Combined hemodynamic-ultrasonic method for studying left ventricular wall stress: Comparison with angiography. Am J Cardiol 35 : 124
4. Brutsaert DL, Sonnenblick EH (1969) Force-velocity-length-time relations of the contractile elements in heart muscle of the cat. Circ Res 24 : 137–149
5. Burch GE, Ray CT, Cronvich JA (1952) Certain mechanical peculiarities of the human cardiac pump in normal and diseased states. Circulation 5 : 504–513
6. Burton AC (1957) Importance of shape and size of heart. Am Heart J 54 : 801–810
7. Downing SE, Sonnenblick EH (1964) Cardiac muscle mechanics and ventricular performance: Force and time parameters. Am J Physiol 207 : 705–715
8. Fallen EL, Elliott WC, Gorlin R (1967) Mechanisms of angina in aortic stenosis. Circulation 39 : 480–488

9. Ford LE (1976) Heart size. Circ Res 39 : 297—303
10. Fry DL, Griggs DM Jr, Greenfield JC Jr (1963) Myocardial meachanics: Tension-velocity-length relationships of heart muscle. Circ Res 14 : 73—85
11. Gault JH, Ross J Jr, Braunwald E (1968) Contractile state of the left ventricle in man. Circ Res 22 : 451—463
12. Geheb F, Janicki JS, Weber KT (1979) The axis of symmetry of the heart and its ventricular chambers. Fed Proc 38 : 1267
13. Glanz S, Hellenbrand WE, Bermann MA, Talner NS (1976) Echocardiographic assessment of the severity of aortic stenosis in children and adolescents. Am J Cardiol 38 : 620—625
14. Gould KL, Lipscomb K, Hamilton GW, Kennedy JW (1974) Relation of left ventricular shape, function, and wall stress in man. Am J Cardiol 34 : 627—634
15. Grant C, Greene DG, Bunnell IL (1965) Left ventricular enlargement and hypertrophy. Am J Med 39 : 895—904
16. Griggs DM, Chen CC, Tchokoev VV (1973) Subendocardial anaerobic metabolism in experimental aortic stenosis. Am J Physiol 3 : 607—612
17. Grossman W, Jones D, McLaurin SP (1975) Wall stress and patterns of hypertrophy in the human left ventricle. J Clin Invest 56 : 56—64
18. Grossman W, Braunwald E, Mann T, McLaurin LP, Green LH (1977) Contractile state of the left ventricle in man as evaluated from end-systolic pressure-volume relations. Circulation 56 : 845—852
19. Gunther S, Grossman W (1979) Determinants of ventricular function in pressure-overload hypertrophy in man. Circulation 59 : 679—688
20. Hefner LL, Sheffiled LT, Cobbs GC, Klip W (1962) Relation between mural force and pressure in the left ventricle of the dog. Circ Res 11 : 654—663
21. Hirshfeld JW, Epstein SE, Roberts AJ, Glancy DL, Morrow AG (1974) Indices predicting long-term survival after valve replacement in patients with aortic regurgitation and patients with aortic stenosis. Circulation 50 : 1190—1199
22. Hood WP Jr, Rackley CE, Rolett EL (1968) Wall stress in the normal and hypertrophied human left ventricles. Am J Cardiol 22 : 550—558
23. Johnson GL, Meyer RA, Schwartz DC, Korfhagen J, Kaplan S (1977) Echocardiographic evaluation of fixed left ventricular outlet obstruction in children. Pre- and post-operative assessment of ventricular systolic pressures. Circulation 56 : 299—304
24. Kennedy JW, Doces J, Stewart DK (1977) Left ventricular function before and following aortic valve replacement. Ciruculation 56 : 944—950
25. Levine ND, Rockoff SD, Braunwald E (1963) An anticardiographic analysis of the thickness of the left ventricular wall and cavity in aortic stenosis and other valvular lesions. Ciruculation 28 : 339—345
26. Linzbach AJ (1960) Heart failure from the point of view of quantitative anatomy. Am J Cardiol 5 : 370—383
27. Maron BJ, Clark CE, Henry WL, Fukuda T, Edwards JE, Mathews EC, Redwood DR, Epstein SE (1977) Prevalence and characteristics of disproportionate ventricular septal thickening in patients with acquired or congenital

heart diseases. Echocardiographic and morphologic findings. Ciruculation 55 : 589—496
28. Marsh JD, Green LH, Wynne J, Cohn PF, Grossman W (1978) Linearity of left ventricular end-systolic pressure-dimension relations in man and sensitivity to inotropic state. Circulation 57 : II—29
29. Paloma AR, Quinones MA, Gaasch WH, Miller RR (1979) Normalized E curves in man: Significance of V_0. Am J Cardiol 43 : 377
30. Pearlman ES, Weber KT, Janicki JS (1979) Fiber alignment and capillary density in normal human heart. Fed Proc 38 : 1267
31. Peterson KL (1978) Instantaneous force-velocity-length relations of the left ventricle: Methods, limitations, and applications in humans. In: Fishman AP (ed) Heart failure. Hemisphere, Washington DC
32. Peterson KL, Uther JB, Shabetai R, Braunwald E (1973) Assessment of left ventricular performance in man. Circulation 47 : 924—935
33. Peterson MB, Lesch M (1972) Protein synthesis and amino acid transport in the isolated rabbit right ventricular papillary muscle. Cir Res 31 : 317—327
34. Reichek N, Devereux RB (1977) Echocardiographic prediction of left ventricular systolic pressure. Circulation 56 : III--26
35. Reichek N, Silverstone P, Wilson J (1978) Non-invasive determination of the left ventricular force-length relationship in man. Am J Cardiol 41 : 435
36. Reichek N, Hishfeld JW, Goldberg S, Wilson JR, Kastor JA (1979) Linearity of the end-systolic force-length relationship in human disease. Clin Res 27 : 198A
37. Sandler H, Dodge HT (1963) Left ventricular tension and stress in man. Circ Res 13 : 91—104
37a. Schlant RC, Felner JM, Heymsfeld SB, Gilbert CA, Shulman NB, Tuttle EP, Blumenstein BA (1977) Echocardiographic studies of left ventricular anatomy and function in essential hypertension. Cardiovasc Med 2 : 477—491
38. Sokolow M, Perloff D (1961) The prognosis of essential hypertension treated conservatively. Circulation 23 : 697—713
39. Sonnenblick EH (1962) Implications of muscle mechanics in the heart. Fed Proc 21 : 975—993
40. Strauer BE (1979) Myocardial 0_2 consumption in chronic heart disease: The role of wall stress, hypertrophy and coronary reserve. Am J Cardiol 44 : 730
41. Streeter DD, Hanna WT (1973) Engineering mechanics for successive states in canine left ventricular myocardium II. Fiber angle and sarcomere length. Circ Res 33 : 656—664
42. Suga H, Sagawa K (1974) Instantaneous pressure-volume relationships and their ratio in the excised, supported canine left ventricle. Circ Res 35 : 117—126
43. Suga H, Sagawa K, Shoukas AA (1973) Load independence of the instantaneous pressure-volume ratio of the canine left ventricle and effects of epinephrine and heart rate on the ratio. Circ Res 32 : 314—322
44. Trenouth RS, Phelps NC, Neill WA (1976) Determinants of left ventricular hypertrophy and oxygen supply in chronic aortic valve disease. Ciruculation 53 : 644—650

45. Weber KT, Janicki JS (1977) Instantaneous force-velocity-length relations: Experimental findings and clinical correlates. Am J Cardiol 40 : 739—747
46. Weber KT, Janicki JS (1977) Myocardial oxygen consumption: The role of wall force and shortening. Am J Physiol 233 : H421—H430
47. Weber KT, Janicki JS (1978) Interdependence of cardiac function, coronary flow, and oxygen extraction. Am J Physiol 235 : H784—H793
48. Weber KT, Janicki JS (1978) Muscle-pump function of the intatct heart. In: Fishman AP (ed) Heart failure. Hemisphere, Washington DC, pp 29-41
49. Weber KT, Janicki JS (to be published) The metabolic demand and 0_2 supply of the heart: Physiological and clinical considerations. Am J Cardiol
50. Weber KT, Janicki JS (to be published) The dynamics of ventricular contraction: Force, length and shortening. Fed Proc
51. Weber KT, Janicki JS, Reeves RC, Hefner LL (1976) Factors influencing left ventricular shortening in isolated canine heart. Am J Physiol 230 : 419—426
52. Weber KT, Janicki JS, Hefner LL (1976) Left ventricular force-length relations of isovolumic and ejecting contractions. Am J Physiol 231 : 337—343
53. Wilson JR, Reichek N, Keller CA, Hirshfeld J, Kastor JA (1979) Non-invasive assessment of load manipulation in chronic asymptomatic aortic regurgitation. Am J Cardiol 43 : 410
54. Woods RH (1892) A few applications of a physical theorem to membranes in the human body in a state of tension. J Anat Physiol 26 : 326—370

Effect of Systemic Vasoconstriction on Left Ventricular Function: Implications Regarding Hypertension and Heart Failure[1]

J.N. COHN AND J.A. FRANCIOSA

A high impedance to left ventricular ejection (aortic input impedance) is a hallmark of hypertension. Cardiac output and stroke volume remain normal, despite this increased impedance, and arterial pressure therefore rises. The ability of the left ventricle to withstand this increased impedance is probably dependent on both acute and chronic compensatory mechanisms. The acute response probably involves primarily an increase in end-diastolic fiber length (Frank-Starling mechanism) that allows the left ventricle to maintain its stroke volume against a higher outflow resistance. The more chronic response involves myocardial hypertrophy, which tends to restore left ventricular wall stress to normal despite the increased systolic pressure [1]. At a later stage ventricular dilation supervenes, wall stress rises again, and heart failure may develop.

The above course of events can explain the natural history of hypertensive heart disease. Since antihypertensive therapy has been so effective in preventing and treating left ventricular failure in hypertensive subjects [2], it may be assumed that any induced reduction of impedance can arrest or reverse the process of hypertrophy and dilation that leads to decompensation.

The natural history of myocardial disease (ischemic or nonischemic) without hypertension has been less clear. In recent years it has become apparent that impedance is increased in this syndrome as well. The absence of hypertension can be explained by the observation that such patients have lost the normal compensatory mechanisms (fiber length, hypertrophy) that allows them to maintain cardiac output as impedance rises. Consequently, the high impedance in heart failure is accompanied by a variably depressed cardiac output that accounts for a blood pressure which may range widely from low to moderately elevated levels.

In the past few years impedance reduction therapy has been widely employed in normotensive patients with left ventricular failure in an effort to improve cardiac function [3]. The acute response to vasodilator therapy has confirmed the thesis that in patients with heart failure cardiac output is impedance limited.

---

1 Supported in part by Grant HL 22977 from the National Heart, Lung and Blood Institute

Therefore, during intravenous infusion of sodium nitroprusside or after oral administration of hydralazine, isosorbide dinitrate, prazosin, trimazosin, phentolamine, or converting enzyme inhibitor, a marked improvement in left ventricular performance can be demonstrated: left ventricular filling pressure falls, stroke volume and ejection fraction rise, and arterial pressure is only slightly reduced.

This salutary acute hemodynamic response to vasodilator drug therapy has naturally led to attempts to utilize this treatment on a chronic basis in patients with severe heart failure. These innovative therapeutic efforts have raised a number of theoretical and practical questions that must be addressed before the place of vasodilator treatment of heart failure can be established. Some of these questions include the following:

1. Are the hemodynamic effects of various vasodilator drugs importantly different?

2. What is the mechanism of the high impedance in heart failure?

3. Would specific interference with the vasoconstrictor mechanism be more effective than nonspecific vasodilation?

4. Does tolerance develop to vasodilator therapy?

5. Is exercise capacity increased by vasodilator therapy?

6. Is the natural history of the disease altered by vasodilator therapy?

7. At what point in the course of the disease, if any, is it appropriate to introduce vasodilator drugs?

The answers to these questions are only now beginning to emerge:

1. Vasodilator drugs vary in their relative effects on arterial and venous smooth muscle and on their relative potency in dilating different regional vascular beds. Drugs with considerable venous effects, such as the nitrates, prazosin, and trimazosin, redistribute blood into the capacitance vessels and result in a considerable reduction in ventricular filling pressure. Drugs with a predominant arterial effect, such as hydralazine, reduce aortic impedance and increase cardiac output with a lesser effect on ventricular filling pressure. How important these differences are in chronic management is not yet certain. Furthermore, the differences in the effect of these drugs on specific regional vascular beds such as the renal, splanchnic, and skeletal muscle circulations is as yet poorly understood.

2. The high impedance in heart failure is multifactorial. In most patients the sympathetic nervous system apperars to be involved, since the plasma concentration of norepinephrine is elevated [4]. In many patients the renin-angiotensin system is probably involved because of markedly elevated plasma renin activity (PRA) [5]. Neither of these factors appears to be entirely responsible for the high systemic vascular resistance, however, and other humoral, metabolic, or mechanical factors probably play a role.

3. The possibility of selective vasodilator therapy based on the specific mechanism of vasoconstriction is attractive. The first reasonable attempt has been with the use of converting enzyme inhibitors to treat patients with high-renin heart failure [5]. Although the initial hemodynamic response to teprotide (Fig. 1) and captopril appears to be closely related to PRA, the more chronic response may depend on actions of the drug other than to prevent formation of angiotensin II. Therefore, chronic therapy with a converting enzyme inhibitor may not necessarily test the efficacy of selective vasodilation. Further studies are needed.

4. Although tolerance to chronic nitrate therapy has long been suspected, recent studies have failed to demonstrate the appearance of an important degree of tachyphylaxis during several months of regular treatment with oral isosorbide dinitrate. In our own studies isosorbide dinitrate's acute vascular effects were still demonstrable after 3 months of continuing administration [6]. Similar data have been shown for hydralazine [7]. In contrast, some investigators have demonstrated tolerance developing early during therapy with prazosin [8]. The importance and frequency of this apparent tachyphylaxis have not yet been established.

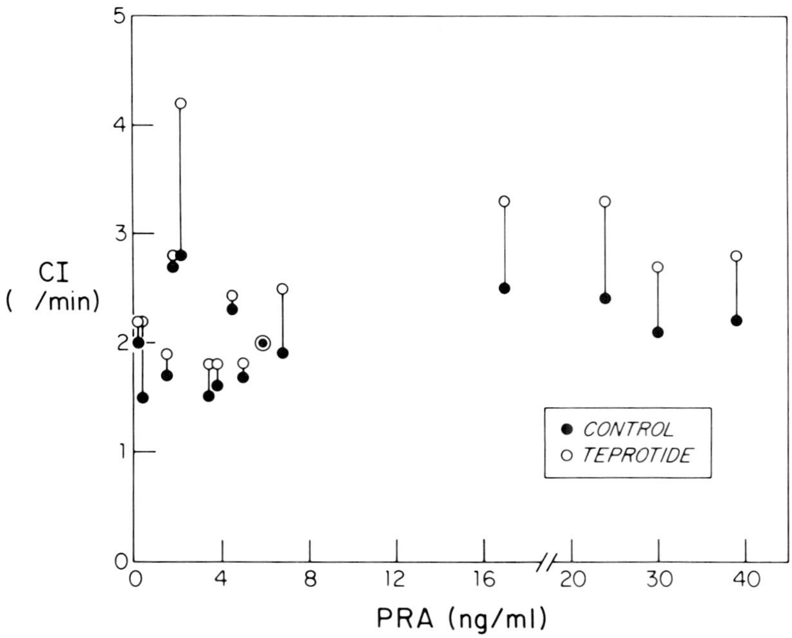

Fig. 1. Response of cardiac output to infusion of the converting enzyme inhibitor teprotide in patients with congestive heart failure. Patients with high control renin acitvity (*PRA*) have a more consistent response than those with lower PRA. Note the wide range of PRA in these patients all of whom had moderate to severe congestive heart failure

5. Despite the marked improvement in resting hemodynamics that occur after acute adminstration of a vasodilator drug, maximal exercise tolerance is not significantly improved after a single dose of either isosorbide dinitrate or the combination of nitrate and hydralazine [9, 10]. In contrast, after chronic therapy with these drugs maximal exercise capacity and oxygen consumption are significantly augmented [11]. Whether this gradual improvement relates to improved mechanical and/or metabolic performance of the left ventricle to improved peripheral utilization of oxygen remains to be established. Nonetheless, it implies that the syndrome of congestive heart failure involves a positive feedback mechanism that may take some time to reverse.

6. No studies of vasodilator drug therapy have been carried out long enough or in a large number of subjects to assess its impact on mortality. Such a study is urgently needed.

7. Most therapeutic attempts up to the present time have involved patients with severe heart failure not controlled with conventional therapy. It is an attractive possibility, however, that high impedance to left ventricle ejection is a factor in the progression of heart failure from its beginning as mild left ventricular dysfunction [12]. If so, vasodilator therapy introduced at an earlier stage of the disease may be more effective than late intervention in altering morbidity and mortality. Studies of such patients with mild disease will be difficult, lenghty, and expensive.

Vasodilator drug therapy in the patient with heart failure is physiologically rational. However, proof of efficacy must await the results of carefully controlled randomized propective therapeutic trials.

References

1. Sandler H, Dodge HJ (1963) Left ventricular tension and stress in man. Circ Res 13 : 91
2. Veterans Administration Cooperative Study Group on Antihypertensive Agents (1967) Effect of treatment on morbidity in hypertension: Results in patients with diastolic blood pressure ranging from 115—129 mm Hg. JAMA 202 : 1028
3. Cohn JN (1978) Vasodilator therapy for heart failure: The influence of impedance on left ventricular performance. Circulation 48 : 5
4. Cohn JN, Taylor N, Vrobel T, Moskowitz R (1978) Contrasting effect of vasodilators on heart rate and plasma cathecholamines in patients with hypertension and heart failure. Clin Res 26 : 547A
5. Curtiss C, Cohn JN, Vrobel T, Franciosa JA (1978) Role of the reninangiotensin system in the systemic vasoconstriction of chronic congestive heart failure. Circulation 58 : 763
6. Franciosa JA, Cohn JN (1978) Sustained hemodynamic effect of nitrates without tolerance in heart failure. Circulation [Suppl II] 58 : II—28

7. Chatterjee K, Ports T, Rubin S, Massie B, Arnold S, Brundage B, Parmley W (1978) Sustained beneficial hemodynamic effects during long term hydralazine therapy in patients with chronic heart failure. Circulation [Suppl II] 58 : II—28
8. Packer M, Meller J, Gorlin R, Herman MV (1979) Hemodynamic and clinical tachyphylaxis to prazosin-mediated afterload reduction in severe chronic congestive heart failure. Circulation 59 : 531
9. Franciosa JA, Cohn JN (1979) Effect of isosorbide dinitrate on response to submaximal and maximal exercise in patients with congestive heart failure. Am J Cardiol 43 : 1009
10. Franciosa JA, Cohn JN (1979) Immediate effects of hydralazine-isosorbide dinitrate combination on exercise capacity and exercise hemodynamics in patients with left ventricular failure. Ciruculation 59 : 1085
11. Franciosa JA, Nordstrom LA, Cohn JN (1978) Nitrate therapy for congestive heart failure. JAMA 240 : 443
12. Cohn JN (1973) Blood pressure and cardiac performance. Am J Med 55 : 351

Ventricular Function and Coronary Hemodynamics Under the Influence of Vasodilating Agents[1]

D.W. BEHRENBECK, M. TAUCHERT, V. HOMBACH AND H.H. HILGER

Vasodilatatory drugs reduce the afterload and preload of the ventricles. Their different effects may be explained by the variable effect in mainly reducing pre- or afterload, or both [3, 4]. Thus vasodilatators can be used in additon to the conventional therapy in emergency treatment of complicated myocardial infarction and congestive heart failure [1, 2, 5, 6, 8, 9]. Thera are two types of vasodilatory nitrates:

1. Sodium nitroprusside (NPN) as the drug with the major effect on hypertensive patients.

2. Nitroglycerin (NTG) or Isosorbide dinitrate (ISDN) as antianginal drugs.

Arterial blood pressure and heart rate are important determinants of myocardial oxygen consumption. Pressure load of the heart results in considerably higher amounts of myocardial oxygen consumption than volume load. According to the investigations of Sonnenblick and Skelton [10], the inotropic state and myocardial wall tension are further significant factors in regulating myocardial oxygen consumption. Holmberg [7] could show that myocardial blood flow during maximal physical exercises increased four to five times the resting control values, whereas the coronary arteriovenous difference of oxygen content revealed only insignificant changes. The corresponding augmentation of myocardial oxygen demands revealed a linear relationship with cardiac work, which can be approximately determined by the product of heart rate and systolic blood pressure. The aim of our study was to evaluate the influence of chronic pressure overload of the heart on coronary hemodynamics as well as the effect of lowering arterial blood pressure on the myocardial oxygen consumption by vasodilatory drugs.

In patients with fixed arterial hypertension in a compensated state, the following measurements were performed during diagnostic renal arteriography: Myocardial blood flow by the argon method, cardiac output by dye dilution technique, and pressures and oxygen saturations in the aorta, pulmonary artery, and the coronary sinus.

---

1 Supported by the Deutsche Forschungsgemeinschaft, SFB 68, Cologne

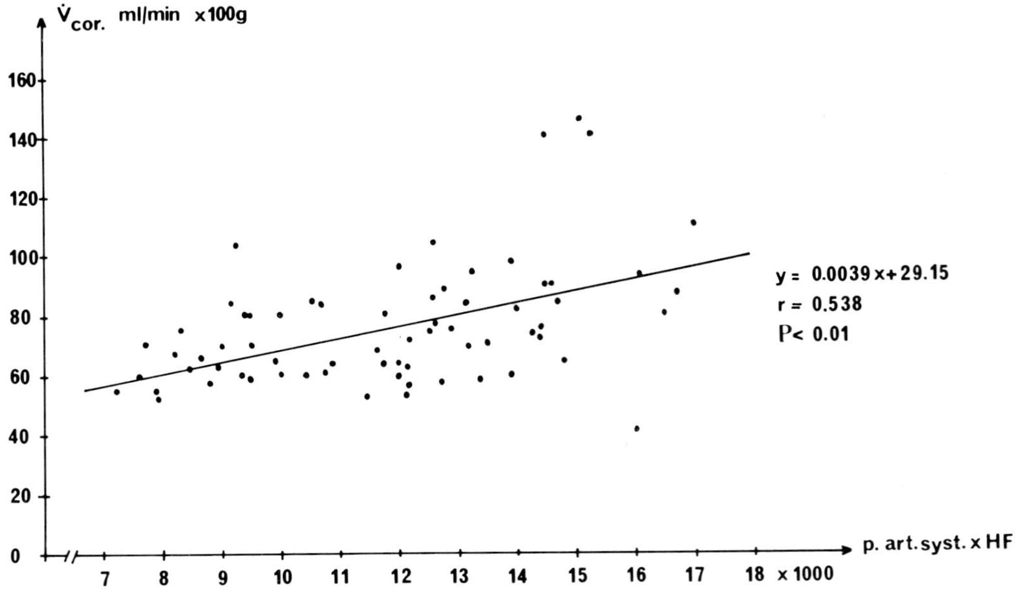

Fig. 1. Myocardial blood flow measured by argon method. V_{cor} (myocardial blood flow) (ml/min. 100 g) in 74 patients related to the amount of cardiac work determined by the product of heart rate and systolic blood pressure. *HF*, heart rate

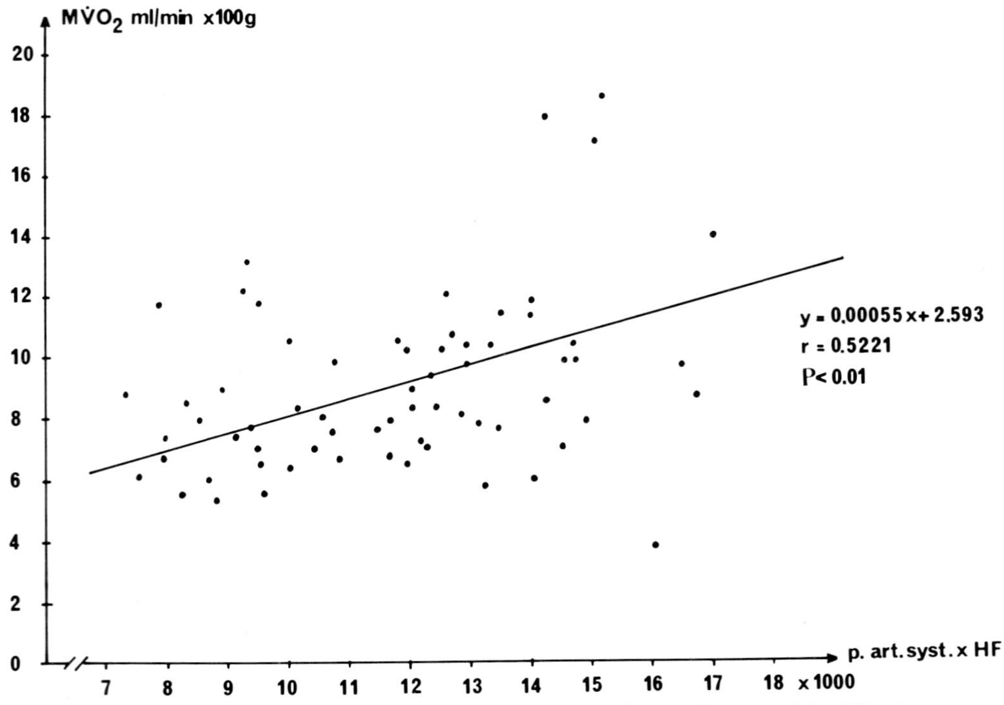

Fig. 2. Myocardial oxygen consumption in 74 patients depicted in Fig. 1

A group of 74 patients revealed only a minor correlation between systolic arterial pressure and myocardial blood flow related to the heart weight. A comparison of the amount of myocardial blood flow with the amount of cardiac work, as estimated from the product of systolic arterial blood pressure and heart rate, gives a better correlation. However, even at a large amount of cardiac work there is only a small increase of myocardial blood flow (Fig. 1).

Myocardial oxygen consumption related to 100 g heart weight revealed a significant correlation with the arterial pressure, yet there was considerable variance of this correlation. When the amount of cardiac work estimated from systolic arterial pressure and heart rate is compared to the weight-related myocardial oxygen consumption, there is a good correlation. In contrast to myocardial blood flow, with an increase of cardiac work a significant increase of myocardial oxygen consumption could be documented (Fig.2).

In a series of five patients with fixed arterial hypertension the above-mentioned hemodynamic measurements were performed after discontinuation of treatment and during controlled gradual lowering of arterial blood pressure (Fig. 3). The

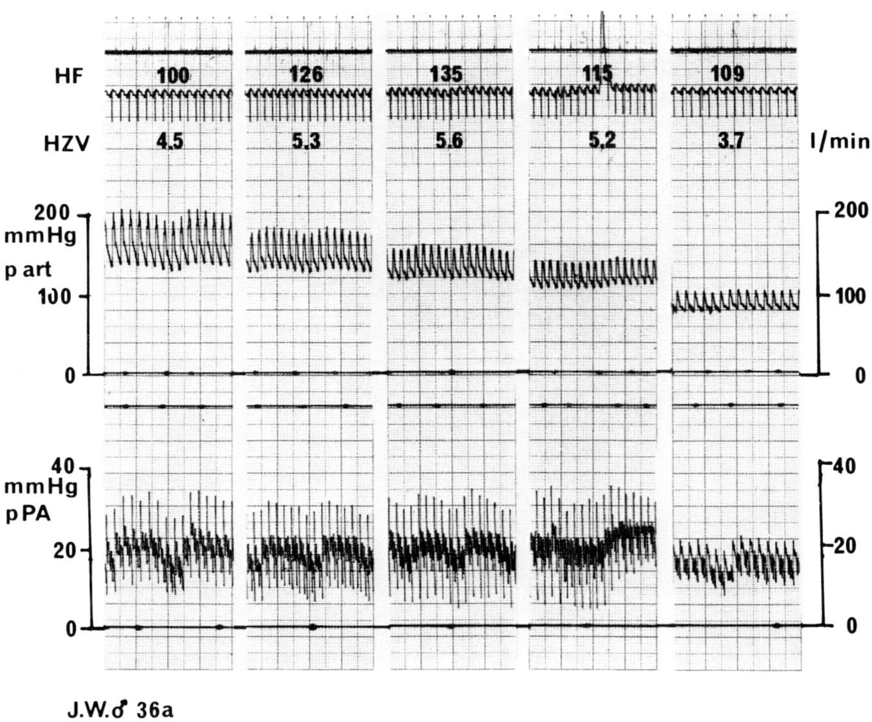

Fig. 3. Measurements performed in a 36-year-old patient with fixed arterial hypertension in a compensated state before and during controlled gradual lowering of arterial blood pressure (P_{art}) by intravenous infusion of sodium nitroprusside (NPN) in steps of about 20 mm Hg. *HF*, heart rate; *HZV*, cardiac output; *pPA*, pulmonary artery pressure

blood pressure decreases were accomplished by intravenous infusion of sodium nitroprusside in steps of about 30 mm Hg. When attaining steady-state conditions at the instant level of blood pressure, after 20—30 min, the measurements were repeated. Sodium nitroprusside was infused in an initial dose of 10 μg/min by means of a precision pump. The infusion rate was then enhanced to reach the next desired lower blood pressure level, which was monitored by direct intravascular pressure control.

We provide the example of a 45-year-old patients with an elevated systolic blood pressure of 240 mm Hg during resting control conditions whose blood pressure was graded reduced to 175, 150, and 100 mm Hg (Fig.4). The heart rate, which was slightly increased at rest, furthermore slightly increase during these maneuvers. The left ventricular end-diastolic pressure, measured as the pulmonary arterial diastolic pressure, remained constant until a pressure level of 150 mmHg, with a value at the upper limit of 12 mm Hg. Only at the lowest pressure level of 100 mm Hg did the end-diastolic left ventricular filling pressure decrease to 9 mm Hg. Cardiac output, which was within normal limits at rest (4.4 liter/min), continuously increased to a maximum of 6.0 liter/min at the pressure levels of 175 and 150 mm Hg. During the lowest pressure level of 100 mm Hg, cardiac output considerably decreased to 3.7 liter/min. Coronary blood

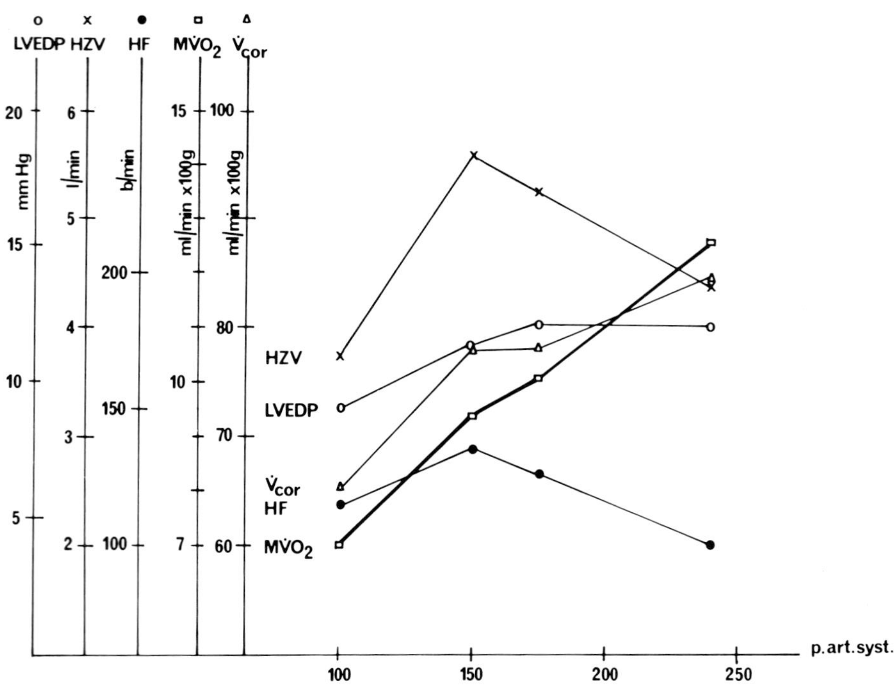

Fig. 4. Measurements performed in 45-year-old paitent depicted in Fig. 3. V_{cor}, myocardial blood flow; MVO_2, myocardial oxygen consumption; *LVEDP*, left ventricular end-diastolic pressure; *HF*, heart frequency; *HZV*, cardiac output

flow, which was 83 ml/100 g x min during control at rest, only insignificantly decreased to 78 ml/100 g x min at the initial diminished pressure levels. After attaining a systolic blood pressure level of 100 mm Hg, myocardial blood flow decreased significantly to 65 ml/100 g x min. Control myocardial oxygen consumption at rest was 12.6 ml/100 g x min and decreased thereafter to 10.1 ml/100 g x min, 9.5 ml/100 g x min, and 7.0 ml/100 g x min at the corresponding pressure levels.

In the total of six patients a decrease of systolic arterial blood pressure was generally associated with a reduction of myocardial blood flow, but these changes were rather small (Fig.5). Only in the case of high initial flow rates was a fall of blood pressure to the lowest level accompanied by a considerable reduction of myocardial blood flow to normal levels. The same holds true for the pressure heart rate product when compared with the myocardial blood flow rates. The decrease of myocardial blood flow with reduction of cardiac work was most marked in those cases with high initial control flow rates.

In all patients control myocardial oxygen consumption was enhanced by the initial hypertension levels and decreased gradually thereafter according to the

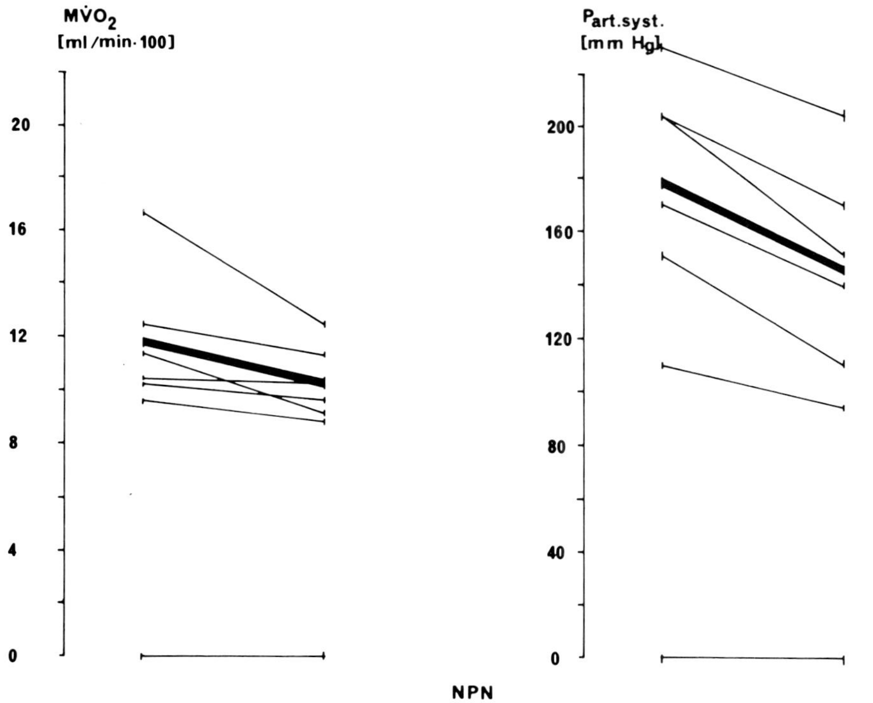

Fig. 5.Myocardial oxygen consumption and arterial blood pressure in six patients with fixed arterial hypertension in a compensated state before and during gradual lowering of arterial blood pressure by *NPN* (sodium nitroprusside). MVO_2, myocardial oxygen consumption

instant plateau phase of blood pressure decline. Again, the higher initial blood pressure values were the more pronounced the greater the reduction of myocardial oxygen consumption. Thus, with a mean reduction of cardiac work by 63% myocardial oxygen consumption was diminshed by 48% (Fig. 6).

These results indicate that myocardial blood flow per unit muscle mass may not be enhanced in all cases with arterial hypertension at comparable pressure levels and might remain within normal limits even in patients with systolic blood pressures of 200 mm Hg. Myocardial oxygen demands will generally be reduced by lowering blood pressure. In relation to cardiac work the oxygen-saving effect of a simple blood pressure decline is most pronounced. At resting conditions myocardial oxygen consumption was enhanced, especially in those patients with elevated left ventricular filling pressures. We are considering this phenomenon as a sign of a beginning cardiac pump failure. Thus, in patients with chronic arterial pressure overload myocardial oxygen consumption per unit muscle would be enhanced by an increase of left ventricular preload. By means of a simple peripheral vasodilatation, such as that induced by sodium nitroprusside, cardiac work declines proportionally and, hence, reduces myocardial oxy-

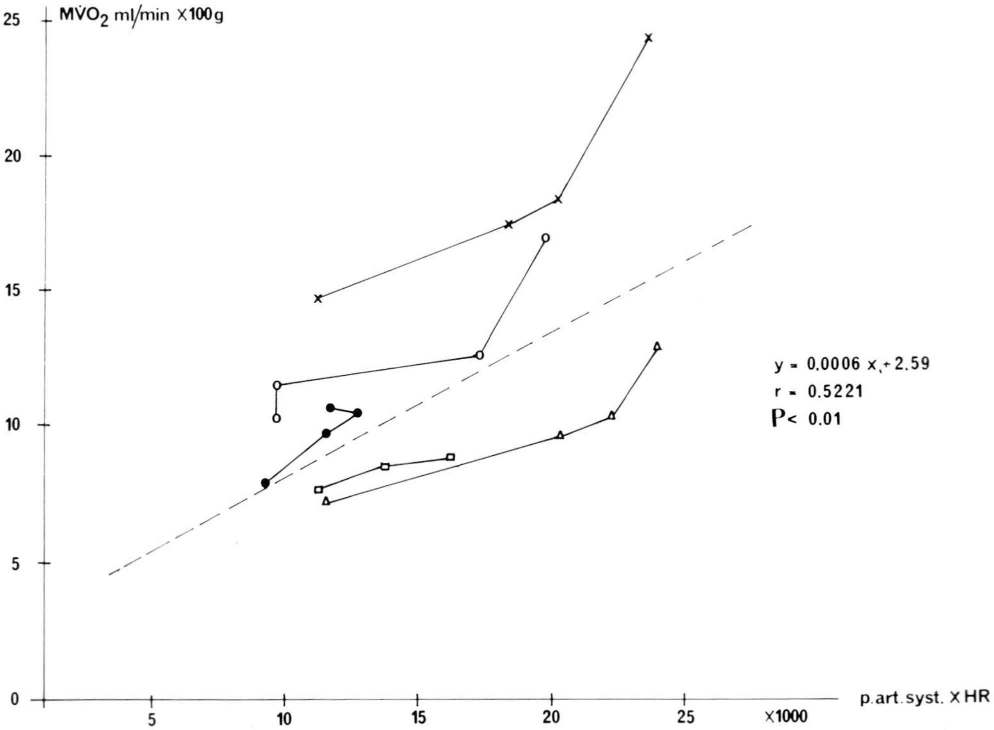

Fig. 6. Myocardial oxygen consumption in six patients depicted in Fig. 5 — before and during gradual lowering of arterial blood pressure by NPN — related to the amount of cardiac work. *Broken line* is the regression of Fig. 2. MVO_2, myocardial oxygen consumption

gen demands. Therefore the oxygen-saving effect depends strictly on the initially prevailing amount of cardiac work load. In compensated patients, small reductions of arterial blood pressures and peripheral resistance increases cardiac output, but concomitantly with a decline of left ventricular filling pressure, myocardial performance, i.e., cardiac output, will decrease.

A forty-six-year-old man had suffered from a nontransmural myocardial infarction and revealed instable angina during his admission to our clinic. Coronarographic examinations of the left ventricle revealed a hypokinetic zone in the anterior wall and a critical stenosis in LAD. During the hemodynamic studies the patient suffered an attack of angina pectoris. The LVFP increased at this time and was reduced to normal levels after administration of NTG (Fig. 7). Some time later during the same study the patient suffered a second angina attack with elevation of the systolic and diastolic left ventricular pressure; with the reduction of this left ventricular pressure by sodium nitroprusside, the patient's angina pectoris ceased (Fig. 8). This therapeutic effect could be reproduced again during a third angina attack half an hour later.

Sodium nitroprusside mediated pressure relief of the heart results in a reduction of myocardial oxygen demands in each case. Thus, in acute cardiac emergency situations, such as myocardial infarction, a controlled lowering of blood pressure merely in the arterial circuit may be helpful in reducing oxygen demands of the myocardium. But, actually, left ventricular filling pressures should not be lowered beyond 12 mm Hg, since decreases of cardiac output have to be expected.

After 0.8 mg nitroglycerin (NTG) sublingual or 5 mg ISDN we found in six patients with coronary artery disease a small increase in the heart rate, a decrease

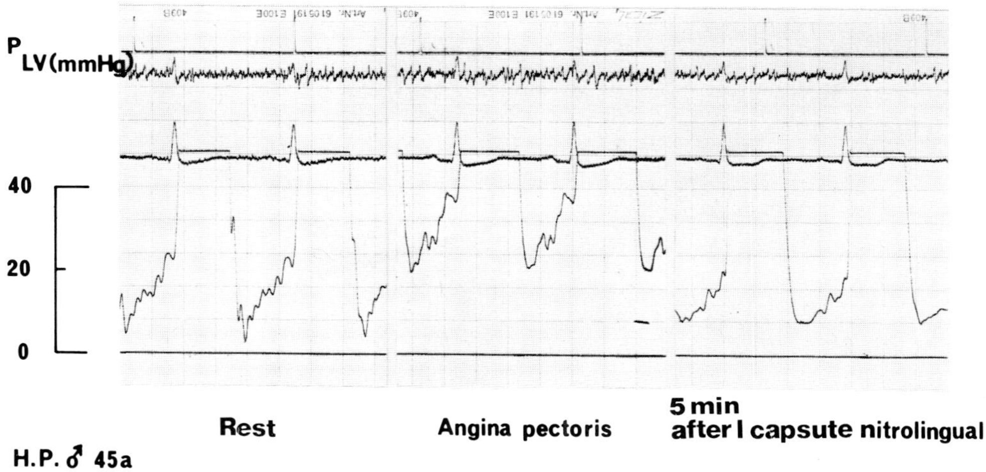

Fig. 7. ECG and LVEDP in a 45-year-old patient during rest, angina attack, and after administration of NTG

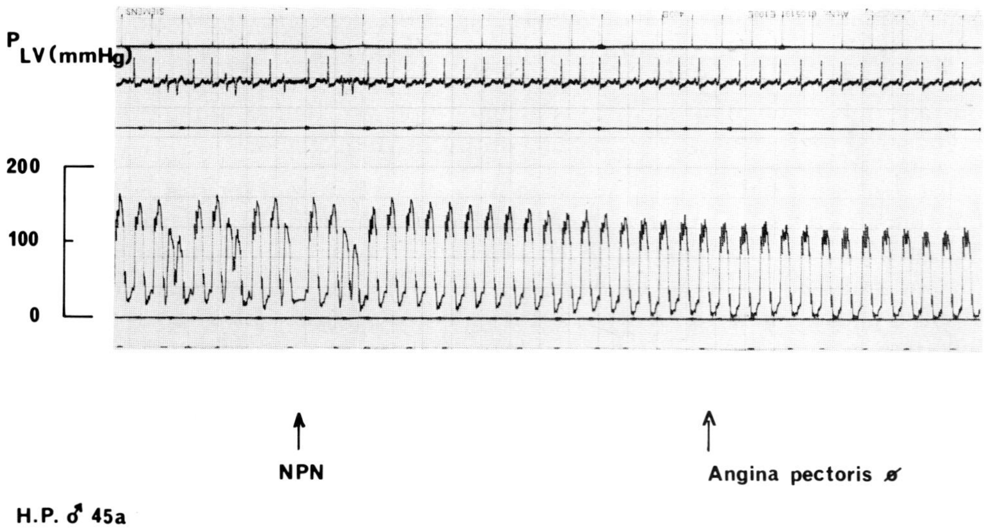

Fig. 8. ECG and LV-pressure (P_{LV}) in the same patient as in Fig. 7 during angina attack and during infusion of NPN (sodium nitroprusside, start and end of infusion)

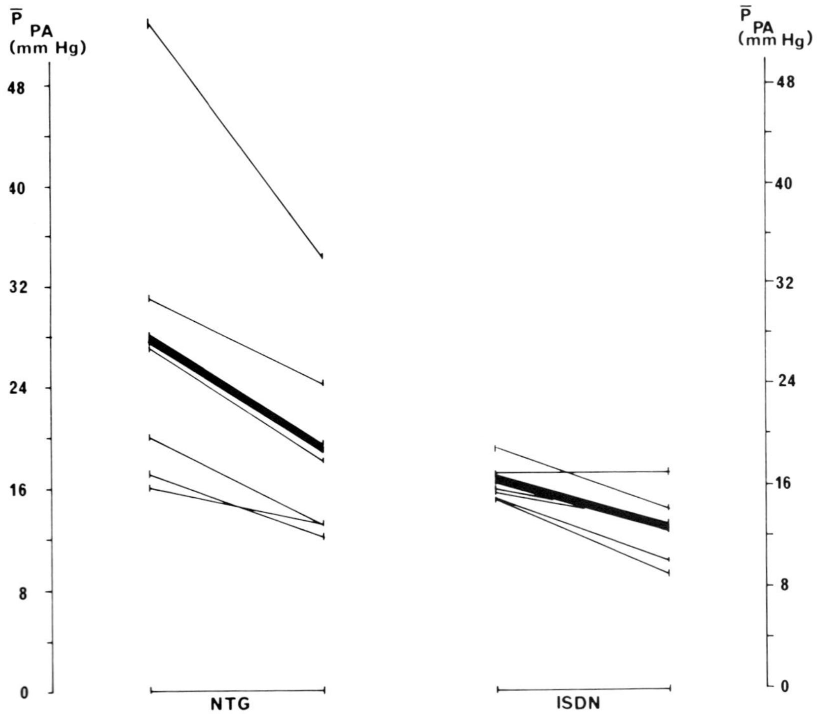

Fig. 9. Pulmonary artery pressure in six patients before and after sublingual administration of 0.8 mg nitroglycerin (NTG) or in six other patients before and after buccal administration 5 mg isosorbide dinitrate (ISDN)

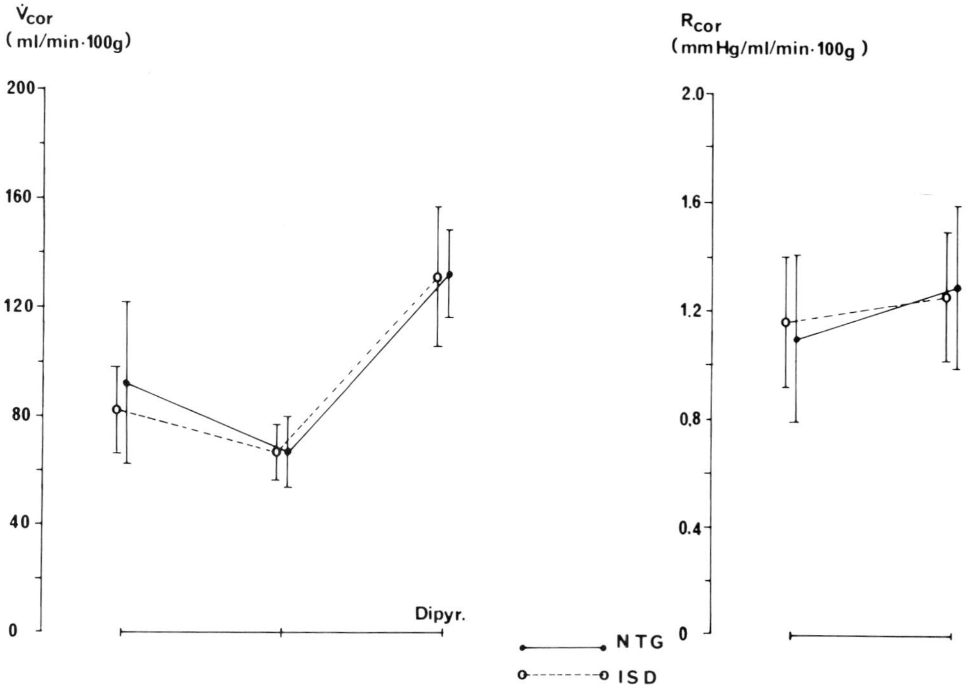

Fig. 10. Myocardial blood flow (V_{cor}) and coronary vascular resistance (R_{cor}) in six patients before and after administration of NTG or NPN (sodium nitroprusside) (like Fig. 9) and after administration of 0.5 mg/kg body wt. dipyridamol

in cardiac output as measured by the dye dilution method, a decrease in the systolic and diastolic arterial pressure, and the well-known lowering effect on the pulmonary arterial pressure (Fig. 9).

Coronary blood flow as measured by the argon method decreases after administration of both NTG and ISDN in the range of 20% to 24% (Fig. 10). To estimate the vasodilatory capacity of the coronary arteries, we measured myocardial blood flow again after intravenous administration of dipyridamol (0.5 mg/kg body wt.). During maximal vasodilatation (coronary reserve) we found an increase of myocardial blood flow of about 50%. An increase of the coronary vascular resistance of 9% and 16% was induced by NTG and ISDN, respectively (Fig. 10). The myocardial oxygen consumption decreased about 26% and 24% after NTG and ISDN, respectively (Fig. 11).

Thus, the reduction of myocardial oxygen consumption is in part induced by lowering the arterial blood pressure, which reduces the left ventricular afterload. However, we found a significant reduction of the preload, as indicated by the pulmonary arterial pressure, as well as left ventricular filling pressure and left ventricular afterload with the fall or arterial blood pressure and the decrease in cardiac output. These hemodynamic effects of the vasodilatatory drugs caused a reduction in myocardial oxygen consumption.

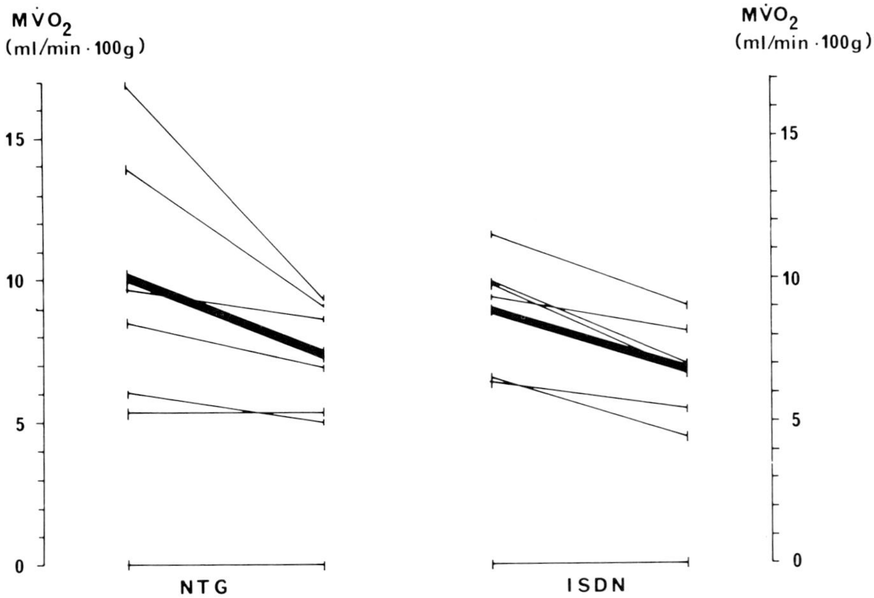

Fig. 11. Myocardial oxygen consumption in six patients before and after administration of 0.8 mg nitroglycerin (NTG) sublingual and in six patients before and after 5 mg isosorbide dinitrate (ISDN) buccal

In conclusion, nitrates are beneficial when used in addition to conventional therapy in the emergency treatment of heart failure. The derivatives of nitrates induced a different hemodynamic response, which was dependent on the patient's initial hemodynamic status.

To obtain optimal effects on cardiac output, the hemodynamic parameters of pre- and afterload have to be controlled very precisely. In cases without hypertension, however, NTG or ISDN results may have a greater benefit than sodium nitroprusside at a given decrease in systemic pressure.

References

1. Armstrong PW, Borcomand K, Parker JO (1976) Nitroprusside in acute myocardial infarction: correlation effects on hemodynamics and precordial mapping. Circulation 54 (Suppl II) : 76
2. Awan NA, Miller RR, Vera Z, Demaria AN, Amsterdam EA, Mason DT (1976) Reduction of S-T Segment elevation with infusion of nitroprusside in patients with acute myocardial infarction. Am J Cardiol 38 : 435
3. Behrenbeck DW, Tauchert M, Niehues B, Hilger HH (1976) Der Einfluss einer "afterload"-Verminderung auf den Sauerstoffverbrauch des Myokards. Verh Dtsch Ges Kreislaufforschung 42 : 286—289

4. Behrenbeck DW, Hilger HH (1976) Beeinflussung der Koronardurchblutung und Koronarangiogramm durch Nitrate. In: Rudolph W, Siegenthaler W (eds) Nitrate. Urban und Schwarzenberg, München-Berlin, Wien S. 86
5. Braunwald E, Pagani M, Vatner STF (1976) Hemodynamic characterisation of nitroprusside in conscious dogs. Circulation 54 (Suppl II) : 194
6. Chatterje K, Swan HJC, Kaushik VS (1976) Effect of vasodilator therapy for severe pump failure in acute myocardial infarction on short-term and late prognosis. Circulation 53 : 797
7. Holmberg S (1971) Coronary circulation during heavy exercise in control subjects and patients with coronary heart disease. Acta Med Scand 190 : 465
8. Lejemtel TR, Nelson GR, Sonnenblick EH, Kirk ES (1976) Preload and afterload changes induced by nitroprusside : Beneficial and detrimental effects on ischaemia. Circulation 54 (Suppl II) : 69
9. Magnusson P, Shell WE, Ganz W (1976) Nitrates and other vasodilators in acute myocardial infarction. Herz 1 : 152
10. Sonnenblick EH, Skelton CL (1971) Oxygen consumption of the heart: Physiological principles and clinical implications. Mod Concepts Cardiovasc Dis 40:9

Session D: Central Haemodynamics, Regional Wall Mechanics, and Ventricular Relaxation in Clinical Hypertension

Chairmen: K. Kochsiek/Würzburg (FRG), E.D. Frohlich/New Orleans (USA)

Part I: Central Haemodynamics at Rest and During Exercise

Central Haemodynamics in Hypertension at Rest and During Exercise

W. HUJER, W.D. PURFÜRST, K.H. GÜNTHER, H. SIEWERT, D. STRANGFELD, E. DRESCHER, J. AUSTENAT, G. LINSS AND P.K.H. SCHMIDT

Historical Introduction

Although haemodynamic investigations were performed in hypertensive subjects early in the 1940s based on the introduction of catheterization of the right heart and the determination of cardiac output (CO), stroke volume and peripheral resistance, the present knowledge about the heart in hypertension (HT) is limited. These circulatory parameters are insufficient in characterizing myocardial function as are criteria taken from conventional (clinical) methods. Therefore some 10 years ago, upon turning our attention to hypertensive heart disease, we began to look for reliable techniques for detecting latent heart failure in HT as basis of a differential therapy [2—4].

Methods

By introducing microcatheterization of the pulmonary artery (PA), left ventricular end-diastolic pressure could be obtained indirectly and semi-invasively, i.e., without left heart catheterization, at rest and during exercise. Until now (30 April 1979) altogether 500 hypertensive patients have undergone floating catheterization of the PA at the Charité in Berlin, 242 of them also during exercise. Another important step was to develop radiocardiography (single In^{113m} bolus injection, intravenously) for the determination of the end-diastolic left ventricular volume and that of the ejection fraction (EF) as well, again without left heart catheterization. [4/7] This method can be used also during exercise. By qualifying apex cardiography for calibration the ventricular pulse, so-called contractility criteria ($df/dt_{max}/IF$. f = force) can be measured, but unfortunately only at rest. Echocardiography recently opened a new era of non-invasive investigation of the heart in hypertension, which is promising since this method can provide functional data in relation to the left ventricular mass, again without left heart catheterization.

Haemodynamic Investigations at Rest

In a first study [10, 11] a group of more than 130 non-congestive hypertensives, composed of men and women with a mean age of 44.5 years and without obvious ischaemic heart disease, was investigated haemodynamically at rest. There was an increased cardiac output (CO) in 41%, stroke volume in 37%, total blood volume in 51%, mean ejection rate in 35%, peripheral resistance in 42% and an increased pulmonary resistance in 23%. Mean systolic blood pressure (BP) was 188 mm Hg, and mean diastolic BP 118 mm Hg, i.e., 21% of the cases have had systolic BP above 200 mm Hg, and 32% diastolic BP more than 130 mm Hg. Latent heart failure was supposed in 34% of the cases, based on an elevation of the PA end-diastolic pressure. From the results we learned that although HT may exist over years (the mean in this group was 5.6 years) and left ventricular hypertrophy should be already present, signs of incipient heart failure cannot be detected at rest, except for a relatively small group.

Calibrated Apex Cardiography

Investigations using the calibrated apex cardiography [8, 9] and comprised of more than 100 non-congestive hypertensives and 100 normotensives with a mean age of 40 and 30, respectively, showed significant differences. In HT the T- and a-waves are higher, df/dt_{max} and the quotient $df/dt_{max}/IF$ is increased, and the time interval $t\text{-}df/dt_{max}$ is shortened. That means, as expected, that these contractility criteria of the left ventricle are elevated.

Haemodynamic Investigations During Exercises

The data of all the haemodynamic exercise tests in HT which have been performed at the Charite Hospital since 1974 have not been comprehensively processed hitherto. Two smaller studies will therefore be reported here which very likely represent the whole group. Fifty non-congestive hypertensives were examined at rest and during ergometrical exercise in a supine position. The systolic cuff blood pressure increased from 168 ± 17.0 to 193 ± 19.0 mm Hg at the 50 W level; the radiocardiographically determined CO from 8.4 ± 2.1 to 15.4 ± 3.1 liters per minute. At the same time an increase of the diastolic pulmonary pressure from 9.4 ± 4.5 to 12.9 ± 4.8 mm Hg was observed. Fig. 1 summarizes the percent change of the haemodynamic parameters which were measured. It is remarkable, in addition, that the end-diastolic left ventricular volume does not change during 50 W exercise, and the ejection fraction increases by about 30% as does the stroke volume. (The mean age of this group was 42.7 ± 8.1 years. Changes at rest/50 W: diastolic BP 112 ± 21.0/123 ± 22.5, mean BP 131 ± 14.0/147 ± 15.2 mm Hg).

Haemodynamics in Hypertension Without and with Ischaemic Heart Disease

Though the filling pressure may be accepted as an important indicator of (latent) heart failure in HT as well, one has to consider it critically since, for in-

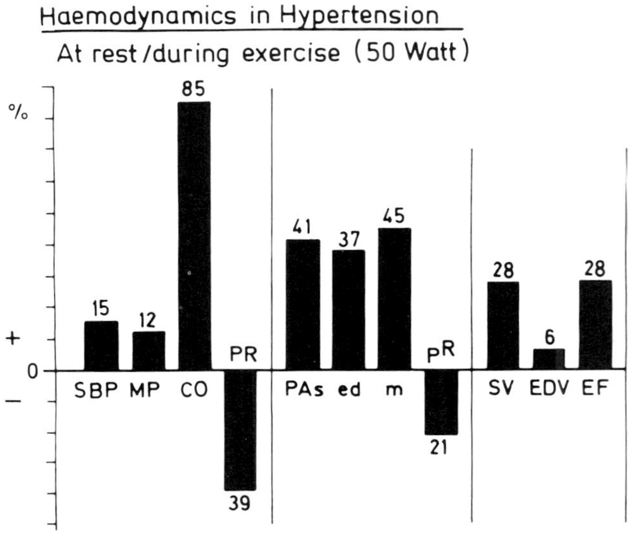

Fig. 1. Changes of the haemodynamic data (percent) in 50 non-congestive hypertensives by 50 W exercise. *SBP*, systolic blood pressure; *MP*, mean blood pressure; *CO*, cardiac output; *PR*, peripheral resistance, *PA*, pulmonary artery pressures; *ed*, end-diastolic, indicator of the left ventricular filling pressure; *s*, systolic; *m*, mean; *pR*, pulmonary resistance; *SV*, stroke volume; *EDV*, left ventricular end-diastolic volume; *EF*, ejection fraction

stance, the filling pressure may be influenced by change of the compliance of the ventricle due to ischaemic heart disease (IHD). Therefore, two groups were compared haemodynamically, one without and one with suspected ischaemic heart disease (based on a "typical" angina pectoris and/or depression of the ST segment equal to or more than 0.1 mV in the left precordial leads of the exercise ECG). As Fig. 2 shows, there is a trend of the HT and IHD group to higher blood pressures, lower CO and similar ejection fractions, the differences being, however, not significant. If one compares then the exercise loads step by step, the "pure" hypertensives reveal a small increase of the filling pressure even at 25 W and reach a pressure plateau, although the load is increased further. None of those stopped the test prematurely. On the other hand, the hypertensives suspected of having ischaemic heart disease indicated a higher increase of the left ventricular filling pressure and half of them stopped the exercise test at 50 W (Fig. 3). It should be emphasized, however, that some of those cases did not interrupt the test earlier but reached at a higher exercise load similar levels of the filling pressure as did the "pure" hypertensives. The explanation of this behavior may be that the clinical diagnosis of ischaemic heart disease is doubtful in those subjects. And for the whole study one might imagine that the doubtful cases are responsible for some overlapping of the two groups, i.e., those without and with ischaemic heart disease, for instance, of the insignificant differences of the ejection fractions. If, indeed, the trends can be confirmed, based

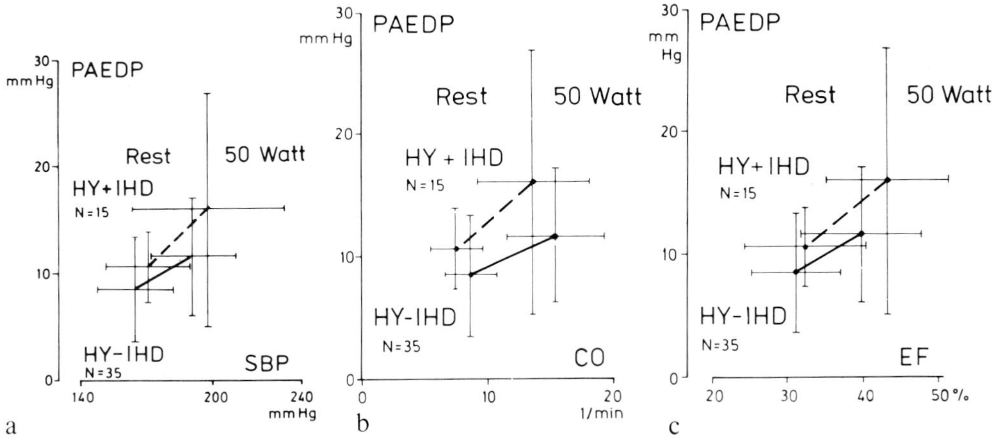

Fig. 2a—c. Haemodynamic changes during 50 W ergometrical exercises in hypertensive cases (*HY*) with suspected ischaemic heart disease (*IHD*) (*HY + IHD*) and without (*HY − IHD*). *PAEDP*, pulmonary artery end-diastolic pressure; other abbreviations see Fig. 1. (Note: The ejection fraction (*EF*) is not yet correlated against background, so the percent values are not real. Compare only the groups and the change from rest to stress)

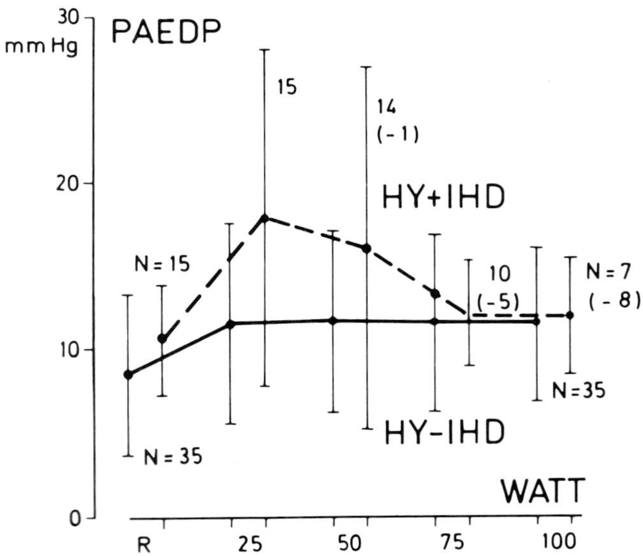

Fig. 3. Comparison of cases with suspicion of ischaemic disease (*IHD*) and those without during the exercise testing step by step. The "pure" hypertensives (*unbroken line*) tend to an increase in the filling pressure (*PAEDP*) by starting the stress, whereas the IHD-suspected cases (*broken line*) tend to have a higher increase of the filling pressure with starting exercise (25 W), some interrupt the test prematurely, and the rest narrow the "pure" hypertensives by increasing the load

on all the haemodynamic exercise tests in HT performed during the last years, the different pattern of the haemodynamic data may render possible the separating of hypertensive cases which are involved at the same time in incipient ischaemic heart disease.

Echocardiography in Relation to Filling Pressure

Finally, a third study can be mentioned in relation to an echocardiographic diagnosis of latent left heart failure in HT. Using the time-motion technique (Echokardiovisor, Organon) 30 non-congestive hypertensive males, WHO stages I—III and mean age 46 ± 7 years, were investigated. Seventeen did not have elevated filling pressure at rest (cuff BP 162 ± 12.3/107 ± 10.5 mm Hg) and the other 13 exhibited increased filling pressure with a mean of 17 from 11 to 25 mm Hg (cuff BP 166 ± 14.4/105 ± 7.8 mm Hg). As expected the group with elevated filling pressures revealed significantly lower values of the so-called mean velocity of circumferential fibre shortening (mVCF), and the ejection fraction was found to be somewhat diminished although insignificantly perhaps to the small number of cases. In additon, this group, which was suspected of having latent heart failure, in comparison to the group with normal filling pressures indicated lower values for the posterior wall amplitude (N.S.), the mitral closing rate ($P <$ 0.05), the PQ-AC time interval, and higher values for left atrium/aorta relation (LA:Ao, N.S.), the end-diastolic diameter (N.S.) and the distance E-IVS ($P < 0.01$). Again this group comprised significantly ($P < 0.01$) more cases with pathological stress ECG (ST depression $\geqslant$ 0.1 mV).

Summary

Since 1969 more than 500 microcatheterizations of the pulmonary artery including more than 240 during ergometrical exercises have been performed at the Charité Hospital in Berlin/DDR to look for a latent heart failure in hypertension. These semi-invasive investigations were generally combined with non-invasive methods, such as radiocardiography (CO, SV, LVEDV) and calibrated apexcardiography ($df/dt_{max}/IF$, $t\text{-}df/dt_{max}$), and recently, echocardiography. An elevation of the left ventricular filling pressure (mostly slight) was found in about one-third of the cases at rest and in two-thirds when using exercise testing (50 W in general). Additionally, higher filling pressures can be seen in hypertensives suspected of having ischaemic heart disease. The latter tend towards smaller ejection fractions and echocardiographic alterations, even at rest. Whether these haemodynamic changes may be due to incipient cardiac insufficiency or to other pathogenetic factors (ischaemia) cannot be decided yet. Pharmacological studies with "well-known" drugs may further elucidate this problem and indicate an additional cardiac therapy in hypertension.

References

1. Drescher E, Günther KH, Austenat J, Hujer W, Purfürst WD (1980) Echocardiographic and haemodynamic investigations of heart function in hypertension. Cor Vasa 22 : 41
2. Günther KH, Schmidt PKH, Strangfeld D, Bohm R, Rademacher I, Günther H, Lucas D, Siewert H (1972) Incipient cardiac failure in hypertensive heart disease. Rev Esp Cardiol (abstr.)
3. Günther KH, Linss G, Strangfeld D, Schmidt PKH, Siewert H, Dieterich WR (1974) Non-invasive estimation of heart function in hypertension. VII World Congress of Cardiology, Buenos Aires (abstr)
4. Günther KH, Schmidt PKH, Linss G, Strangfeld D (1975) Die Beurteilung der Herzfunktion bei Hypertonie-Methoden und Kriterien. In: Baumann R, Schchwazabaja JK (eds) Probleme der kardiovaskulären Regulation. Abhandlungen der Akademie der Wissenschaften der DDR, Jg. 73, Akademie-Verlag, Berlin, p 309, see also Linss et al. 1975; Schmidt et al. 1975
5. Günther KH, Hujer W, Purfürst WD, Strangfeld D, Drescher E, Austenat J, Siewert H (1978) Prevention of heart failure in hypertension. Proceed. VIII World Congress of Cardiology, Tokyo 1978. Excerpta Med S 844
6. Hujer W, Purfürst WD, Strangfeld D, Günther KH (1976) Herzfunktionsuntersuchungen unter Belastung bei Hypertonikern mit und ohne ischämische Herzkrankheit. Ber Ges Inn Med 10 : 305
7. Hujer W, Günther KH, Purfürst WD, Siewert H, Strangfeld D (1979) Möglichkeiten der Früherkennung von Herzfunktionsstörungen bei Hypertonie — eine methodische Übersicht. Dtsch Gesundheitswes 34 : 160
8. Linss G, Strangfeld D, Günther KH, Schmidt PKH (1975) Herzfunktion bei Hypertonie — Untersuchungen mittels quantitativer und differenzierter Apexkardiographie. In: Baumann R, Schchwazabaja JK (eds) Probleme der kardiovaskulären Regulation. Abhandlungen der Akademie der Wissenschaften der DDR, Jg. 73, Akademie-Verlag Berlin, p 313
9. Linss G, Günther KH, Strangfeld D, Dübel HP (1976) The role of calibrated and differential apexcardiography for the estimation of heart function in hypertension. Eur J Cardiol 4 : 399 (abstr.)
10. Schmidt PKH, Günther KH, Strangfeld D, Lucas D, Linss G (1975) Herzfunktion bei Hypertonie — Untersuchungen mittels Rechtsherzkatheterisierung ohne Röntgenkontrolle. In: Baumann R, Schchwazabaja JK (eds) Probleme der kardiovaskulären Regulation. Abhandlungen der Akademie der Wissenschaften der DDR, Jg. 73, Akademie-Verlag, Berlin, p 325
11. Schmidt PKH, Günther KH, Strangfeld D, Lucas D, Linss G, Dieterich WR (1975) Hemodynamic changes of the lesser circulation in hypertension. Prog Respir Res 9 : 243

Arterial Hypertension: Left Ventricular Function at Rest and During Exercise

H. JUST AND P. LIMBOURG

Arterial hypertension is commonly considered a state of circulatory dysregulation with secondary involvement of the heart (Table 1). The term "secondary" implies a more or less passive adaptation of the heart to changes in arterial pressure on the one hand and venous return, on the other. The underlying pathophysiological process is thereby localized peripherally in the vascular system, mostly as a rise of peripheral arteriolar resistance of whatever origin, but probably also with changes in the venous compartment and of circulation blood volume [17, 10]. Adaptation of the heart then consists of an increase in muscle mass through concentric hypertrophy, pressure load being the dominant factor according to conventional understanding. The process of hypertrophy itself leads to depression of myocardial performance, which has been documented in the experimental animal [18—20] for the left and the right ventricle [21, 22], as well as in man [8—10, 23]. With long-standing and/or progression of the process, critical heart weight may be reached and exceeded, a point from which myocardial hyperplasia and fibrosis sets in and heart failure invariably follows.

Table 1. Involvement of the heart in arterial hypertension

1. Hypertrophy: Pressure load, volume load, increased contractile performance, hyperreactivity
2. Dilatation: Pressure and/or volume overload, acute or chronic hypertrophy in excess of critical heart weight
   Myocardial damage (v. i.)
3. Myocardial damage: Advanced hypertrophy, myocardial fibrosis
   Fluid retention (renal disease, heart failure) Catecholamine-myocarditis
   Angiotensin-myocarditis
   Uremia
   Coronary artery disease (v. i.)
4. Secondary complications: Coronary artery disease with or without infarction
   Pericarditis (uremia)
   Aortic dissection
   Pulmonary hypertension (congestive, hyperkinetic)
   Iatrogenic: fluid retention (vasodilators), interference with adrenergic support

Secondary complications such as coronary disease may now further aggravate cardiac involvement [21] (Table 1).

Evidence has been presented, however, which indicates that alterations of cardiac function in arterial hypertension may be more complex. This relates generally to the earlier stages of the disease, where a rather wide spectrum of change of cardiac function may be found, while after long-standing hypertension a more uniform picture, well in accord with the "secondary" role of the heart as outlined above, is seen.

As early as 1939 Wezler described that in hypertension elevation of blood pressure is frequently caused by increased cardiac output and stroke volume in the face of normal or even low vascular resistance [24]. This has been confirmed later on by several investigators [2—6]. Brod [1] demonstrated convincingly that such hyperdynamic dysregulation in the early stages of essential hypertension may be present at rest or only during exercise. The response to physical or mental exercise was exaggerated even if resting behavior was normal. He likened this condition in early or „borderline" essential hypertension to a state of "constant readiness for severe muscular exercise" and considered it characteristic of this phase of the disease. Hyperdynamic circulatory dysfunction at rest or with inappropriate increases of cardiac pumping in response to different stressful stimuli or situations has been shown during the past 10 years to be present in many different forms of hypertension, both in humans and in the experimental animal [12,], and is probably characeristic of the onset phase of most forms of hypertension in man. The hyperreactive state may be found with stimuli such as cold, tilt, mental stress, dynamic, or isometric exercise, and hypoglycemia.

Sannerstedt was the first author to show that physical exercise in hyperdynamic hypertensives was inappropriatedly augmented [17]. From his figures a considerable and likewise inadequate increase in contractile performance can be deduced (large increase of stroke volume without or with only mild increment of left ventricular filling pressure). An increasing body of data is currently being accumulated which shows that augmentation of contractile performance of the left ventricle accompanies the state of increased cardiac pumping under the conditions described above [17]. Direct measurements of the contractile properties of the heart, however, have only very occasionally been presented [21]. The underlying causes are still obscure. A possible causative role or contributory effect in the process of hypertensive disease has not been defined. A specific form of hypertension may originate from the heart itself, namely, early postoperative hypertension after aortocoronary bypass procedures. Here a reflex-type hypertension may arise from stimulation of the afferent limb of a cardiosympathetic reflex, the afferent area of perception being localized in the vicinity of the left anterior descending branch of the coronary artery. Apart from this exceptional and still not fully proven situation the role of the heart in hypertension can still be considered secondary. Yet its involvement in the process would seem complex and not just merely a result of altered output impedance and augmented venous filling.

Guyton [7] has proposed the so far most complete hypothesis concerning the development of arterial hypertension, wherein the heart is considered entirely dependent upon primary changes which take place in the regulation of total body water and/or sodium as a result of altered pressure diureses mechanism in the kidneys in the first place. Increased plasma volume leads to increased venous return to the heart. Sometimes the mechanism is enhanced or solely represented through altered distribution of circulating blood volume into the central, i.e., pulmonary, compartment. Thereby cardiac filling leads to increased output. Increased cardiac pumping evokes a fall in peripheral vascular resistance with resultant excess organ blood flow. This in turn through organ-specific autoregulatory processes is followed by vasoconstriction. Fluid volume is shifted into the extravascular compartment and extracellular fluid volume rises. Vascular resistance remains high and continues to rise as the process continues. With increasing pressure load through elevated resistance, cardiac output is reduced. With progressive hypertrophy and myocardial damage it may fall below normal and yet, in the face of elevated resistance, pressure will remain high. The interplay of variable cardiac output and variable peripheral resistance will allow all kinds of combinations from normal pressure with high flow and low resistance over high pressure with high flow and normal resistance to excessive pressure with high flow and high resistance to high pressure with normal flow and high resistance as well als high pressure with low flow and very high or excessive resistance.

In all instances, however, at the outset of the disease, whatever the primary alteration may be, as long as it involves retention of sodium or fluid or redistribution of circulating blood volume in favor of the central compartment, increased cardiac filling will induce the above outlined sequence of events. The hyperdynamic state of circulation will characterize the early phase of the disease, which is well in accord with clinical observation and which is equally found in those forms of experimental hypertension which are considered most akin to human hypertension.

Guyton has calculated that through the described cascade effect a 2% increase in extracellular fluid volume will lead to a 35%–65% increase in mean arterial pressure. This value is reached with a 5%–10% augmentation of cardiac output and a total peripheral resistance 25%–50% above normal [7]. The validity of the concept is fostered and not contradicted by the behavior of the adaptive reflexes of the circulation, especially the baroreceptor system. The finite gain of the reflex system allows it to reset at any pressure level as long as the time constant of the change is sufficiently long, very much unlike the renal fluid volume system. The baroreceptor reflex will correct each pressure change by a proportionate amount, but never completely. The renal fluid volume system with infinite gain will correct pressure changes slowly but completely to the present level and in accordance with total body fluid. The state of the kidney and the fluid volume will determine the pressure level to which blood pressure will be adjusted.

Here the heart is, indeed, merely passively involved, and although most of the single steps in the process can well be explained and most of the clinical observations be fitted to the sequence of events outlined, it remains unclear why the

Table 2. Hyperkinetic or high output hypertension

1. Early, labile, or borderline essential hypertension
2. Certain forms of sustained essential hypertension
3. Early renal hypertension, especially glomerulonephritis
4. Primary aldosteronism
5. Pheochromocytoma
6. Hypertension with anemia (uremic)
7. Hypertension under vasodilator therapy

contractile state of the myocardium should be augmented in the early stages of the disease being discussed. Depression of contractility is easily explained of course with progression of hypertensive heart disease. And it remains to be explained why such inappropriate increases in cardiac pumping and myocardial contractility are regularly observed in the hyperkinetic forms of hypertension (Table 2). Here the sympathetic system will have to be invoked, although a number of aspects will not be explicable by enhanced sympathetic or decreased vagal tone.

The hypercontractile hyperkinetic state should be accompanied by increased heart rate. This, however, is not seen [12]. Increased liberation of adrenalin and noradrenalin is observed in its most pronounced fashion in pheochromocytoma and here excess increase in contractility is found until catecholamine-induced myocardial damage limits cardiac performance or contraction of plasma volume secondarily reduces cardiac filling and output. In most instances of hyperkinetic hypertension, augmented catecholamine levels will be seen, but are as a rule not very pronounced, thereby only incompletely explaining the hyperreactive cardiocirculatory response. Possibly increased sensitivity of the heart toward endogenous catecholamines will have to be invoked. The well-known mechanism of increased stroke volume in response to increased filling with increased end-diastolic fiber length (Frank-Straub-Starling mechanism) may well explain increased pumping of the heart within certain limits, but will certainly not explain any augmentation of the myocardial contractile state as mentioned above and as will be demonstrated below. Afterload-dependent compensatory mechanisms such as homeometric autoregulation (Anrep effect) and myocardial hypertrophy itself may enable the heart to maintain stroke volume in the wake of elevated or rising aortic impedance, but will never explain augmented contractility at rest or hyperreactive response to exogenous stimuli. It would seem reasonable, therefore, to assume that the role of the heart in arterial hypertension is not entirely that of a slave of changes in the arterial and venous system and/or blood and fluid volume. It must be more intimately linked to the basic underlying process, most likely some more or less specific alteration of the sympathetic/parasympathetic system with ill-defined participation of the heart and myocardial itself.

The points discussed will be explained further by our own studies aimed at clarification of the heart's performance in hyperkinetic forms of hypertension.

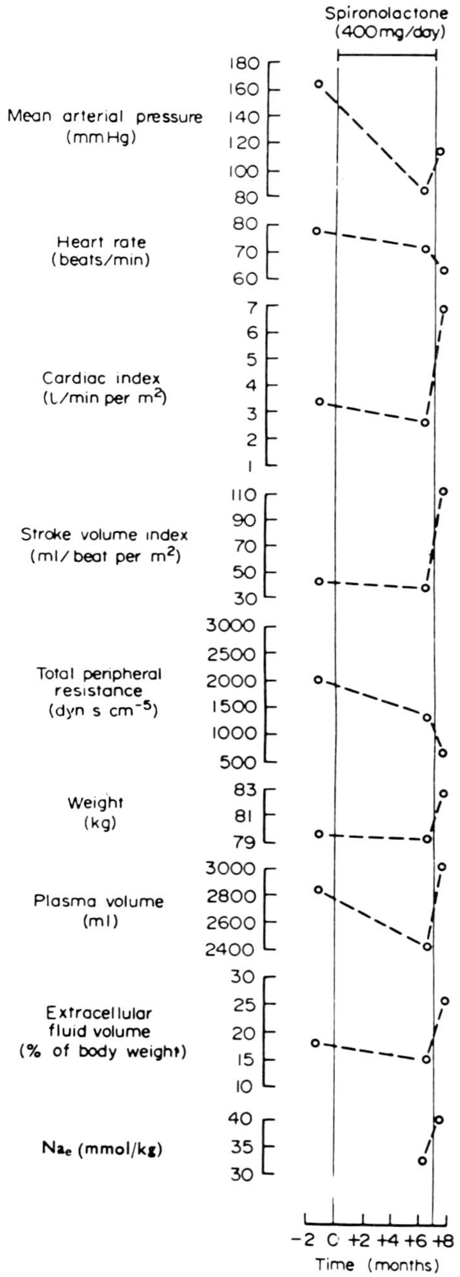

Fig. 1. Changes of hemodynamics, body weight, plasma volume, extracellular fluid volume, and total exchangeable sodium in a patient with primary aldosteronism before, during, and 10 days after spironolactone therapy. Note that with cessation of aldosterone inhibition extracellular fluid increases and is accompanied by a marked rise of cardiac output. This, however, results in only a mild pressure rise because vascular resistance falls in this early period

Fig. 1 shows hemodynamic data and measurements of plasma and fluid volume as well as total exchangeable sodium in a patient with primary aldosteronism. He was studied before, during, and 10 days after cessation of specific inhibition of the hypertensive process by spironolactone blockade of the aldosterone effect [2]. It can be seen that this patient was severely hypertensive and had normal heart rate, normal stroke and cardiac indexes, and a high total peripheral resistance.

After 6 months of spironolactone therapy he was restudied. Pressure was normalized: cardiac index, stroke index, and heart rate still were nomal, yet resistance had decreased together with or as a consequence of extracellular fluid and plasma volume. Ten days after omission of spironolactone blood pressure had again risen to hypertensive values. Now this is found to be due to an excessively increased cardiac index and stroke volume. The heart rate was even somewhat reduced, which at this early stage could be due to baroreceptor-mediated response to the rising pressure. Peripheral vascular resistance had fallen below normal, but extracellular fluid volume, as consequence of aldosterone-dependent sodium retention — increase in exchangeable sodium — had risen considerably. The sequence of events or the pattern of change is entirely in accordance with the previously mentioned theory advanced by Guyton. Measurements of contractility were not made in this patient. Identical studies where, however, performed in six patients with primary aldosteronism and with and without spironolactone therapy, and identical alterations were found [2]. In accordance with other publications on this topic, it can therefore be considered reasonably certain that the initial step, i.e., resetting of the renal fluid volume system through the action of excess aldosterone with progressive increase in total body sodium and water, constitutes a pure example of a form of hypertension which develops through a hyperkinetic phase with low resistance into a sustained phase of high pressure with high resistance and normal or low cardiac output. The sequence is reversible as long as no major damage to the heart or vascular system has occurred.

Contractile behavior of the left ventricle in arterial hypertension was studied in conjunction with diagnostic renal arteriography in 32 patients with essential hypertension of varied severity and duration. Three groups were formed. Group 1 was composed of 14 patients with mild or labile hypertension and for the most part with normal blood pressure at rest at the time of study. Group 2 consisted of 11 patients with established, moderate hypertension. Group 3 had 7 patients with severe long-standing hypertension and advanced hypertensive heart disease, in part involving coronary disease, yet without infarction. These were compared with the behavior of 23 normal persons under identical conditions of study, on the one hand, and, on the other hand, with the response of patients with clear-cut damage to the left ventricle and depressed left ventricular function due to coronary disease with or without infarction and cardiomyopathy, respectively.

Left ventricular pressure and isovolumic velocity-related indexes of contractility were measured directly by catheter-tip manometer and recorded at high paper speed. Baseline measurements were obtained without sedation in the resting supine fasting state after the effects of arterial puncture had subsided. Renal arteriography was done after contractility measurements had been completed. Following the recording at rest the patients underwent isometric exercise by pressing a balloon dynamometer at 0.4 kp/cm^2 for 2 min. Measurements were repeated at the height of the load. The results were compiled and analyzed by conventional statistical methods.

The results are given in Figs. 2—4 (see also 13—16). As can be seen in Fig. 1, systolic pressure, end-diastolic left ventricular pressure, and contractility are within normal limits. Only in a few cases were these values found to be outside the normal at-rest values. Even the response to isometric exercise is normal, albeit at the upper limits. It can be concluded that regulation of ventricular and peripheral vascular dynamics is normal in these cases and that intermittent pressure elevation, which had led to the diagnosis, had not yet led to alterations of ventricular functional or morphological properties (hypertrophy which could express itself, for example, in altered compliance or contractility). In Group 3 sys-

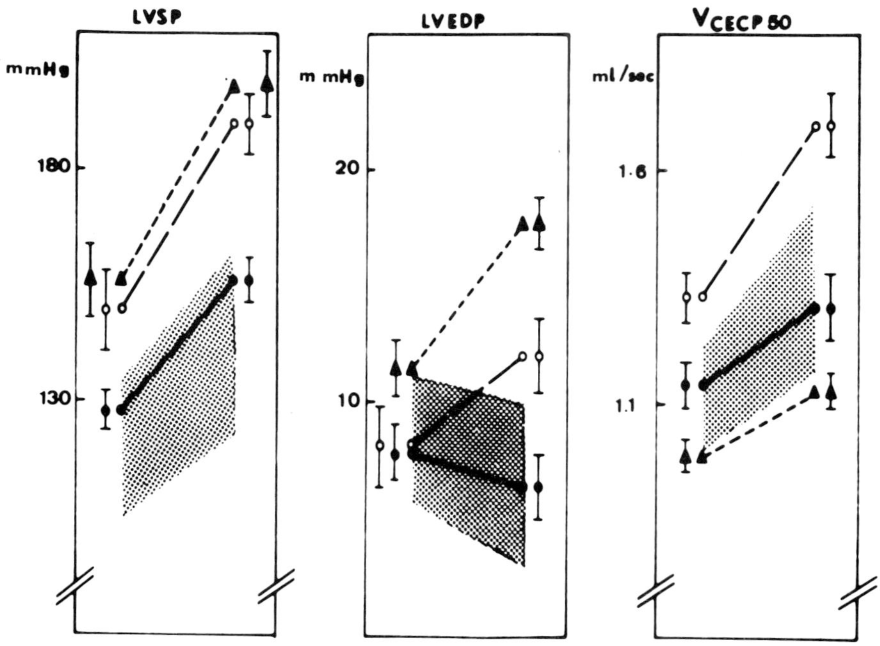

Fig. 2. Behavior of systolic arterial pressure. Left ventricular systolic pressure (*LVSP*), left ventricular end-diastolic pressure (*LVEDP*), and contractility, i.e., velocity of circumferential fiber shortening at developed pressure of 50 mm Hg (V_{CECP50}), at rest (*left*) and during isometric exercise sustained handgrip (*right*). Three groups of patients with arterial hypertension are depicted: *dots*, labile hypertension, eight patients, normotensive at the time of study; *open circles*, early established hypertension, seven patients; *triangles*, advanced hypertension without cardiovascular complications, but with hypertensive heart disease, 10 patients; *shaded area*, range of normal. Note the hyperdynamic response in group 2 (*open circles*)

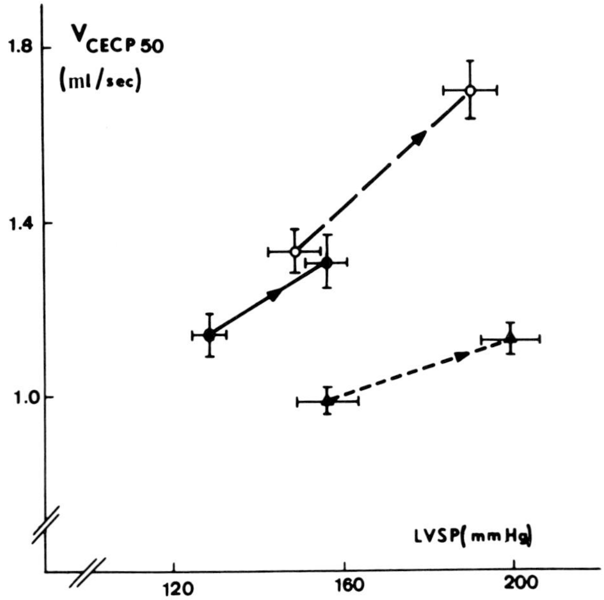

Fig. 3. Relation of developed systolic pressure rise with isometric handgrip exercise and left ventricular contractility. Identical groups of patients as in Fig. 2. In group 2 (*open circles*) contractile performance is already augmented at rest. Systolic pressure rise is effected through an inordinate increase in contractility far above normal. The statistically identical pressure increment in advanced hypertension is evidently reached with only slight increase in contractility, but with marked augmentation of peripheral vascular resistance (values not shown here)

tolic pressure is already high at rest. This holds also for end-diastolic pressure, implying severe hypertrophy with decreased compliance in the absence of failure. The absence of heart failure was ascertained in every case. In these patients with advanced hypertension end-diastolic pressure rises with isometric exercise, indicating that systolic pressure increment can only be achieved by activation of compensatory mechanisms and not through increased contractility, which is shown here in the only minimal increase of V_{CEP50}. This has to be considered an element of early or latent heart failure. The fact that contractile performance is already below normal at rest shows the well-known myocardial depression of advanced and long-standing hypertrophy. Although a morphological correlate cannot be demonstrated for our patients, the aforementioned conclusion as to a morphological defect seems permissible.

Group 2 patients are distinctly different from those of groups 1 and 3: Systolic pressure is elevated at rest and increases strongly with exercise. This is accomplished from a normal left ventricular filling pressure which, although rising with exercise, barely leaves the normal range. The patients of this group are clearly

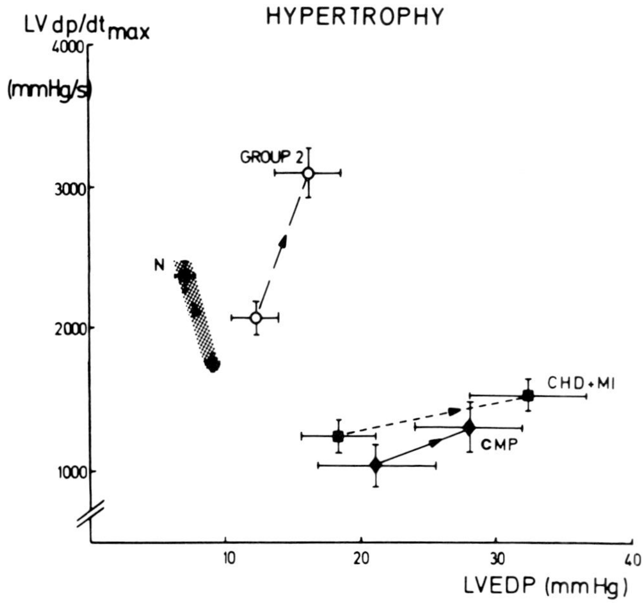

Fig. 4. Relation of left ventricular contractility ($LVdp/dt_{max}$) and left ventricular end-diastolic pressure (*LVEDP*) in patients with early, established hypertension (group 2, as in Fig. 2). For comparison, normal behavior is given (*N*) in the *shaded area* to the left as well as conditions with depressed left ventricular function in patients with coronary artery disease, with or without old myocardial infarction (*CHD + MI*) or cardiomyopathy (*CMP*). As in Figs. 2 and 3, the relation is given at rest and during isometric handgrip exercise (*arrow* indicates direction from resting to exercise value). Again the hyperdynamic, hypercontractile behavior of the patients with early established arterial hypertension is evident (see also Figs. 2 and 3)

hyperkinetic in terms of their contractile performance: the isovolumic contractility index is definitely above normal at rest and increases inordinately with isometric exercise far beyond the response in the other two groups. Cardiac output was not determined in our patients. It would seem, however, that our group 2 patients with augmented contractile performance would belong to hypertensives showing hyperkinetic behavior in terms of increased cardiac pumping.

Figure 3 shows the relation between peak systolic pressure and contractility at rest and during exercise. As can be seen, the hyperkinetic group 2 patients are located at rest at a point identical to that achieved by isometric exercise in the group 1 patients, i.e., those with labile, mild hypertension. Isometric exercise leads then in our hyperkinetic group to the hypertensive response, which can be attributed to the high level of ventricular performance and its augmentation with the stress reaction of our exercise. In contrast, in group 3 systolic pressure increases to the same level, yet without significant increase of contractility. It must be concluded that here the peripheral vascular response with increase in resistance is responsible for the pressure rise. This is accomplished by the hypocontractile ventricle through elevation of end-diastolic pressure, i.e., the Frank-Straub-Starling mechanism.

The hyperkinetic hypertensive patients with augmented contractile performance at rest and strong inotropic response to isometric exercise are nevertheless "below" normal as shown in Fig. 4. Here the relation of contractility to left ventricular end-diastolic pressure is depicted. Normal hearts respond to isometric exercise with a mild but significant reduction in filling pressure. This is not the case in hypertensive hearts. Here the large increase in contractility affords maintenance or even increase of filling pressure. It can be concluded that the systolic pressure rise with exercise results from inotropic stimulation and intense vascular response, i.e., rise in resistance. The heart, performing above normal at rest, requires intense inotropic stimulus, and in a number of patients probably hypertrophy is advanced to a point where a compliance defect accounts for elevated filling pressure and/or possibly activation of the Frank-Straub-Starling mechanism. All this takes place at a level far above and to the left of the conditions prevailing in hypertrophied hearts with left ventricular damage (coronary disease, cardiomyopathy).

In conclusion, the role of the heart in arterial hypertension would seem more complex than heretofore believed. Although largely under passive control of change in venous return, circulating blood volume and its distribution as well as aortic impedance and/or peripheral vascular resistance, an additional factor or contribution of the heart to the hemodynamic pattern or response of the cardiovascular system in hypertension can be found at both ends of a spectrum. In early manifest or borderline labile hypertension as well as in a subset of manifest hypertension, occasionally advanced hypertension hyperkinetic states may be found. This occurs in essential hypertension, renal and renoprival states, and in primary aldosteronism and pheochromocytoma. Under these conditions with increased cardiac pumping, augmentation of myocardial contractile state can be identified. This is accompanied by a hyperreactive response to stressful stimuli and could in our studies be demonstrated for the case of isometric exercise of mild intensity. The reason for the hypercontractile hyperreactive condition should be sympathetic in origin. Detailed information, especially as far as a possible hypersensitivity towards sympathetic outflow is concerned, is lacking and clarification is needed.

On the other hand, in advanced hypertension left ventricular hypertrophy and myocardial damage due to a variety of hypertension-linked processes will lead to a progressive reduction of cardiac performance. Compensatory mechanisms enable the heart to maintain adequate output over a long, although of course variable, period of time. Blood pressure remains elevated here due to high peripheral resistance. Under the conditions of exercise the diminished cardiac reserve can be unmasked in these cases.

The identification of the state of the heart and the circulation, especially the recognition of the hyperkinetic dysregulation, would seem to be of the greatest clinical importance, namely, in therapeutic decisions. Vasodilating drugs will certainly not be indicated nor will they be effective in a situation with already normal or low peripheral resistance and high cardiac output. Hyperkinetic hyperresponders will instead benefit from beta-adrenergic blockade. Standard clinical evaluation of the hypertensive patient should make more use of hemodynamic measurements and cardiac performance should be paid more attention than has been done in the past, if nowadays the more refined therapeutic armament is to be used with the full potential it provides.

References

1. Brod J, Fencl V, Hejl Z, Jirka J, Ulrych M (1962) General and regional hemodynamic pattern underlying essential hypertension. Clin Sci 23 : 339
2. Distler A, Just H, Philipp T (1973) Studies on the mechanism of aldosterone-induced hypertension in man. Clin Sci 45 : 743
3. Esler M, Nestel PJ (1973) Renin and sympathetic nervous system responsiveness to adrenergic stimuli in essential hypertension. Am J Cardiol 32 : 643
4. Ewing DJ, Irving JB, Kerr F, Kirby BJ (1973) Static exercise in untreated hypertension. Br Heart J 35 : 413
5. Finkelman S, Worcel M, Agrest A (1965) Hemodynamic patterns in essential hypertension. Circulation 31 : 356
6. Frohlich ED, Tarazi RC, Dustan HP (1969) Hyperdynamic β-adrenergic circulatory state. Arch Intern Med 123 : 1
7. Guyton AC (1977) Personal view on mechanisms of hypertension. In: Genest J, Koiw E, Kuchel O (eds) Hypertension. McGraw-Hill, New York, pp 384–393
8. Innuoe K, Smulyan H, Young GM, Gierson AL, Eich RH (1973) Left ventricular function in essential hypertension. Am J Cardiol 32 : 264
9. Julius S, Conway J (1968) Hemodynamic studies in borderline blood pressure elevation. Circulation 38 : 282
10. Julius S, Pascal AV, London R (1971) Role of parasympathetic inhibition in hyperkinetic type of borderline hypertension. Circulation 44 : 413
11. Just H, Horbach L, Nicolescu RF, Rosenthal J, Brod J, Wolff HP (1973) Veränderungen der Hämodynamik und Reninaktivität bei physiologischer Orthostase. Cardiol Bull 6 : 191
12. Kuchel O, Cuche JC, Barbeau A, Brecht M, Boucher R, Novaczynski W, Genest J (1970) The relative excess of nor-adrenaline over and dopamin renin hyperresponsiveness in hyperkinetic circulation. J Clin Invest 49 : 53a–54a
13. Limbourg P, Fiegel P, Just H, Lang KF (1974) Kreislaufumstellung und Funktion der linken Kammer während isometrischer Belastung bei Hochdruckkranken. In: Distler A, Wolff HP (eds) Hypertension. Thieme, Stuttgart
14. Limbourg P, Just H, Kobitzsch I, Lang KF (1975) Linksventrikuläre Funktion bei koronarer Herzerkrankung. Verh Dtsch Ges Kreislaufforsch 41 : 176
15. Limbourg P, Fiegel P, Just H, Lang KF (1975) Effect of diazoxide on left ventricular performance in hypertension. Eur J Clin Pharmacol 8 : 387

16. Limbourg P, Just H, Lang KF (1976) Einfluß von Herzfrequenz, Vor- und Nachbelastung auf die maximale systolische Druckanstiegsgeschwindigkeit des linken Ventrikels. Verh Dtsch Ges Kreislaufforsch 42 : 143
17. Sannerstedt R (1966) Hemodynamic response to exercise in patients with arterial hypertension. Acta Med Scand [Suppl] 180 : 458
18. Sasayama S, Ross J Jr, Franklin D, Bloor CM, Bishop S, Dilley RB (1976) Adaptations of the left ventricle to chronic pressure overload. Circ Res 38 : 172
19. Spann JF, Covell JW, Eckberg DC, Sonnenblick EH, Ross J Jr, Braunwald E (1967) Contractile performance of the hypertrophied and chronically failing cat ventricle Circulation Res 21 : 341
20. Spann JF, Buccino RA, Sonnenblick EH, Braunwald E (1967) Contractile state of cardiac muscle obtained from cats with experimentally produced ventricular hypertrophy and heart failure. Circ Res 21 : 341
21. Strauer BE (1979) Das Hochdruckherz. Springer, Berlin Heidelberg New York
22. Tarazi RC, Farrario CM, Dustan HP (1977) The heart in hypertension. P 738. In: Genest J, Koiw E, Kuchel O (eds) Hypertension. McGraw-Hill, New York
23. Taylor SH, Donald KW, Bishop JB (1957) Circulatory studies in hypertensive patients at rest and during exercise. Clin Sci 16 : 351
24. Wezler K, Böger A (1939) Die Dynamik des arteriellen Systems. Der arterielle Blutdruck und seine Komponenten. Ergeb Physiol 41 : 292

Assessment of Left Ventricular Muscle Mass with ^{201}Thallium Myocardial Imaging[1]

U. BÜLL AND B.E. STRAUER

In cardiovascular nuclear medicine, ^{201} Thallium (^{201} TL) is mainly employed to detect and to assess coronary artery disease. Therefore, ^{201} TL myocardial scintigraphy is sometimes characterized as myocardial perfusion imaging. This term is incomplete, since it does not reflect the three determinants of myocardial ^{201} TL uptake which are myocardial blood flow, myocardial metabolism, and myocardial mass.

The present study was undertaken to compare the relation of myocardial ^{201} TL uptake to myocardial muscle mass in the cat and in man. In man, we additionally sought to differentiate normal from hypertrophied left ventricle (LV). Moreover, this study was designed to determine whether an asymetric hypertrophy could be seperated from a global one.

Material and Methods

Experimental Studies

Studies were carried out under artificial ventilation with room air in 42 healthy cats (1.8—4.2 kg) which were anesthesized with pentobarbital (25 mg/kg IP). Heparine (Liquemin) (600 IU/kg) was administered. Reinjections (100 IU/kg) were given at 30-min intervals. Aortic pressure was measured through fluid-filled catheters connected to Statham transducers (P 23 Db). Left ventricular pressure was obtained by a steel catheter which had been introduced through the carotid artery retrogradely into the LV. This catheter was connected with a P 23 Gb Statham transducer.

Following a constant distribution period of ^{201} TL of 20 min in each experiment the chest was opened widely and the heart was removed. Then the coronary artery system was perfused with Krebs-Ringer solution of 30 s in order to completely wash out the radioactive intracoronary blood pool. This procedure proved efficient, since at the end of coronary perfusion the ventricular effluent had counts per minute (CPM) less than 0.01% of mean LV count rate.

---

1 Supported by the Deutsche Forschungsgemeinschaft

The LV, including the intraventricular septum, was separated from the right ventricle (RV). From both sides of the heart, tissue specimens with a large range of different mass were obtained: the RV was dissected across the ventricular wall. Tissue specimens from the LV were taken (a) from the inner layer of the free wall, i.e., from the subendocardium up to 1—1.2 mm midwall depth; (b) from the outer layer of the free wall, i.e., from the subepicardium up to 1—1.5 mm midwall depth; and (c) from the LV papillary muscles. Both muscle mass and counts per min (measured in well counter and related to the injected dose) were then determined for each specimen.

Correlations were performed for: (a) the relationship between total muscle mass and count rate per injected dose, (b) the relationship between muscle mass and count rate, with special reference, to the site of tissue biopsy (LV: subendocardium, subepicardium, and papillary muscle, and RV), and (c) for the ratio of count rate per injected dose and the regional muscle mass.

Clinical Studies

Forty-five patients are included in this study. Of these, 24 complained of non-specific angina but revealed normal findings in ECG (rest and exercise), the coronary arteriogram, and left ventriculography (normal group). Ten patients had and asymmetric hypertrophy of the intraventricular septum (ASH) in cineventriculography, seven patients had essential hypertension, and four patients revealed aortic incompetence (degree III/IV).

Quantitative Ventriculography. Left ventriculograms (50 frames/s) were obtained with multiple-whole catheters using power injections (Contrac) and 40—60 ml 76% meglumine sodium diatrizoate. The projection was 30° in the right anterior oblique view (RAO). Calculations of LV volumes were made from single plane ventriculograms. Wall thickness (d) was taken frame by frame as the average thickness of a 4-cm segment of the free wall on the anterior projection one—third of the distance from the apex. Left ventricular mass (LVMM) determinations were made from end-diastolic chamber dimensions, i.e., from end-diastolic measurements of wall thickness and volume. These calculations are based on the determinations of shell volume created by adding lateral wall thickness to calculated ellipsoidal dimensions and subtracting adjusted chamber volume. Shell volume was converted to mass by multiplying by the specific gravity of heart muscle: It should be noted that RAO volumes and diameters regularly overestimate biplane data calculated by area-length methods by 20%—25%. However, since this error seems to be relatively constant, RAO measurements provide a useful technique for the evaluation of dynamic geometry of the LV, i.e., for calculations of LV volumes and mass indexes. Quantitative ventriculography was carried out as described elsewhere, enabling calculation of LVMM indexes.

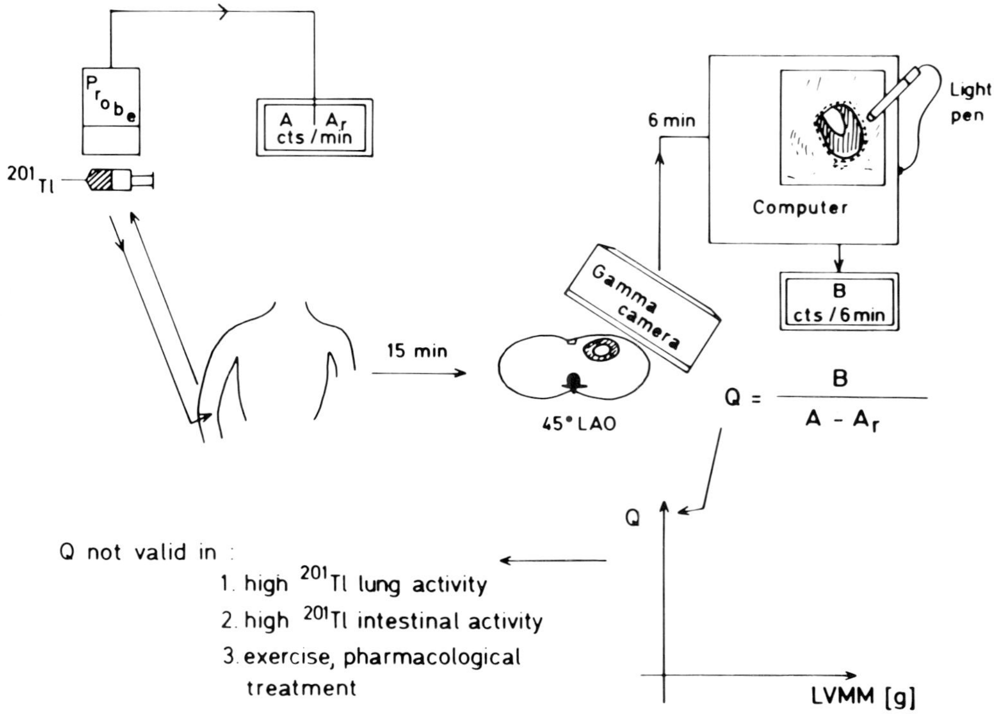

Fig. 1. Scheme to illustrate determination of Q in man. Injected ^{201}TL counts (*A*, counts/min before, *Ar*, counts/min after injection) were used to establish Q by dividing *B* (counts within the LV-region) by A minus A_r. *LVMM* = LV mass

Myocardial imaging was done as illustrated in Fig. 1. A calibrated dose of 1.5 mCi ^{201}TL was injected intravenously; 15 min thereafter the LV was imaged with a wide-field gamma camera, positioned in 45° LAO. Data were on-line fed into a minicomputer for 6 min. Total counts in the LV (B) were determined by a light-pen. From B a ratio Q was calculated by division with ^{201}TL injected counts [counts/min before (A) minus counts/min after injection (A_r)] as measured beneath a probe. This ratio Q was used to graduate the ordinate of a correlative graph. It must be emphasized that values of Q are different from laboratory to laboratory since they additionally depend on the sensitivities of the probe and gamma camera. Therefore, the values of Q may change systematically within a definite parallel range. This allows employment of Q values, individually determined for each laboratory, as a correlate for the LV muscle mass, invasively calculated by the method of Sandler and Dodge without any change of the correlation coefficient.

Myocardial imaging in patients with ASH was done as shown above. Total LV counts were not determined. Distribution of ^{201}TL in the interventricular sep-

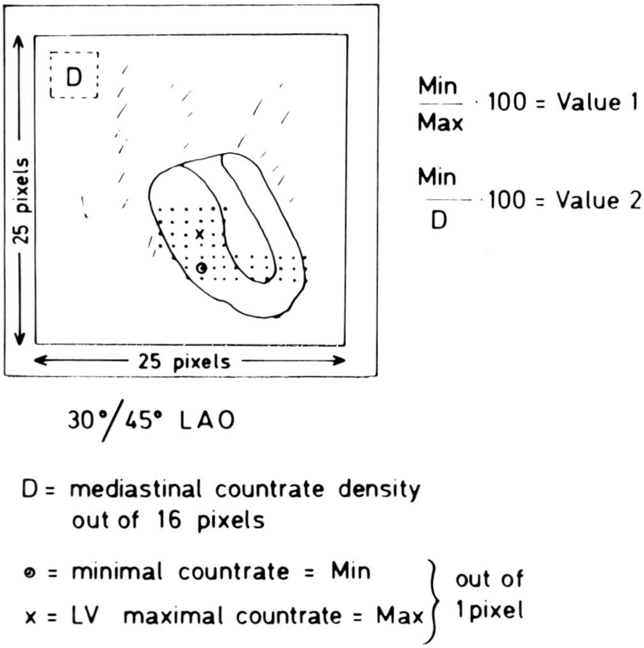

Fig. 2. Scheme to illustrate determination of minimal regional LV ^{201}TL uptake values, either related to LV maximal count rate or to mediastinal count rate density within a matrix of 25 x 25 pixels (^{201}TL scintimetry)

Table 1. Relative minimum ^{201}TL uptake ($x \pm s_x$) (%) in the interventricular septum in one projection (30° LAO) in 15 normal patients and in ten patients with asymmetric septal hypertrophy and IHSS

Reference values:	n	Myocardial max.[a]	Mean mediastinal TL-201 uptake [c]
Normal values	15	78.3% ± 4.7[b]	228.9% ± 30.6[d]
ASH	10	83.4% ± 2.9[b]	283.4% ± 43.4[d]

[a] 100% = maximum ^{201}TL uptake in the LV myocardium
[b] $P < 0.005$
[c] 100% = mean mediastinal ^{201}TL uptake
[d] $P < 0.0025$

tum was computed by a scintimetric method, already published in detail [1]. In short (Fig. 2), LV image was stored within a computer matrix containing 25 x 25 picture elements (pixels). The computer program determined (a) maximum myocardial uptake (cts) in one pixel and expressed (b) minimum uptake in each anatomically defined LV area as a percentage of (a) (value 1 in Fig.

2). Moreover, the mean mediastinal uptake was expressed as count rate density out of a region of interest (D in Fig. 2) placed in the mediastinal area. Minimal septal ^{201}TL uptake was expressed as percentage of this mean mediastinal uptake (value 2 in Fig. 2) to enable computation of septal ^{201}TL minimal uptake in relation to a nonmyocardial ^{201}TL uptake area within the same patient. Values 1 and 2 were compared with the values obtained from the normal group (Table 1).

Results

Experimental Studies

There was a linear and highly significant correlation between the LVMM and the myocardial ^{201}TL concentration (Fig. 3). A 3% ^{201}TL accumulation of the whole injected dose was detected in the LV.

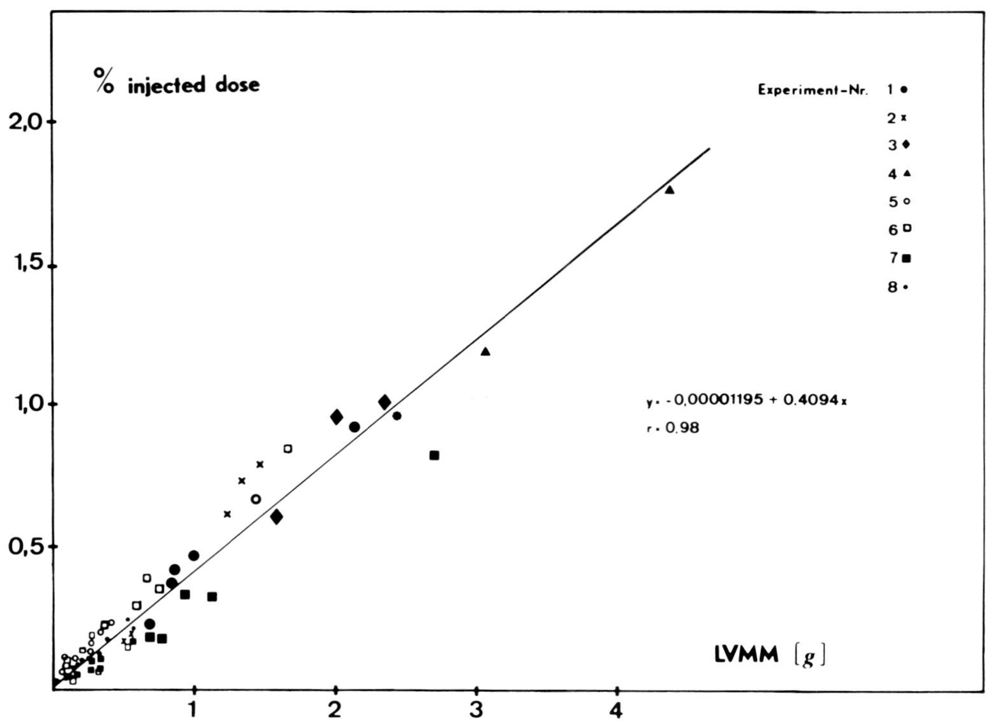

Fig. 3. Relationship between left ventricular muscle mass (*LVMM*) and the LV ^{201}TL concentration as expressed in percent of radioactivity of the injected dose in the cat heart. All data from LV specimens from eight experiments. A linear and highly significant relationship was found between both variables

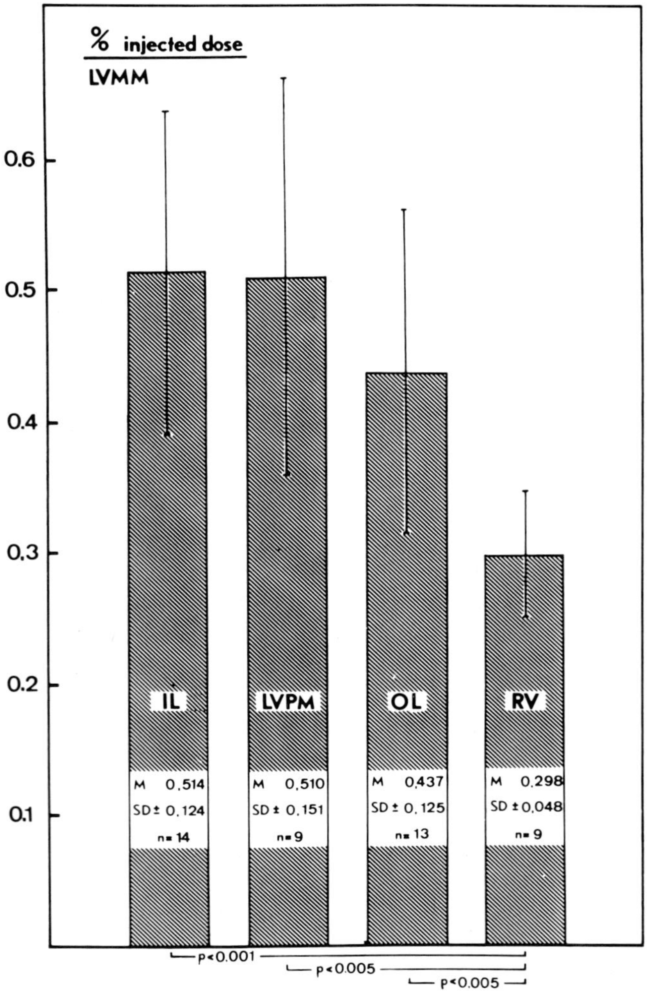

Fig. 4. Ratio of myocardial ^{201}TL accumulation (in terms of percentage of injected dose) and the left ventricular mass (*LVMM*) in grams with regard to the regional site within the LV wall. *IL*, inner layer (subendocardium); *OL*, outer layer (subepicardium); *LVPM*, left ventricular papillary muscle; *RV*, right ventricle. Note that ^{201}TL accumulation is increased in the inner layer and in the papillary muscles when compared with the outer layer and also that ^{201}TL accumulation is markedly lower in the RV when compared with the LV

There was quite an inhomogeneous ^{201}TL distribution in the heart when separately considering the inner and outer layer of the LV, the papillary muscle, and the RV. The largest ^{201}TL concentration per gram muscle weight was found in the inner LV layer as well as in the LV papillary muscle, whereas the outer layer contained 10%—15% less radioactivity per gram in comparison with the inner layer (Fig. 4). A 40% decrease in ^{201}TL accumulation was found in the RV when compared with the radioactivity of the whole LV.

Clinical Studies

The correlation of LV mass in grams and Q ^{201}TL in man is illustrated in Fig. 5. The correlation coefficient *r* was 0.89. The line of identity did not match the ordinate at zero since the LV ^{201}TL uptake values include radioactivity derived from areas in front and beyond the LV (i.e., ^{201}TL stored in lungs and muscles). There was no significant difference of a high LV mass in essential hypertension from aortic incompetence (Figs. 6, 7). On the other hand, there was a difference in LV size (Figs. 4, 5) in the two groups. This difference could be derived from LV ^{201}TL images which allowed assessment of the LV size by determination of number of pixels (NX in Fig. 8) included in the LV region of interest.

Relative (minimal) ^{201}TL uptake in the interventricular septum in patients with ASH was significantly higher than in normals (Table 1). This was true for both reference values (myocardial maximum ^{201}TL uptake and mean mediastinal uptake). The LV ^{201}TL images revealed additional information by illustrating size and exact location of the hypertrophied septal area (Fig. 9).

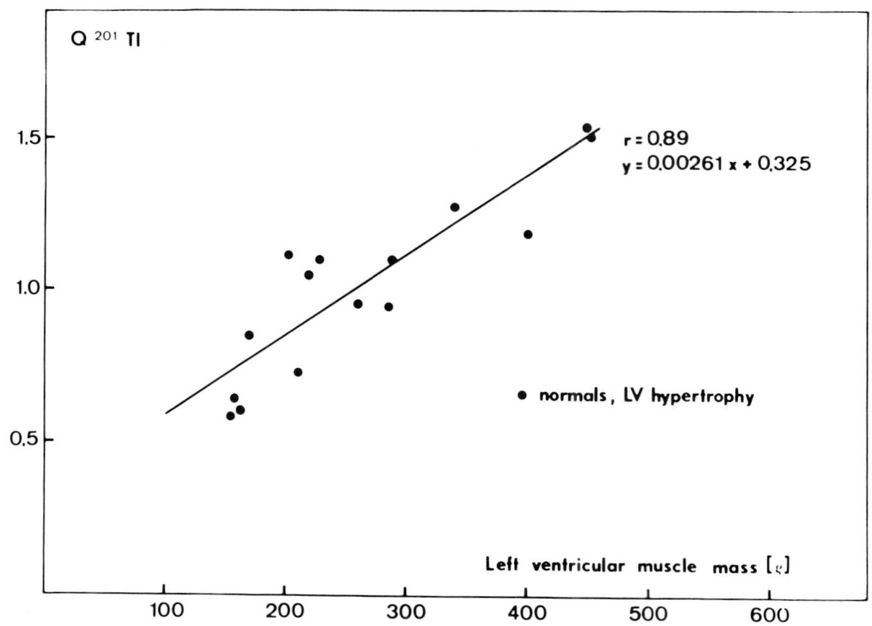

Fig. 5. Correlation of Q (see Fig. 1) with LVMM in man (normals and LV hypertrophy in essential hypertension and aortic incompetence)

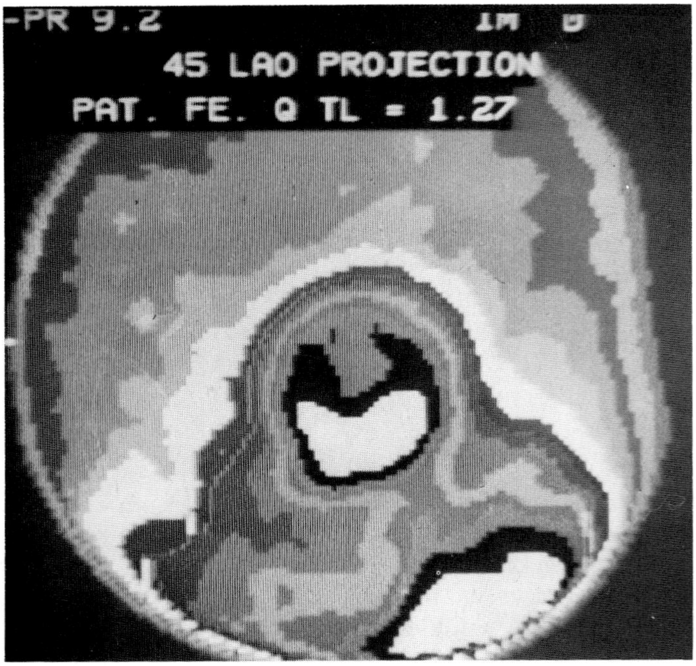

Fig. 6. LV hypertrophy in essential hypertension (LVMM 330 g; Q = 1.27). Note the relatively small LV with thick walls

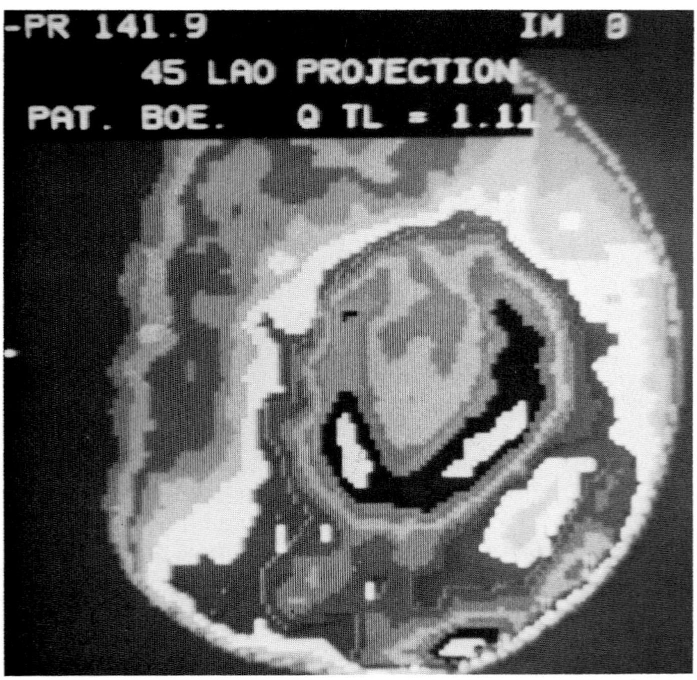

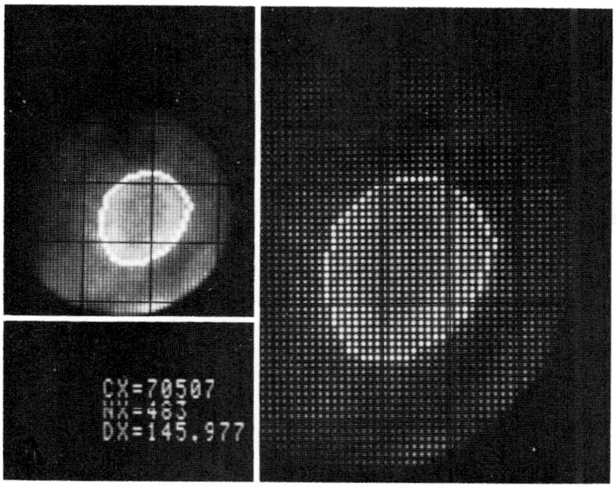

Fig. 8. Region of interest including the LV to indicate NX (number of LV pixels within a 64 x 64 matrix) as a measure for the LV size

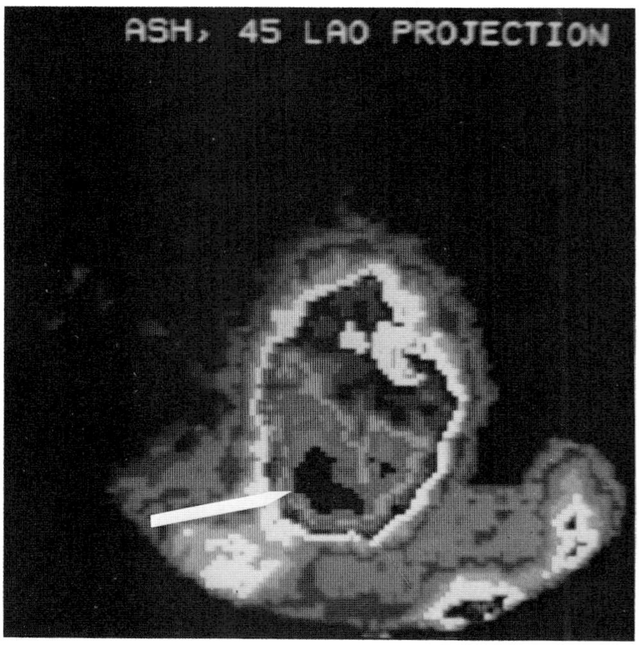

Fig. 9. Asymmetric septal hypertrophy (ASH) (45° LAO projection) to illustrate imaging of ASH by ^{201} TL (*arrow* indicates *hot spot* with the interventricular septum). Note difference in comparison to LV shape given in Figs. 6 and 7

◂ Fig. 7. LV hypertrophy in aortic incompetence (LVMM 300 g; Q = 1.11). Note the large LV with relatively thin walls

Discussion

The results of this study (Figs. 3, 5) demonstrate that the LV muscle mass, except for myocardial flow and metabolism, is one of the major determinants of ^{201}TL uptake. The excellent relationship between experimentally determined muscle mass of the cat LV and the ^{201}TL uptake (Fig. 3) underlines the importance of the amount of viable LVMM for ^{201}TL accumulation. However, homogeneous distribution of ^{201}TL seems not to be present in the whole LV, since the inner LV layers as well as the LV papillary muscle accumulate more ^{201}TL than the outer layers (Fig. 4) and the RV [8].

It may be reasonable to relate this different ^{201}TL uptake at constant mass to different myocardial perfusion and/or metabolism. ^{201}TL uptake at constant mass is related to altered cardiac metabolism and, hence, to altered mechanical function. Systolic wall stress has proved to be a major determinant of myocardial oxygen consumption in animal experiments as well as in human studies, and a correlation exists between peak systolic wall stress and the oxygen consumption of the LV in man. Comparative studies on stress measurements in thin-walled and thick-walled ellipsoidal ventricles have shown transmural (endoepicardial) decrease in wall stress by 10%—25%. This means that systolic stress is greater by 10%—25% in the subendocardial layers than in myocardial areas near the subepicardium. Accordingly, a proportional decrease in regional myocardial oxygen consumption from subendocardial to subepicardial layers ought to be expected. Data concerning regional oxygen consumption are not yet available. However, regional flow may be greater in the inner layers than in the subepicardial myocardium, a mechanism which may be the consequence of increaesed oxygen consumption of the subendocardial myocardium. Conversely, the reduced ratio between ^{201}TL and RV mass may be related to decreased energy demand per gram of RV weight. Systolic wall stress is not easily determined in the double cone-shaped RV. However, assuming equal intraventricular volume and shape in both ventricles, the peak systolic stress in the RV wall could be approximately one half of the LV stress. This may help to explain the decreased RV energy demand per mass unit and, hence, decreased ^{201}TL uptake.

Evaluation of ^{201}TL myocardial uptake in man is mainly done by visual inspection which allows detection of regional changes of normal distributtion. If data are stored in a minicomputer, some information is easily obtained from quantitative analysis of LV ^{201}TL images (Figs. 1,2). As to that , we have demonstrated the validity of scintimetric analysis to describe coronary artery disease and changes in total and regional ^{201}TL uptake at rest and after exercise or dipyridamole [7]. Moreover, the simple procedure of relating LV ^{201}TL global count rates to injected ^{201}TL dose (Fig. 1) showed considerable results in discriminating myocardial mass from LV total mass (Fig. 10). This could be done since nonviable myocardium does not take up ^{201}TL in the same amounts as a viable one. Therefore, LV areas of nonviable myocardium are included in the invasively determined LV mass but do not contribute to the LV ^{201}TL count rate. This result is demonstrated in Fig. 10, where badly or nonperfused

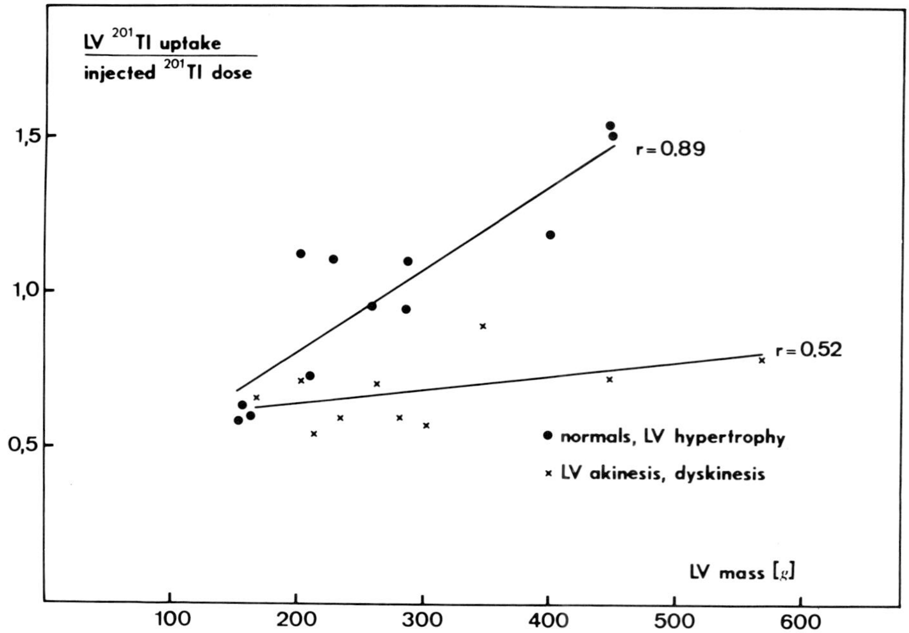

Fig. 10. Relationship between left ventricular mass (*LVMM*) and the ^{201}TL concentration in patients without (•) and with (x) wall motion abnormalities

areas due to myocardial infarction have significantly lower ^{201}TL uptake than normal or hypertrophied myocardium.

The increase of minimal ^{201}TL uptake in IHSS is just the reverse and the consequence of increased LV muscle mass and, hence, of increased total LV oxygen consumption, whereas oxygen consumption per 100 g of LV weight was normal in these seven patients (mean: 8.9 ml/min x 100 g). Thus, increased LV ^{201}TL uptake results from increases in LVMM at normal LV oxygen consumption per mass unit. This supports the importance of LVMM as a determinant of ^{201}TL uptake, since — at constant myocardial oxygen consumption per mass unit — doubling of muscle mass doubles total LV oxygen consumption. Metabolically induced changes in ^{201}TL uptake of the heart thus may be accomplished by an increase in myocardial oxygen consumption per mass unit (hypertensive hypertrophy, aortic incompetence) and/or by augmentation of muscle mass to constant LV oxygen consumption per mass unit (IHSS). In contrast, patients with CAD plus severe wall-motion abnormalities have low minimal ^{201}TL uptake due to injury or loss of muscle mass. Muscle mass is regionally reduced, and minimal ^{201}TL uptake, which takes areas of minimum ^{201}TL uptake into account, is significantly diminished. ^{201}TL is therefore appropriate for both detecting and quantifying regions of reduced ^{201}TL uptake and viable LVMM, especially in cardiac hypertrophy [essential hypertension (Fig. 6), valve lesions (Fig. 7), etc] or in coronary artery disease with wall motion abnormalities [1, 2]. Thus, evaluation of total LV muscle mass may be noninvasively performed by quantifying ^{201}TL techniques (Fig. 5). The progression or regression of LV hypertrophy may be followed by this procedure. On the other hand, if left ventriculography is available, the comparative assessment of both techniques enables the differentiation of viable from nonviable muscle mass, as in scars due to coronary artery disease.

References

1. Büll U, Niendorf HP, Strauer BE, Hast B (1976) Evaluation of myocardial function with the ^{201}thallium-scintimetry in various diseases of the heart. Eur J Nucl Med 1 : 125
2. Büll U, Strauer BE, Hast B (1976) Ergebnisse der ^{201}Thallium-Szintimetrie des Herzens bei der koronaren Herzkrankheit. Dtsch Med Wochenschr 101 : 1088
3. Bürger S, Strauer BE, Büll U (1977) Determinanten der ^{201}Thallium-Speicherung. Z Kardiol [Suppl] 3
4. Bunnell I, Grant C, Greene DG (1965) Left ventricular function derived from the pressure-volume diagram. Am J Med 39 : 881
5. Dodge HT, Sandler H, Baxley WA, Hawley RR (1966) Usefulness and limitations of radiographic methods for determining left ventricular volume. Am J Cardiol 18 : 10
6. Strauer BE (1979) Myocardial oxygen consumption in chronic heart disease: Role of wall stress, hypertrophy and coronary reserve. Am J Cardiol 44 : 730
7. Strauer BE, Büll U, Bürger SB (1978) Clinical studies concerning the determinants of myocardial ^{201}thallium uptake. Basic Res Cardiol 73 : 365
8. Strauer BE, Büll U, Bürger SB (1978) Multifactorial determination of ^{201}thallium uptake of the heart: An experimental study concerning the influence of ventricular mass, perfusion and oxygen consumption. Basic Res Cardiol 73 : 298

Part II: Noninvasive Assessment of Ventricular Contraction and Relaxation

Detection of Abnormal Left Ventricular Performance During Early Systole in Patients with Chronic Pressure Overload Due to Systemic Arterial Hypertension

J.S. KARLINER

There is considerable controversy concerning left ventricular performance in hypertrophied states. Previous data have suggested that ventricular function is depressed as a result of the hypertrophic process per se [1—5]. However, more recent experiments suggest that in the absence of overt congestive cardiac failure left ventricular performance is normal [6—10]. Because systemic arterial hypertension is a common cause of left ventricular hypertrophy, we have characterized the functional state of the left ventricle in 18 patients with left ventricular hypertrophy produced by systemic arterial blood pressure [11]. In these patients we used echocardiography to assess left ventricular performance. Patients receiving digitalis glycosides, reserpines, or guanethidine were excluded, and only one patient was taking propranolol. Patients with a history of angina pectoris or previous myocardial infarction also were excluded from the study. Two patients who had recently recovered from an episode of congestive cardiac failure associated with accelerated hypertension, but no other patients had a history of heart failure, and none had signs of left ventricular decompensation such as pulmonary rales or a third heart sound at the time of study. At the time of study systolic arterial pressure averaged 170 mm systolic (range 130—200 Hg) and 104 mm Hg diastolic (range 75—140 mm Hg). The heart rate averaged 66 beats/min (range 50—79). Each patient had left ventricular hypertrophy as defined by electrocardiographic and vectorcardiographic cirteria.

Data were obtained by standard M-mode echocardiography employing a 2.25 MHz transducer focused at 7.5 cm with a repetition rate of 1000 impulses/s. Standard analyses of left ventricular function were performed and, in addition, a new method recently developed by Dr. Robert Slutsky in our laboratory for measuring left ventricular performance during the first third of systole by echocardiography was also employed [12]. To further substantiate the diagnosis of left ventricular hypertrophy, the average ratio of wall thickness to end-diastolic radius was measured and was 0.56 ± 0.03 (SE). This value is significantly greater than that observed in 29 normal subjects (0.34 ± 0.02, $P < 0.00001$, unpaired t test). Wall thickness measurements were also increased, averaging 14.6 ± 0.6 mm in the left ventricular posterior wall. In 17 of 18 patients this value exceeded 11 mm, which is the upper limit of normal in our laboratory. Interventricular septal thickness averaged 12.7 ± 0.8 mm and exceeded the upper limit or normal of 11 mm in 12 of 16 patients in whom it was measured.

In the basal state left ventricular performance was normal, the mean rate of circumferential fiber shortening (Vcf) averaging 1.27 ± 0.06 diameter/s (range 0.71 to 1.79 diameters/s). The mean Vcf of only two patients fell below the lower limits of normal, which in our laboratory is 1 diamter/s. Similarly, the mean velocity of posterior wall shortening was also normal. Ejection fraction averaged 75 ± 2.4% (range 47 to 91%), and only three patients had reduced values. The percent change in internal diameter averaged 37 ± 1.8% with a range of 20%—50%, and only two patients had reduced values for this measure (< 28%) (Fig. 1). The end-diastolic diameter was normal in all but two patients (< 56 mm).

However, when first third measurements were considered, ejection fraction during first third of systole was reduced in half the patients (< 0.25), and the per-

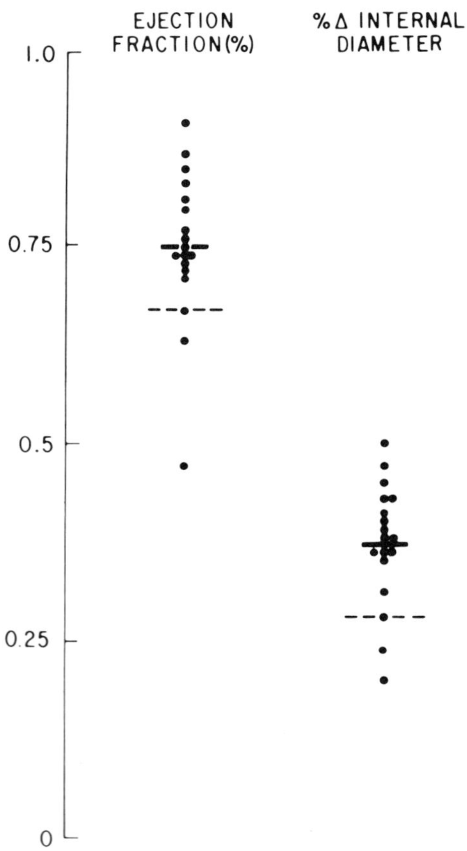

Fig. 1. Ejection fraction and percent of diameter shortening are shown. Most of the patients exhibit normal values in the basal state

cent of fractional shortening was reduced in eight patients and was borderline in two individuals (Fig. 2). This was so despite the fact that calculated end-diastolic wall stress values at rest in 18 patients with left ventricular hypertrophy averaged 167 ± 8.7 g/cm^2, a value not significantly different from that obtained in 29 normal subjects (1.72 ± 6.6 g/cm^2).

The results of the present study indicate that the mechanical performance of the hypertrophied heart in the basal state remeins within the normal range in patients with left ventricular hypertrophy when all of systole is considered. However, when early systolic shortening is taken into account, half the patients showed abnormal values. Although we did not measure wall stress early in systole, it is likely that the increased systemic pressure generated by these patiens is not adequately compensated for by wall thickeness and that a "mismatch" [13] between the extent of shortening and the afterload occurs, resulting in reduced shortening early in systole. However, one this physiological obstacle is overcome, the remainder of shortening appears to be adequate, and the

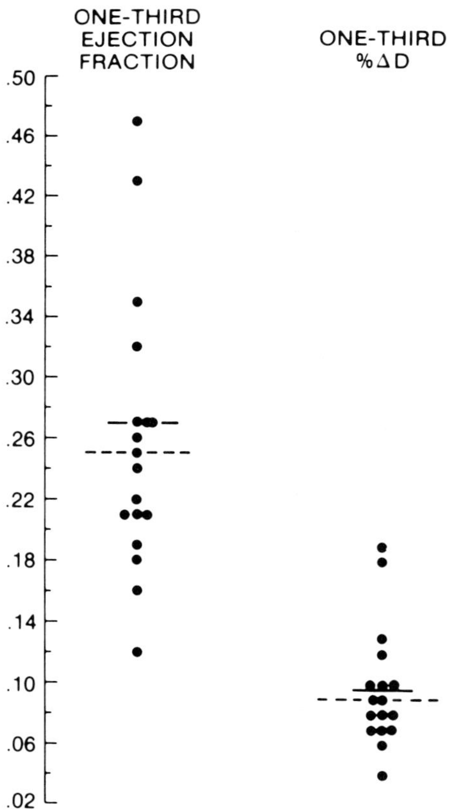

Fig. 2. When ejection and the percent of shortening during the first one-third of systole are calculated, half the patients exhibit depressed left ventricular performance

total amount of shortening and the time required for shortening appear to be within the normal range, thus allowing the hypertrophied heart to generate a normal cardiac output at rest and often in response to the stress of exercise.

Currently, we are uncertain of the significance of this observation but it likely represents a subtle abnormality in left ventricular performance resulting from hypertrophy. Whether this abnormality identifies patients in whom congestive cardiac failure will occur earlier compared with patients without early systolic abnormalities remains a subject for future investigation.

References

1. Spann JF Jr, Buccino RA, Sonnenblick EH, Braunwald E (1967) Contractile state of cardiac muscle obtained from cats with experimentally produced ventricular hypertrophy and heart failure. Circ Res 21 : 341
2. Bing OHL, Matsushita S, Fanburg BL, Levine HJ (1971) Mechanical properties of rat cardiac muscle during experimental hypertrophy. Circ Res 28 : 234
3. Spann JF, Covell JW, Eckberg DL, Sonnenblick EH, Ross JJr, Braunwald E (1972) Contractile performance of the hypertrophied and chronically failing cat ventricle. Am J Physiol 223 : 1150
4. Gunning JF, Cooper G IV, Harrison CE, Coleman HN III (1973) Myocardial oxygen consumption in experimental hypertrophy and congestive heart failure due to pressure overload. Am J Cardiol 32 : 427
5. Mehmel HC, Maxxoni S, Krayenbuehl HP (1975) Contractility of the hypertrophied human left ventricle in chronic pressure and volume overload. Am Heart J 90 : 236
6. Cooper G IV, Puga FJ, Zujko KJ, Harrison CE, Coleman HN III (1973) Normal myocardial function and energetics in volume-overload hypertrophy in the cat. Circ Res 32 : 140
7. Ross JJr (1974) Adaptations of the left ventricle to chronic volume overload. Circ Res [Suppl II] 34/35 : 64
8. Williams JFJr, Potter RD (1974) Normal contractile state of hypertrophied myocardium after pulmonary artery constriction in the cat. J Clin Invest 54 : 1266
9. Sasayama S, Ross JJr, Franklin D, Bloor CM, Bishop S, Dilley RB (1976) Adaptations of the left ventricle to chronic pressure overload. Circ Res 38 : 172
10. LeWinter M, Engler R, van Nyhuis L, Karliner J (1977) Effects of increased arterial pressure on left ventricular systolic function in conscious dogs with chronic volume overload. Circulation [Suppl III] 56 : 53
11. Karliner JS, Williams D, Gorwit J, Crawford MH, O'Rourke RA (1977) Left ventricular performance in patients with left ventricular hypertrophy due to systemic arterial hypertension. Br Heart J 39 : 1239
12. Slutsky R, Karliner JS, Naylor R, Gordon D, Peterson KL (1978) Analysis of early ejection: A new echo approach to identifying left ventricular dys-

function in coronary artery disease. In: 51st Scientific Sessions of the American Heart Association, November 13—16, 1978, Dallas, Texas. Circulation 58, part II, II—41
13. Ross JJr (1976) Afterload mismatch and preload reserve: A conceptual framework for the analysis of ventricular function. Prog Cardiovasc Dis 18 : 255

Quantitative Echocardiographic Analysis of Pharmacological Stress Testing in Essential Hypertension

A. KMENT, D. ANTONI, C. ANGERMANN, D. HÖSS AND G. AUTENRIETH

Essential hypertension is the most common cause of left ventricular hypertrophy. Changes in blood pressure, ventricular diameters and wall thickness lead to alterations of left ventricular afterload and performance [10, 19, 23]. In contrast to earlier studies [2, 5, 7], recent reports on the performance of the hypertrophied left ventricular myocardium indicate normal myocardial function in compensated essential hypertension at rest [14, 18, 24]. However, resting state conditions in normals and patients with essential hypertension are not comparable in terms of blood pressure. Therefore, characterization of left ventricular function should take into account the actual level of blood pressure as well as estimation of actual wall stress or afterload of the individual heart.

Left ventricular performance and especially the functional reserve of the myocardium can be evaluated by pharmacological stress testing [1, 4, 15, 21]. In this study we aimed at comparing left ventricular function of normals and patients with uncomplicated essential hypertension at rest, at comparable levels of blood pressure and finally at comparable levels of wall stress.

Methods

We studied 23 subjects, 12 of whom were healthy volunteers (ages 19—35, mean 29 years); the others were patients with stable or borderline hypertension (ages 16—55, mean 36 years). The patients had neither symptoms or signs of heart failure nor coronary artery disease. They were receiving no drugs.

After a resting period, referred to as control (C), angiotensin II (Hypertensin-Ciba) was infused by a infusion pump (Perfusor, Braun Melsungen) into a cubital vein at two subsequent infusion rates. It was started at 910 ng/min, subsequently referred to as A1. After stabilization of blood pressure the infusion rate was raised to 2280 ng/min, subsequently referred to as A2.

Blood pressure was measured every minute by cuff. M-Mode echocardiograms were recorded and evaluated as reported earlier from our laboratory [1]. We used an Echokardiovisor (Fa. Organon Teknika, B.V., Oss Holland) and M-mode-echocardiograms were recorded on light-sensitive paper at a paper speed of 50 mm/s using an 2.25 MHz unfocused ultrasound transducer.

Before starting the infusion, an optimal record was obtained for each patient's left ventricle, demonstrating only minimal remnants of mitral valve motion. It served as a standard for the recordings during the test.

Left ventricular diameter was measured as the distance between septal and posterior wall endocardium and was taken at the time of the maximum distance of diastole [pre-ejection diameter (PED)] and at the earliest point of minimum distance in systole (ESD). Mid-systolic diameter (MSD) was measured in the middle of the ejection time (ET), which was measured as the length of time from PED to ESD.

Systolic left ventricular wall thickness (intraventricular septum, posterior wall) was measured at the time of ESD; diastolic wall thickness (intraventricular septum, posterior wall) was measured just before the atrial contraction was identifiable at the left ventricular posterior wall.

Table 1 presents the variables taken from the echocardiographic recordings and the parameters of left ventricular function derived from these measurements. The calculation of circumferential wall stress was based on the modified formula of Sandler and Dodge [20, 23]. In this study ventricular afterload was calculated at the time of aortic valve opening where pressure (P) represented the diastolic pressure in dyn/cm^2 [20].

For paired observations statistical analysis was based on the t-test and the U-test according to presence or absence of normal distribution. For regression analysis normal distribution was asserted by the David test; linear regression lines were calculated and regression coefficients (r) were compared using standard methods [22].

Results

Left Ventricular Wall Thickness

As a consequence of the left ventricular hypertrophy in the patients, their mean values for wall thickness of left posterior wall and interventricular septum were significantly higher than in normals, both during systole and diastole (Table 2). Since left ventricular diameters tended to be even lower than in normals, average ratio of wall thickness to diameter during diastole as well as during systole was significantly higher in patients with essential hypertension (Table 2).

Mean Arterial Pressure and Heart Rate

Comparison of mean arterial pressures and heart rates for normals and patients at control and both levels of stress at A1 and A2 is shown in Table 3. Heart rate was at the same level for normals and patients at rest. During infusion of angiotensin heart rate was significantly different in A2 due to a slight decrease of heart rate in normals ($P < 0.01$). Mean arterial pressure was significantly

Table 1. Left ventricular variables determined by echocardiography [20]

Measured	Derived
Diameters	
Pre-ejection D (PED)	1. Fractional syst. shortening of int. diameter (Δ Ds %)
End-systolic D (ESD)	2. Fractional shortening of int. diameter during first half of systole (Δ Ds/2%)
Mic-systolic D (MSD)	
Time intervals	3. Mean normalized rate of int. diameter shortening (VΔDs, PED/s)
Ejection time (ET)	4. Circumferential wall stress at beginning of ejection (σ) $\sigma = \frac{P \cdot D/2}{h} \; 1 - \frac{D}{8(D+h)}$
Left ventricular wall thickness	
Post. wall end-diast. (LVWT d)	
Post. wall syst. (LVWT s)	
Intravent. septum end-diast. (IVS d)	
Intravent. septum syst. (IVS s)	

Table 2. Comparison of left ventricular wall thickness (cm) between normals (N) and patients with essential hypertension (PEH)[a]

	N	PEH	N	PEH
	$LVWT_{syst}$	$LVWT_{syst}$	IVS_{syst}	IVS_{syst}
C	1.16 ± 0.13	1.53 ± 0.31	1.1 ± 0.17	1.4 ± 0.15
	$LVWT_{diast}$	$LVWT_{diast}$	IVS_{diast}	IVS_{diast}
C	0.79 ± 0.15	1.11 ± 0.24	0.82 ± 0.15	1.11 ± 0.1
	WT/PED_{diast}	WT/PED_{diast}	WT/ESD_{diast}	WT/ESD_{diast}
C	0.3 ± 0.045	0.44 ± 0.08	0.7 ± 0.11	0.93 ± 0.15

[a] WT_{diast}/PED = average ratio of wall thickness to diameter during diastole; WT_{syst}/ESD = average ratio of wall thickness to diameter during systole; IVS_{syst} = intravent. septum syst.; $LVWT_{syst}$ = post wall syst.; and $LVWT_{diast}$ = post wall end-diast. Mean ± standard deviation, *P* always < 0.001 (N vs. PEH)

Table 3. Mean values for normals and patients during control and stages of stress

	HR (min^{-1}) N	*P*	PEH	MAP (mm Hg) N	*P*	PEH
C	63 ± 8	n.s.	63 ± 10	83 ± 8	$P<0.005$	110 ± 21
A1	54 ± 8	$P<0.05$	63 ± 11	104 ± 9	$P<0.001$	140 ± 26
A2	53 ± 10	$P<0.01$	64 ± 9	116 ± 11	$P<0.0005$	155 ± 23
	Δ Ds (%) N	*P*	PEH	Δ Ds/2 (%) N	*P*	PEH
C	39.3 ± 3.9	n.s.	36.4 ± 4.9	25.4 ± 5.8	$P<0.01$	19.2 ± 3.8
A1	35.9 ± 3.9	$P<0.02$	30.6 ± 4.9	23.0 ± 3.7	$P<0.01$	16.2 ± 6.0
A2	34.7 ± 4.0	$P<0.0005$	25.8 ± 4.2	22.6 ± 5.8	$P<0.0005$	12.9 ± 3.3
	VΔDs (PED/s) N	*P*	PEH	σ ($10^3 \cdot$dyn/cm^2) N	*P*	PEH
C	1.2 ± 0.18	n.s.	1.41 ± 0.25	279 ± 51	n.s.	243 ± 61
A1	1.03 ± 0.15	$P<0.02$	1.24 ± 0.34	365 ± 56	n.s.	335 ± 62
A2	1.0 ± 0.16	n.s.	1.03 ± 0.14	411 ± 76	n.s.	399 ± 89

[a] PEH = hypertensive patients; N = normals; C = control resting period; A1 = 910 ng/min infusion rate; A2 = 2280 ng/min infusion rate

higher in patients at rest (C) as well as during all steps of investigation (A1, A2). The same was true for the diastolic blood pressure. For the purpose of functional comparison of patients and normals, it is important to note that the mean arterial pressure of patients at control was not statistically different from that of normals during A1 as well as A2.

Calculation of Wall Stress

When afterload was calculated in terms of circumferential wall stress, no statistical difference between patients and normals could be found at all steps of the test (Table 3). However, wall stress was increased in normals as compared to patients when mean arterial blood pressure was comparable ($P < 0.0001$, comparing patients at C versus normals at A1 as well as A2).

Relationship Between Wall Stress and Ventricular Geometry

Figure 1 correlated the ratio of wall thickness radius at beginning of systole to the calculated level of wall stress for patients at control and normals at A1 (i.e. at comparable levels of blood pressure). The inverse relationship between these two parameters demonstrates a decrease of wall stress with the increase of left ventricular hypertrophy. The shaded area of this graph stands for "isobaric conditions" in the pressure range of 80—90 mm Hg. Similar lines could be constructed for other levels of blood pressure, for instance an isobaric area for the range of 95 to 100 mm Hg with higher wall stress.

Fractional Systolic Diameter Shortening (Δ Ds)

The Δ Ds was not different between groups at control, but was significantly higher in normals at A1 and A2 (Table 3). Differences were not significant when patients at control were compared to normals at comparable blood pressure (A1, A2; Fig. 2).

Fractional Diameter Shortening During First Half of Systole (Δ Ds/2)

The Δ Ds/2 of normals exceeded the Δ Ds/2 of patients at all steps of investigation. When control values of patients were compared to normals at A1 the difference was still significant ($P < 0.025$), but at A2 normals could not be distinguished from patients at rest statistically (Table 3).

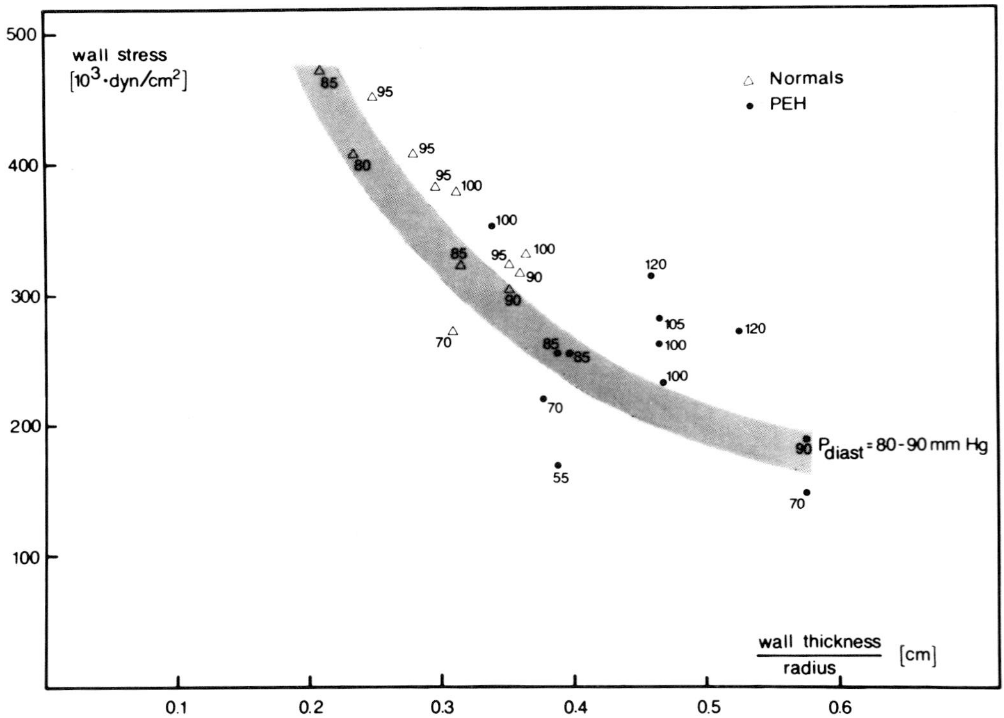

Fig. 1. Relationship between the wall thickness to radius ratio and circumferential wall stress at comparable levels of blood pressure [normals at A1 (910 mg/min infusion rate) vs. patients at C (control resting period)]. *Shaded area* comprises values for diastolic pressures from 80—90 mm Hg with one exception. A similar area could be determined for values between 90 and 100 mm Hg or 70 mm Hg. *PEH*, hypertensive patients; P_{diast}, diastolic pressure

Mean Normalized Velocity of Diameter Shortening (V Λs)

The differences in VΔ Ds at comparable levels of the test reached statistical significance at A1 only ($P < 0.02$). However, VΔ Ds was significantly higher in patients at comparable levels of blood pressure (patients at C versus normals at A1/A2, $P < 0.001$), that is when wall stress was considerably higher in normals (Table 3).;

Relationship Between Wall Stress and Fractional Systolic Diameter Shortening

Indirect calculation of wall stress allows comparison of left ventricular function without additional consideration of blood pressure. Therefore, all values of normals and patients were correlated to analyse fractional systolic shortening as a function of wall stress (Fig. 3). It is evident that there is a considerable scatter

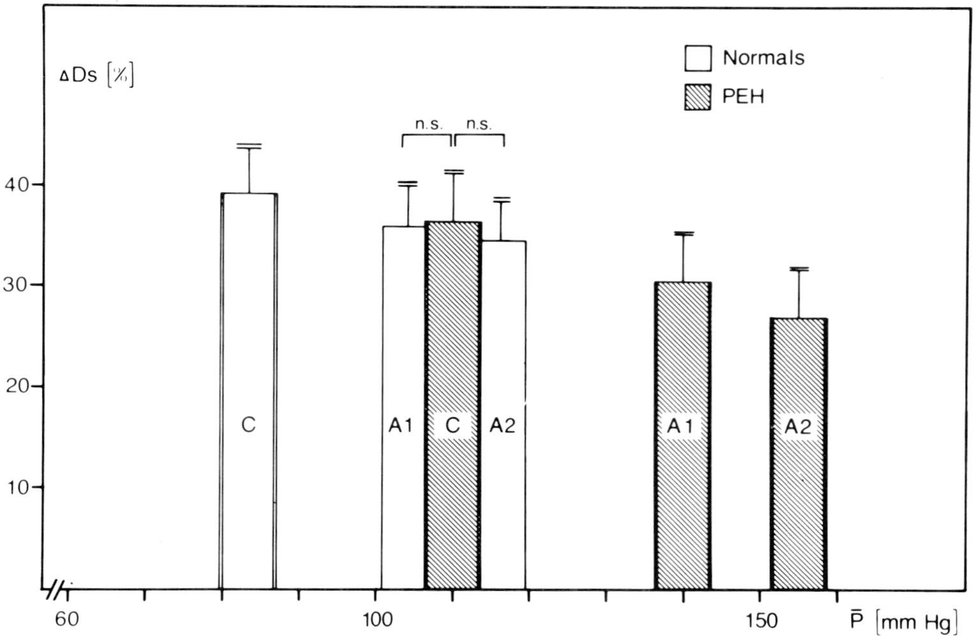

Fig. 2. Changes in fractional systolic diameter shortening (ΔDS) and mean arterial pressure ($\bar{P}$) in normals (*open bars*) and patients (*hatched bars*) for control (C) and both levels of angiotensin infusion ($A1$, $A2$). n.s., not significant

for normals and patients. No statistical correlation could be found for normals ($n = 36; P < 0.01; r = -0.281$). For patients there was a significant but rather poor linear correlation ($n = 32; P < 0.001; r = 0.613$). Nevertheless, this mathematically indicates the tendency for the hypertrophied myocardium to lessen systolic shortening at a given level of wall stress when wall stress was increased above 250×10^3 dyn/cm^2. All values of diameter shortening below the lowest value of normal subjects were obtained from patients during infusion of angiotensin (7 of all 11 patients).

Discussion

Heart Rate

Infusion of angiotensin II had virtually no effect on heart rate in hypertensive patients (PEH). Therefore, rate-sensitive parameters of left ventricular function such as VΔ Ds remain comparable between rest and both levels of the stress test, since rate-induced simulation of a positive inotropic effect does not occur.

On the other hand, the decrease in heart rate in normals indicates some decrease in adrenergic tone by baroreceptor reflex in this group. Subnormal baroreflex

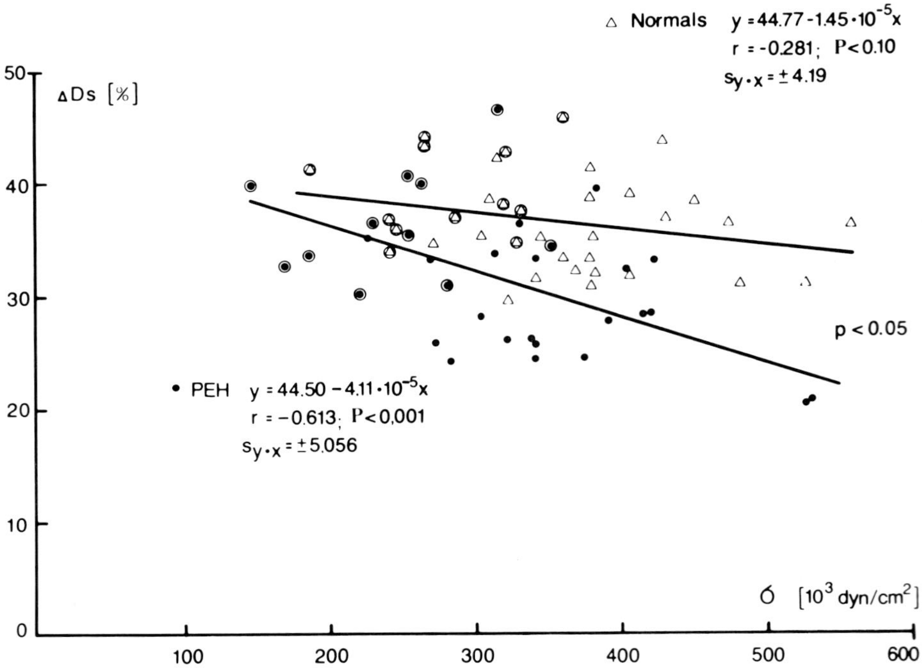

Fig. 3. Relation between wall stress (afterload) and fractional systolic diameter shortening at rest and during all levels of stress. Resting values are encircled. *Open triangles*, normals; *full circles*, patients (PEH)

responiveness is known in subjects with borderline hypertension [6]. Thus, adrenergic stimulation cannot be invoked for explanation of any superior ventricular performance in normals during infusion of angiotensin II. Reflex bradycardia and its prevention by atropine is a well known effect of angiotensin [3, 17].

Arterial Blood Pressure

Mean arterial blood pressure as well as systolic and diastolic pressures were expectedly higher in PEH when compared to normals at all steps of the test. While the absolute increase of mean pressure was significantly higher in PEH, there was a remarkable similarity in the relative rise in normals (+ 25% at A1, + 39% at A2) when compared to that in PEH (+ 27% at A1, + 41% at A2). Infusion of angiotensin II raised arterial pressure in normals to values which were statistically comparable to the resting level of PEH. This gives the opportunity to compare ventricular performance in normals and PEH at comparable levels of blood pressure (i.e. normals at A1 and A2 versus PEH at C).

Comparison of Left Ventricular Function at Rest

The conventional echocardiographic parameters of left ventricular function Δ Ds and VΔ Ds indicated normal ventricular performance in both groups during resting conditions. This is not only in agreement with the clinical state of these patients but also with numerous studies which found no evidence of depressed ventricular function in the compensated state of essential hypertension [5, 14, 25].

Comparison of Left Ventricular Function at Comparable Levels of Blood Pressure

The stepwise increase in blood pressure caused the values of VΔ Ds and ΔDs to decrease in both groups. This would be expected, since acute changes of blood pressure must influence afterload-dependent parameters.

The VΔ Ds at C in PEH was higher than VΔ Ds in normals at comparable levels of blood pressure. Since VΔ Ds is very sensitive to heart rate [16], the slight decrease in heart rate of normals might have contributed to this effect.

Therefore, it does not seem appropriate to attribute this difference to superior left ventricular performance in PEH. Δ Ds in normals did not fall below the shortening fraction of PEH at rest when the pressure of normals was raised. On the other hand, Δ Ds of PEH fell with increasing pressure to values significantly below those of normals at the same levels of angiotensin infusion. Thus, PEH showed larger reductions in fractional shortening when blood pressure increased in a similar percentage as in normals. Whether this is evidence of diminished left ventricular reserve can only be determined when blood pressure is related to ventricular geometry, i.e. when the resulting wall stress is considered.

Comparison of Left Ventricular Function at Comparable Levels of Wall Stress

Myocardial function is determined by heart rate, inotropic state, pre-load and afterload. In our study heart rate was constant in PEH and fell slightly in N. Taking heart rate as an indicator of sympathetic tone, no appreciable change in inotropic state has to be anticipated in patients, while normals may have some slight decrease. Pre-load has not been assessed in this study since left ventricular diastolic pressure cannot be measured non-invasively.

However, no increase in diastolic ventricular dimension occurred. The main change induced by the test was an increase in blood pressure leading to an increase in afterload.

Afterload is best expressed in terms of circumferential wall stress. We determined it according to the method of Ratshin et al. from echocardiographic dimension of the left ventricle and diastolic blood pressure [20]. Good agreement of such estimates with invasively determined values has been shown by these authors.

Left ventricular hypertrophy in PEH kept calculated circumferential wall stress as low as in normals during all steps of the test, although blood pressure was significantly higher in patients (Table 3). At comparable afterload one should expect comparable ventricular function. However, as a group PEH exhibited significantly smaller fractional systolic shortening than normals at A1 and A2 (Table 3). The mean decrease of Δ Ds for patients was 10.6%, whereas it was only 4.6% in normals.

This indicates that the contractile reserve of the left ventricle is diminished on the average in patients with clinically compensated essential hypertension. The same conclusion can be reached by analysing the relationship of Δ Ds to actual wall stress in individual subjects (Fig. 3). When the lowest value of Δ Ds of a normal subject is taken as the lower limit of normal, 7 of our 11 patients fell below it, all of them during angiotensin infusion. This indicates diminished contractile reserve of PEH with clinically compensated essential hypertension during afterload stress. Since the difference is not explained by higher wall stress in PEH, different intrinsic properties of the left ventricle have to be assumed.

Our results do not agree with findings of other authors, who found a superior performance of the left ventricle in similar patients. However, ventricular function was not compared in respect to wall stress. In addition, a physical exercise such as treadmill exercise [24] or handgrip exercise [12] has been used. However, increased plasma catecholamine levels have to be anticipated in physical exercise in patients with hypertension [9].

Pattern of Left Ventricular Contraction

Diminished fractional shortening during first half of systole was present in PEH at rest and during infusion of angiotensin II. Its total decrease with increasing afterload was also greater in PEH than in normals — 6.2% vs. — 2.8%; see Table 3).

This indicates a diminished velocity of diameter shortening at the beginning and an increased velocity during the second half of systole during resting conditions, since total Δ Ds was normal. Decreased ejection fraction during the first third of systole by angiography has been considered a very sensitive indicator of functional impairment in patients with coronary artery disease [8, 11]. By echocardiography in an earlier study our group has shown diminished Δ Ds/2 in patients with coronary artery disease [1], and Karliner and co-workers have presented the finding of diminished first third shortening during this symposium (see session D, Part II). If these findings can be substantiated in the future, Ds/2 will be the most sensitive indicator for altered ventricular function in PEH since the development of functional class (NYHA) and conventional echocardiographic parameters for this group of patients.

References

1. Autenrieth G, Angermann C, Goss F, Bolte HD (1977) Echocardiographic evaluation of myocardial performance during infusion of angiotensin and handgrip-exercise. In: Myocardial failure. Springer, Berlin Heidelberg New York, p 220
2. Bing OHL, Matsushita S, Fanburg BL, Levine HJ (1971) Mechanical properties of rat cardiac muscle during experimental hypertrophy. Circ Res 28 : 234
3. Brod J, Hejl Z, Hornyeh A, Jirka J, Slechta V, Burianova B (1969) Comparison of hemodynamic effects of equipressor doses of intravenous angiotensin and noradrenaline in man. Clin Sci 36 : 161
4. Cyran J, Bolte HD (1976) Zur diagnostischen Aussagefähigkeit des Angiotensin-Infusionstestes als Funktionsprüfung des Ventrikelmyokards. Verh Dtsch Ges Kreislaufforsch 42 : 147
5. Dunn FG, Chandraratna P, de Carvalho JGR, Basta LL, Frohlich ED (1977) Pathophysiologic assessment of hypertensive heart disease. Am J Cardiol 39 : 789
6. Eckberg DL (1979) Carotid baroreflex function in young men with borderline blood pressure elevation. Circulation 59 : 632
7. Frohlich ED (1973) Clinical-physiologic classification of hypertensive heart disease in essential hypertension. Hypertension: Mechanisms and management. Grune & Stratton, New York, p 181
8. Gibson DG, Doran JH, Traill TA, Brown DJ (1978) Abnormal left ventricular wall movement during early systole in patients with angina pectoris. Br Heart J 40 : 758
9. Grobecker H (1979) Catecholamines in experimental and essential hypertension. In: International symposium: The heart in hypertension, Munich, June 1979, p 13
10. Hood WP, Thompson WJ, Rackley CE (1969) Comparison of calculations of left ventricular wall stress in man from thin-walled and thick-walled ellipsoidal models. Circ Res 24 : 575
11. Johnson LJ, Ellis K, Schmidt D, Weiss MB, Cannon PJ (1975) Volume ejected in early systole. A sensitive index of left ventricular performance in coronary artery disease. Circulation 52 : 378
12. Just H (1979) Arterial hypertension: Left ventricular function at rest and during exercise. In: International symposium: The heart in hypertension. Munich, June 1979, p 54
13. Karliner JS (1979) Detection of abnormal left ventricular performance during early systole in patients with chronic pressure overload due to systemic arterial hypertension. In: International symposium: The heart in hypertension. Munich, June 1979, p 56
14. Karliner JS, Williams W, Gorwit J, Crawford MH, O'Rourke RA (1977) Left ventricular performance in patients with left ventricular hypertrophy caused by systemic arterial hypertension. Br Heart J 39 : 1239
15. Linhart JW, Hildner FJ, Barold SS, Samet P (1969) Myocardial function in patients with coronary artery disease. Am J Cardiol 23 : 379

16. De Maria AN, Neumann A, Schubart PJ, Lee G, Mason DT (1979) Systemic correlation of cardiac chamber size and ventricular performance determined with echocardiography and alterations in heart rate in normal persons. Am J Cardiol 43 : 1
17. Nolan JP, Cobb LA, Thompson JI (1967) Circulatory responses to angiotensin in man. Clin Pharmacol Ther 8 : 235
18. Pfeffer MA, Pfeffer JM, Frohlich ED (1976) Pumping ability of the hypertrophying left ventricle of the spontaneously hypertensive rat. Circ Res 38 : 423
19. Rackley CE, Hood WPJr, Rolett EL (1970) Left ventricular end-diastolic pressure in chronic heart disease. Am J Med 48 : 310
20. Ratshin RA, Rackley CE, Russel RO (1974) Determination of left ventricular preload and afterload by quantitative echocardiography in man. Circ Res 34 : 711
21. Regan TJ, Levinson GE, Oldewurtel HA, Frank MJ, Weisse AG, Moschos CB (1969) Ventricular function in noncardiacs with alcoholic fatty liver: Role of ethanol in the production of cardiomyopathy. J Clin Invest 48 : 397
22. Sachs L (1972) Statistische Auswertungsmethoden, 3rd edn. Springer, Berlin Heidelberg New York, pp 254, 341
23. Sandler H, Dodge HT (1963) Left ventricular tension and stress in man. Circ Res 13 : 91
24. Strauer BE (1978) The heart in hypertension. I. Left ventricular function at rest and during exercise. Z Kardiol 67 : 375
25. Toshima H, Yoshinosi K, Haruki Y, Toshinori A, Nobovu K (1975) Echocardiographic classification of hypertensive heart disease. Jp Heart J 16 : 377

Left Ventricular Relaxation and Filling Pattern in Different Forms of Left Ventricular Hypertrophy

P. HANRATH, D. MATHEY, P. KREMER AND W. BLEIFELD

Recent echocardiographic and angiographic studies have shown that hypertrophic obstructive cardiomyopathy (HOCM) is often associated with abnormal left ventricular (LV) relaxation and an abnormal diastolic filling pattern [1—3]. It was the purpose of this study to examine whether these abnormalities are only typical for this special type of LV hypertrophy or whether they can be found in other forms of LV hypertrophy as well [4].

Therefore, the time intervals and dimensional changes during LV relaxation and filling were studied in normal subjects, patients with hypertrophic obstructive cardiomyopathy, and in patients with LV hypertrophy due to chronic pressure overload (CPO).

Patients and Methods

Seventy-six subjects were studied and divided into three groups. Included were 28 persons without evidence of heart disease (N), 24 patients with hypertrophic obstructive and nonobstructive cardiomyopathy, and 24 patients with chronic LV pressure overload due to aortic stenosis or severe arterial hypertension. During the time of the study no patient was on β-blocker or digitalis.

Echocardiograms were recorded in a standard manner and digitized with a hand-controlled crosswire cursor according to a computerized method previously described [5]. With this method the time and dimensional measurements described below were performed.

Measurements of Time Intervals

Time intervals were referred to the peak of the R-wave (R) of the first QRS complex as a zero reference point. With respect to this reference point, the occurence of the time point of the different LV dimensions within the cardiac cycle could be exactly determined.

Time parameters of particular interest for this study were the time point of mitral valve opening and the left ventricular filling period (cycle length minus time point of mitral valve opening). The time point of end-systole was defined as minimum LV dimension, where its normalized first differential $\frac{dD}{dt \times D}$ was zero.

Measurements of LV Dimensions

End-systolic and end-diastolic dimensions, percentage shortening of the LV minor axis, peak endocardial circumferential fiber shortening ($V_{CF\ max}$) and lengthening velocity, the wall thickness of the interventricular septum, and the LV posterior wall at end-diastole were measured.

The diastolic left ventricular dimension time curve, which is divided into the four phases isovolumic relaxation, rapid filling, slow filling, and filling due to atrial contraction, was analyzed in a way similar to the method first described by Decoodt (Fig. 1)[6].

An approximate measurement of the "isovolumic relaxation period" was obtained from the time difference between the time points of end-systolic dimension (DS) and mitral valve opening [7—10]. This time interval is referred to as relaxation time index. After mitral valve opening, the rapid filling phase begins. Its end was defined as the point where the normalized lengthening rate had decreased to 50% of its peak volume [5]. Similarly, the end of the slow filling period was determined as the point where the last second lengthening peak due to atrial contraction had reached half of its maximum. The dimension increase due to atrial contraction was terminated with the peak of the next R wave.

Only in those cases where a clearly separate peak of the normalized lengthening rate due to atrial contraction was seen was analyzed. This break-point determination enabled a calculation of absolute time periods as well as dimensional changes during each of these different phases (Fig. 1). Furthermore, these absolute time and dimensional values were related to the total LV filling time (t LVF) and the total LV diameter increase during this period and expressed as a percentage according to the following formulas (abbreviations see Fig. 1):

1. $t\ RF\ (\%) = \frac{ERF - MO}{t\ LVF} \times 100$

2. $t\ SF\ (\%) = \frac{ESF - ERF}{t\ LVF} \times 100$

3. $t\ AC\ (\%) = \frac{EAC - ESF}{t\ LVF} \times 100$

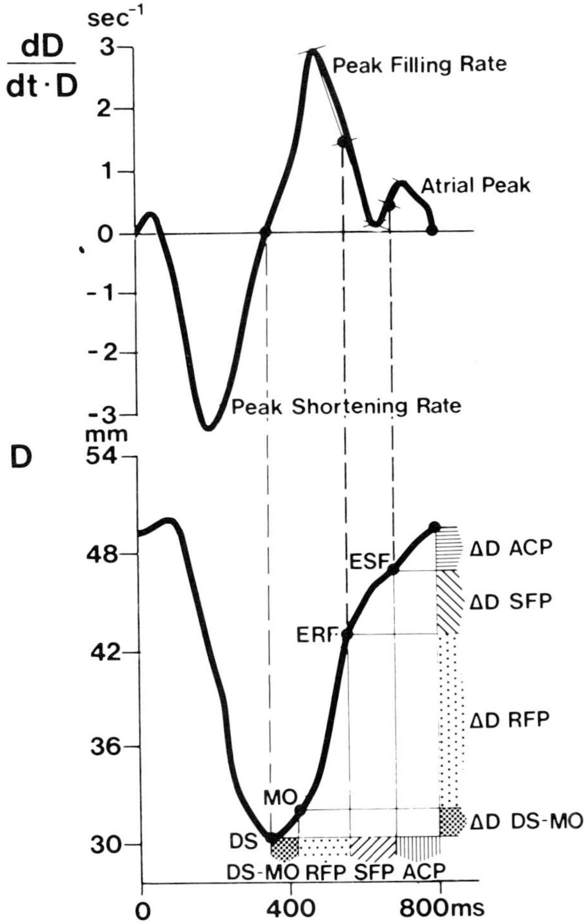

Fig. 1. Dimension time curve and its first normalized derivative for the analysis of the different phases of left ventricular filling. *ACP*, filling phase due to atrial contribution; *DS*, end-systolic dimension; *EAC*, end-point of the filling phase due to atrial contraction which equals end-diastolic dimension; *ERF*, end-point of the rapid filling phase; *ESF*, end-point of the slow filling phase; *MO*, mitral valve opening; *RFP*, rapid filling phase; *SFP*, slow filling phase; and *D*, LV dimension

4. $\Delta D\ RF\ (\%) = \dfrac{\Delta D\ (ERF - MO)}{\Delta D\ (EAC - MO)} \times 100$

5. $\Delta D\ SF\ (\%) = \dfrac{\Delta D\ (ESF - ERF)}{\Delta D\ (EAC - MO)} \times 100$

6. $\Delta D\ AC\ (\%) = \dfrac{\Delta D\ (EAC - ESF)}{\Delta D\ (EAC - MO)} \times 100$

The statistical analysis of the data was performed by Student's t-test.

Results

Normal Subjects

For the whole group of normal subjects mean LV cavity dimension at end-systole and end-diastole were 30.3 ± 4.5 (± 1 S.D.) and 48.5 ± 5.3 mm, respectively, yielding a fractional shortening of LV cavity dimension of 38 ± 5%. End-diastolic septal and posterior wall thickness were 9.5 ± 1.9 and 8.2 ± 1.4 mm, respectively. The sum of the end-diastolic wall thicknesses of the interventricular septum and the LV posterior wall was 17.7 ± 2.4 mm. Mean heart rate was 72 ± 13 min^{-1}.

The time interval between end-systolic LV dimension and mitral valve opening (t DS-MO) was 13 ± 15 ms (range: — 29 to + 35 ms). During this period a mean dimension increase of 0.6 ± 0.5 mm was observed (Fig. 2).

After mitral valve opening, left ventricular dimension increased by 10.7 ± 2.2 mm during the rapid filling phase, which had a duration of 111 ± 32 ms (Fig. 3). In 17 of the 28 normal subjects the dimension time curve could be further separated into a slow filling phase and a filling phase due to atrial contraction. The durations of these two phases were 264 ± 156 ms and 115 ± 44 ms, respective-

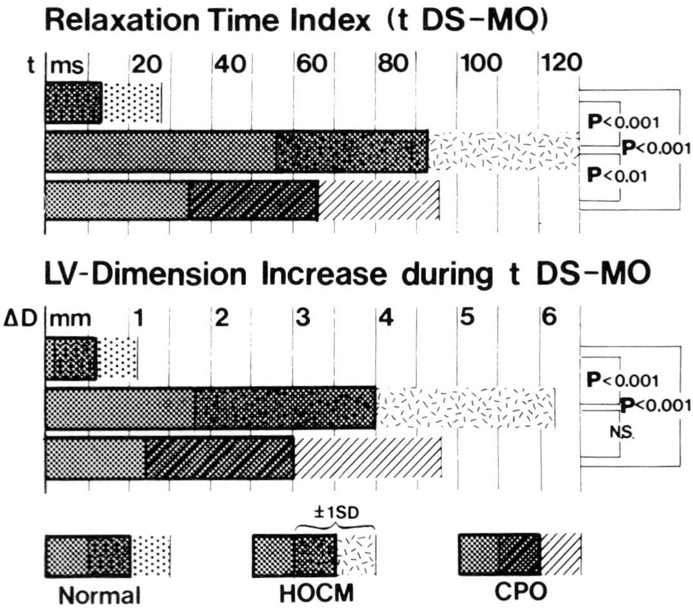

Fig. 2. Relaxation time index [time interval minimal left ventricular dimension (tDS)—mitral valve opening (MO)] and left ventricular dimension increase during this time interval in normal subjects (*normal*), patients with hypertrophic obstructive cardiomyopathy (*HOCM*) and chronic left ventricular pressure overload (*CPO*, mean value ± 1 S.D.)

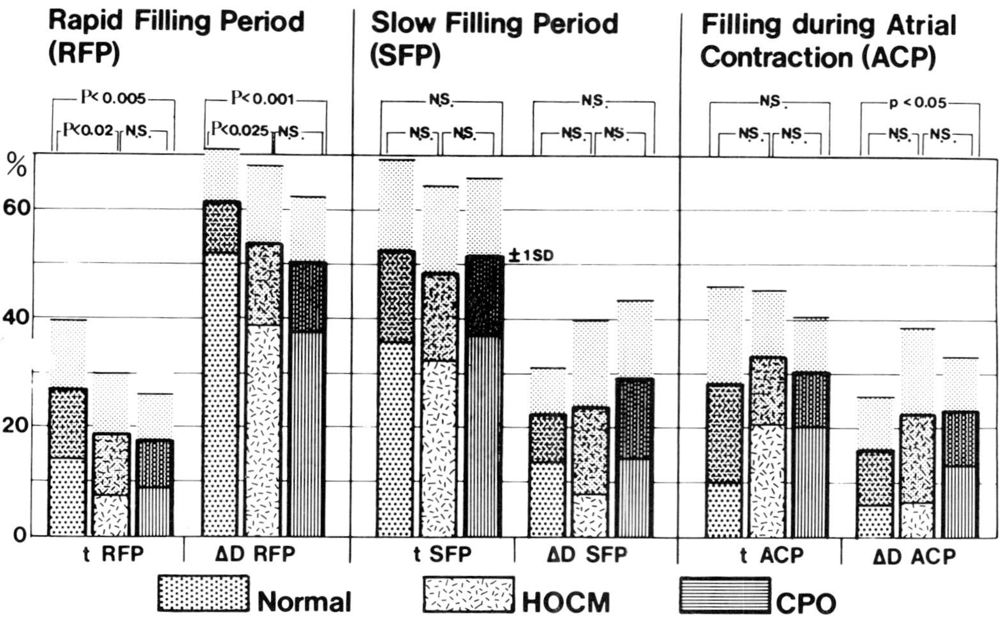

Fig. 3. The relative time interval (t %) and LV dimension increase (Δ D %) during the rapid (RFP) and slow (SFP) filling period as well as during atrial contraction (ACP). Abbrevations see Fig. 2

ly. The absolue dimension increases during these periods were 4.1 ± 1.9 mm and 2.8 ± 1.8 mm, respectively. Duration and change in dimension expressed as a percentage of the total diastolic filling time and dimension increase, respectively, were als follows:

1. Rapid filling time: 27 ± 13%
2. Slow filling time: 52 ± 16%
3. Time of filling due to atrial contraction: 28 ± 18%
4. Dimension increase during rapid filling: 62 ± 10%
5. Dimension increase during slow filling: 22 ± 9%
6. Dimension increase during atrial contraction: 16 ± 10%

Hypertrophic Obstructive Cardiomyopathy

Mean cavity dimensions at end-systole and end-diastole were 24.0 ± 5.0 mm and 42.7 ± 5.9 mm, respectively. Both were significantly smaller than in normals (HOCM→ N: $P < 0.001$). Thus, the fractional shortening of the LV minor axis was greater (44 ±7%, $P < 0.001$) compared with normal subjects. Heart rate was not different from normal (71 ± 14 min^{-1}). Septal and posterior wall thickness at end-diastole were increased (21.9 ± 4.6 and 11.8 ± 2.3 mm, respec-

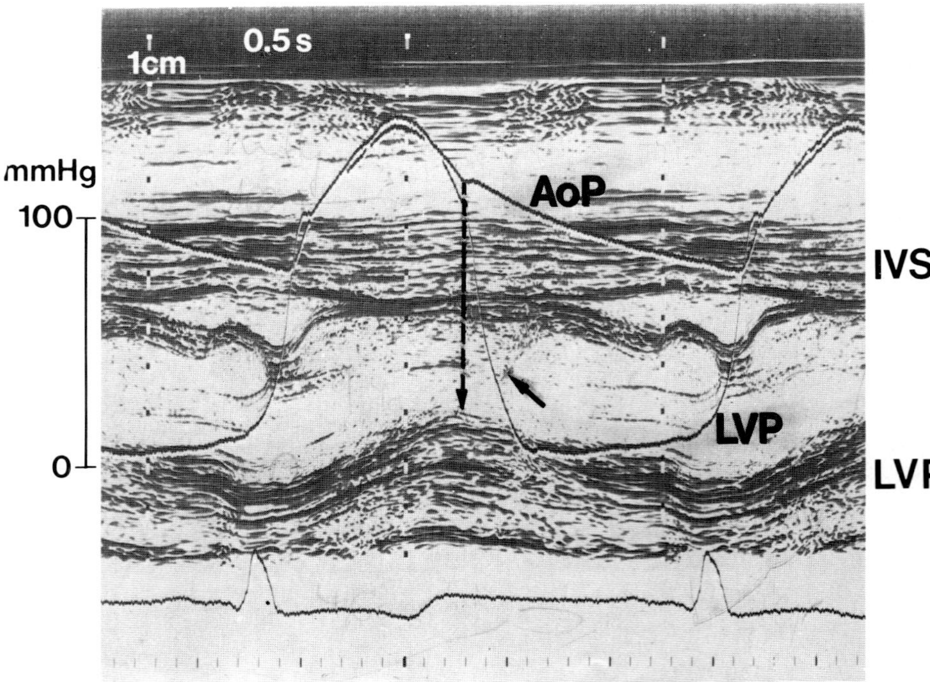

Fig. 4. LV echogram and simultaneous recording of LV and aortic pressure (*LVP*) and *AoP*, respectively) in a patient with hypertrophic cardiomyopathy with no pressure gradient at rest. Mitral valve opening is markedly delayed with regard to minimal LV dimension, which in this case coincides with aortic valve closure

tively, HOCM → N: $P < 0.001$). The sum of the end-diastolic septal and posterior wall thickness was 33.5 ± 5.1 mm (HOCM → N: $P < 0.001$).

The time interval t DS-MO (93 ± 37 ms, HOCM → N: $P < 0.001$) was significantly prolonged. During this time period, left ventricular dimension increased by 4.0 ± 2.2 mm (HOCM → N: $P < 0.001$) (Figs. 2, 4).

The rapid filling period was reduced in absolute (78 ± 45 ms; $P < 0.005$) and relative terms (19 ± 11%; $P < 0.02$) compared with normal subjects. The absolute dimension increase during the rapid period was 7.6 ± 2.7 mm ($P < 0.001$), while the relative dimension increase with respect to the dimension increase during LV filling was 54 ± 15% ($P < 0.025$) (Fig. 3). Concerning the slow filling phase and the filling behavior during atrial contraction, there was no significant difference in absolute and relative terms compared with normal subjects (Fig. 3).

Left Ventricular Chronic Pressure Overload

Mean end-distolic and end-systolic LV dimension in these patients were 48.5 ± 7.9 mm and 26.9 ± 6.1 mm, respectively. The end-diastolic dimension was not

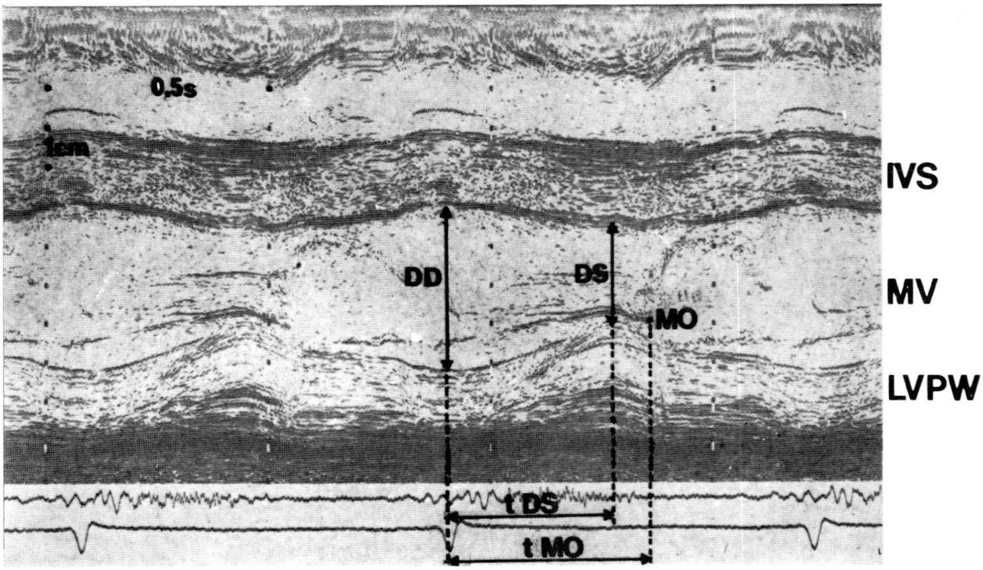

Fig. 5. Echocardiogram of a patient with LV hypertrophy due to valvular aortic stenosis showing septum (*IVS*), posterior wall (*LVPW*) and mitral valve leaflets (*MV*). Mitral valve opening (*MO*) with regard to minimal LV dimension (*DS*) is delayed. *HOMC*, hypertrophic obstructive cardiomyopathy and *CPO*, chronic LV pressure overload

different from normal, but significantly greater than in patients with HOCM ($P < 0.01$). The end-systolic dimension was not different from HOCM, but significantly reduced in comparison with the control group ($P < 0.05$). Fractional shortening of the LV minor axis was 44 ± 8% and significantly greater than in normal subjects ($P < 0.005$). Heart rate (66 ± 11 min^{-1}) was not different from N or patients with HOCM. Septal (16.5 ± 3.5 mm) and posterior (12.5 ± 2.6 mm) wall thickness were significantly greater compared with normals ($P < 0.001$). The septal wall thickness in patients with CPO was smaller than in HOCM ($P < 0.001$). The sum of septal and posterior wall thickness (29.1 ± 4.8 mm) was greater than in normal subjects ($P < 0.001$), but smaller than in HOCM ($P < 0.005$).

The mean time interval t DS-MO in patients with CPO was 66 ± 31 ms and significantly prolonged compared with that of normal subjects ($P < 0.001$) but shorter than in patients with HOCM ($P < 0.01$). During this time period, LV dimension increased significantly by 3.0 ± 1.8 mm (N→ CPO: $P < 0.001$) (Figs. 2, 5).

The rapid filling period in patients with CPO was decreased in absolute (85 ± 42 ms) and realtive (17 ± 9%) terms (CPO→ N: $P < 0.02$ and 0.005, respectively). The shortened rapid filling phase was accompanied by an absolute (9.2 ± 2.9 mm, CPO→N:$P < 0.05$) and relative reduction in LV dimension increase (50.5 ± 11.8%; CPO→ N: $P < 0.001$) (Fig. 3). Concerning the slow filling period there was no difference between the three groups in terms of duration and dimension change. During atrial contraction, LV dimension (4.5 ± 1.5 mm, $P <$ 0.05 and 23.1±9.9%, $P < 0.05$ respectively) was significantly increased in CPO compared with normals. The duration of LV filling due to atrial contraction was not different between the three groups (Fig. 3). Left ventricular dimension time curve with its normalized rate of change in a patient with CPO is illustrated in Figs. 5.

Discussion

In this study, as in previous studies by others and ourselves, the time interval from minimum LV dimension to the onset of mitral valve leaflet separation was considered as an index of the isovolumic relaxation period [2, 3, 7—12].

The time interval thus obtained underestimates true isovolumic relaxation period, especially in normal subjects, because closure of the aortic valve usually precedes minimum LV dimension [3]. Simultaneous recording of the LV echogram and LV as well as aortic pressure revealed that in patients with normal left ventricular function little change in dimension occurs during isovolumic relaxation [13, 14].

LV Relaxation

The relaxation time index (minimum LV dimension to mitral valve opening) was 13 ± 15 ms in normal subjects . This value was only slightly different from those previously mentioned by others using a computerized technique for the evaluation of LV echograms [2, 3, 7—8, 11]. During this time interval, only a small increase of 0.6 ± 0.5 mm in LV dimension was noted. For the whole of the isovolumic relaxation period, Gibson et al. could not demonstrate any significant diameter change in normal subjects either [12]. In contrast to the normal subjects, patients with HOCM as well as patients with CPO showed a significant prolongation of the relaxation time index. This has been previously shown in patients with HOCM [2, 3], but not in CPO. The average value in HOCM was 93 ± 37 ms, which is slightly more than found by Sanderson et al. [2] (76 ms) and Sutton [3] (71 ± 31 ms), who used a similar technique for the analysis of the echocardiogram.

A further abnormality of LV relaxation in patients with different forms of LV hypertrophy concerns LV diameter change, which averaged 0.6 ± 0.5 mm in normal subjects, but 4.0 ± 2.2 mm in patients with HOCM and 3.0 ± 1.8 mm in those with CPO during the relaxation time interval. Since the mitral valve is still closed during this period and no aortic regurgitation was present, this dimension increase by an average of 21% or 14% with respect to the total diastolic dimension change has to be caused by a shape change of the LV cavity during the isovolumic relaxation phase, as has been recently reported by Sanderson et al. using frame by frame analysis in patients with HOCM [1].

The underlying mechanism of the prolonged LV relaxation time and the associated shape change is unknown. It has been suggested that the specific architecture of the myocardial fibers in HOCM might be responsible [1]. From our data, however, this seems unlikely, since we could demonstrate that the same relaxation abnormality was also present to a somewhat lesser degree in CPO, where no such disarrangement of myocardial fibers can be found [14].

LV Filling

In our normal group, percent diameter increase during the three phases of diastolic filling was in the same range as previously reported by Decoodt et al. [5], i.e., 62 ± 10% during the rapid filling phase, 22 ± 9% during the slow filling phase, and 16 ± 10% due to atrial contribution. In HOCM and CPO, we found the percent diameter change during the rapid filling phase equally reduced to 54 ± 15% and 51 ± 12%, respectively. In accordance with Sanderson et al. [2], the duration of the rapid filling phase was significantly shortened by about 30% for both groups. In the absence of any significant difference between the three groups regarding the slow filling phase, the reduced dimension increase during the rapid filling phase was compensated for by a more vigorous atrial "kick" (23 ± 9,9%) in CPO, resulting in a normal end-diastolic left ventricular dimension. In HOCM, however, the end-diastolic dimension remained below "normal", suggesting that compensatory mechanisms during the slow filling phase and during atrial contraction could not fully compensate for the lack in early diastolic dimension increase. This might be due to the inability of thinning of the IVS during atrial contraction which is frequently observed in patients with HOCM.

References

1. Sanderson JE, Gibson DG, Brown DJ, Goodwin JF (1977) Left ventricular filling in hypertrophic cardiomyopathy. An angiographic study. Br Heart J 39 : 661–670
2. Sanderson JE, Traill TA, Sutton MGSJ, Brown DJ, Gibson DG, Goodwin JF (1978) Left ventricular relaxation and filling in hypertrophic cardiomyopathy. An echocardiographic study. Br Heart J 40 : 596–601
3. Sutton MGSJ, Tajik AJ, Gibson DG, Brown DJ, Seward JB, Giuliani ER (1978) Echocardiographic assessment of left ventricular filling and septal and posterior wall dynamics in idiopathic hypertrophic subaortic stenosis. Circulation 57 : 512–520
4. Hanrath P, Mathey D, Siegert R, Bleifeld W (1980) Left ventricular relaxation and filling pattern in different forms of left ventricular hypertrophy. An echocardiographic study. Am J Cardiol 45 : 15–24
5. Krebs W, Hanrath P, Bleifeld W, Effert S (1977) Rechnergestützte Auswertung von M-Mode-Echokardiogrammen. Herz Kreislauf 9 : 519–525

6. Decoodt PR, Mathey DG, Swan HJC (1976) Automated analysis of the left-ventricular diameter time curve from echocardiographic recordings. Comput Biomed Res 9 : 549—558
7. Upton MT, Gibson DG, Brown DJ (1976) Instantaneous mitral valve leaflet velocity and its relation to left ventricular wall movement in normal subjects. Br Heart J 38 : 51—58
8. Upton MT, Gibson DG, Brown DJ (1976) Echocardiographic assessment of abnormal left ventricular relaxation in man. Br Heart J 38 : 1001—1009
9. Gibson DG (1977) Detection of incoordinate left ventricular contraction by echocardiography. In: Bom N (ed) Echocardiology. Nijhoff, The Hague, pp 105—122
10. Gibson DG (1978) The use of M-Mode echocardiography in ischemic heart disease. Acta Med Scand [Suppl] 627 : 137—141
11. Ahmad M, Sanderson JE, Dubowitz V, Hallidie-Smith KA (1978) Echocardiographic assessment of left ventricular function in Duchenne's muscular dystrophy. Br Heart J 40 : 734—740
12. Hanrath P, Siegert R, Bleifeld W, Mathey D, Kupper W (1978) Abnormal left ventricular relaxation and diastolic diameter change in hypertrophic obstructive cardiomyopathy. Trans Eur Soc Cardiol 1 : 87
13. Gibson DG, Brown DJ (1976) Assessment of left ventricular systolic function in man from simultaneous echocardiographic and pressure measurements. Br Heart J 39 : 8—17
14. Caspari PG, Newcomb M, Gibson E, Harris P (1977) Collagen in the normal and hypertrophied human ventricle. Cardiovasc Res 11 : 554—558

Session E: Therapy of Hypertensive Heart Disease

Chairmen: H. Blömer/München (FRG), K.D. Bock/Essen (FRG)

Part I: Therapeutical Management of Hypertrophy and Heart Failure

Impaired Cardiac Performance in Rats with Long-Term Spontaneous Hypertension[1]

J. PFEFFER, M. PFEFFER, P. FLETCHER AND E. BRAUNWALD

Abstract

Cardiac performance was assessed during the progression from moderate to severe left ventricular hypertrophy in ether-anesthetized 6- and 18-month-old female spontaneously hypertensive rats (SHR), in 18-month-old male SHR, and in sex- and age-matched normotensive rats (NORM). Peak pumping ability during volume loading, maximum pressure generation during an aortic occlusion, and passive pressure-volume relationships were determined. Ejection phase indexes of young female SHR were comparable to those of age-matched NORM, i.e., both groups ejected the same peak stroke volumes from similar end-diastolic volumes, so that their indexes of ejection fraction were identical. However, a reduced peak stroke volume was ejected from a normal end-diastolic volume in old female SHR and from a significantly larger end-diastolic volume in old male SHR, so that ejection fraction indexes were moderately and substantially reduced, respectively. Maximum pressure developed during an aortic occlusion was always significantly greater in SHR. Despite elevated systemic arterial blood pressures and moderate cardiac hypertrophy, young female SHR ejected a normal stroke volume from a normal end-diastolic volume. Even though the severity of hypertension did not progress with age, cardiac mass increased markedly in old female and male SHR, and yet systolic function decreased. Therefore, hypertrophic growth of the left ventricle of the SHR is associated with both a compensated and a depressed phase of cardiac performance.

Introduction

The heart responds to a sustained imposition of a pressure over-load by hypertrophic growth in an attempt to maintain its functional capacity. The increased

---

1 Supported in part by funds from the National Institutes of Health Grants HL 20552 and 20572. Dr. J. Pfeffer is a recipient of a Public Health Service Research Fellowship5—F32—HL05477. Dr. P. Fletcher is a John Halliday Overseas Research Fellow of the Life Insurance Medical Research Fund of Australia and New Zealand

functional demands imposed on the heart are often progressive, and cardiac failure may ensue despite rather than because of hypertrophy.

In young and mature SHR we have observed a moderate degree of left ventricular hypertrophy in the presence of marked systemic hypertension (Fig. 1). With increased duration but no further elevation of systemic arterial blood pressures, left ventricular hypertrophy in old SHR was found to be twice that of age-matched normotensive rats. In our previous studies of peak pumping ability in 12-, 24-, and 52-week-old SHR, we noted normal blood flow and reserve capacity despite

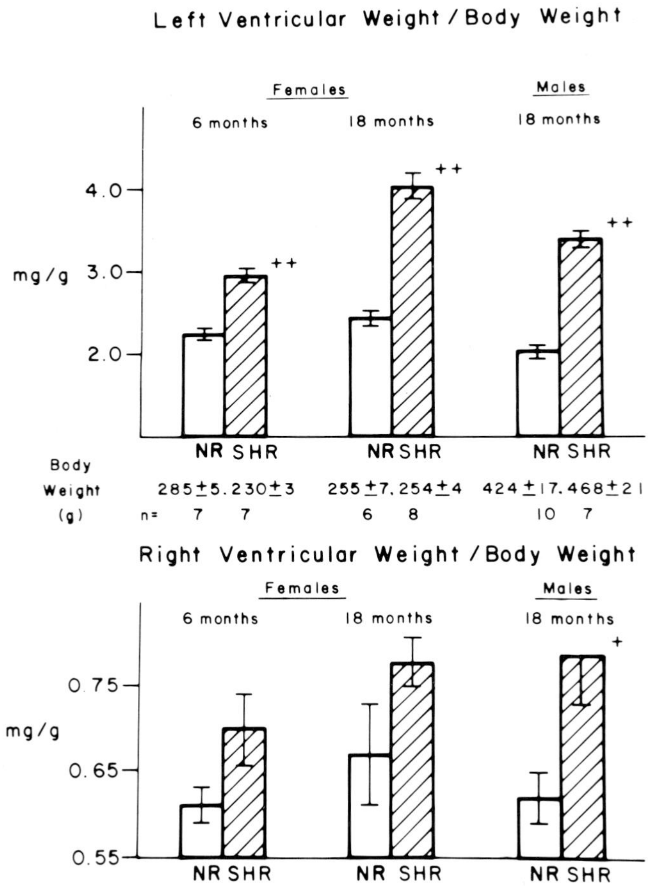

Fig. 1. *Upper*: Left ventricular weight to body weight ratios of 6-month-old female and male spontaneously hypertensive (SHR) and normotensive rats (NR). Presented are the means ± SEM. *Lower:* Right ventricular weight to body weight ratios of 6-month-old female SHR and NR and 18-month-old female and male SHR and NR. Presented are the means ± SEM. Note the increased ratio only of 18-month-old male SHR. † $P < 0.01$, †† $P < 0.001$, SHR versus age-matched NR

severe hypertension [1—3]. In contrast, although blood pressures of 83-week-old SHR were similar to those of younger SHR, peak pumping performance was markedly reduced. Therefore, in this animal model of genetic hypertension, we have found both compensated and depressed phases of cardiac performance: in young rats with moderate left ventricular hypertrophy peak pumping ability was normal, whereas in old rats with longstanding hypertension and marked hypertrophy, decompensation occurred and pumping ability was severely reduced.

In the present study, our objective was to characterize the peak pumping ability, maximum pressure generating capacity, and passive pressure-volume relationships of the intact left ventricle of the SHR during the progression from moderate to severe hypertrophy.

Methods

Experiments were performed on two strains of normotensive rats, the Wistar-Kyoto (WKY) and an American Wistar (NWR), and on the SHR. Female rats were studied at 6 months (seven SHR, seven WKY) and at 18 months (eight SHR, three WKY, seven NWR) of age. Male rats were also studied at 18 months (seven SHR, three WKY, seven NWR). All rats were obtained from our colony of inbred (brother-to-sister) SHR and WKY and randomly bred NWR.

The surgical preparation has been described in detail previously [4, 5]. Anesthesia was induced with ether, and a catheter was advanced via the right carotid artery into the left ventricle for measurements of systolic and end-diastolic pressures and dP/dt and then withdrawn into the aorta for measurements of phasic and mean arterial pressures. A second catheter was inserted into the right jugular vein and advanced into the right atrium for continuous pressure measurements. Ventilation then was provided by a positive pressure respirator connected in series to an ether drip apparatus. The chest was opened to expose the ascending aorta for placement of an electromagnetic flow probe which permitted measurements of blood flow (less coronary flow) and its first derivative, the acceleration of aortic blood flow. Phasic and mean pressures and flow were recorded at 2-min intervals over a stable 10-min period to determine the baseline values for each rat.

A rapid infusion of Tyrode's solution (40 ml/min/kg for 45 s) into a femoral vein produced a prompt rise to a plateau in cardiac output, at which point the continued infusion further elevated venous pressure and yet failed to increase blood flow [1]. The maximum cardiac output and stroke volume attained served as indexes of the peak pumping ability of the intact left ventricle.

When hemodynamic variables returned to baseline levels, the flow probe was removed and the arterial catheter was advanced into the left ventricle for continuous monitoring of intraventricular pressure and its first derivative, dP/dt, and of end-diastolic pressure, which was displayed at a high sensitivity on an additional channel. The ascending aorta then was occluded briefly with a suture to produce isovolumic (except for coronary flow) contractions. Maximum developed left ventricular pressure (peak systolic minus end-diastolic) was calculated from measurements obtained during the first seven beats of aortic occlusion.

The heart then was arrested in diastole with intravenous potassium chloride and a double lumen catheter was inserted into the left ventricular cavity via the aorta and secured into place with a suture around the atrioventricular groove. Within 10 min of arrest and before the onset of rigor mortis, three repeatable pressure-volume curves were determined with saline infused at a rate of 0.68 ml/min over a pressure range of —5 to 30 mm Hg.

An index of ejection fraction was derived from the information on ventricular volumes and peak stroke volumes as follows: In a separate group of normotensive and hypertensive rats, the in vivo volume loading procedure described above was shown to increase left ventricular end-diastolic pressure to 17—20 mm Hg. This pressure range corresponds to a very steep portion of the pressure-volume curve determined in vitro, so that volume changes per mm Hg within that range are minimal. An ejection fraction index for each rat then was obtained by dividing the peak stroke volume determined during volume loading in vivo by the ventricular volume at 20 mm Hg from that rat's pressure-volume curve determined in vitro.

Since no differences were found between WKY and NWR, the data from these two normotensive groups were pooled and termed NORM for comparison with age-matched SHR. For all variables, except peak stroke volume (where males and females were analyzed separately), a one-way analysis of variance of the six groups of rats was performed. When the difference between groups was significant (Fisher's F-ratio), the pooled error mean square was used to test the significance of the mean difference of the three planned comparisons between age- and sex-matched SHR and NORM (Student's unpaired t-test) [6]. Data are expressed as mean ± standard error of the mean within the group.

Results

Left ventricular weight to body weight ratio in 6-month-old female SHR was significantly increased by 31% compared to age-matched female NORM of similar body weight (Fig. 1). Although arterial blood pressure had remained stable from 6 to 18 months of age, the amount of left ventricular hypertrophy had more than doubled in both female (+ 64%) and male (+ 55%) SHR (Fig. 1). Right ventricular weights of the old female SHR were not significantly increased, although tending to be so when expressed either as absolute values or in relation to body weight (Fig. 1). However, in the old male SHR right ventricular weights were significantly increased.

In all age groups of SHR arterial blood pressures were significantly elevated compared to NORM (Table 1). Yet left ventricular end-diastolic pressures were normal in both the young and old female SHR, but were moderately, though

Table 1. Prethoracotomy hemodynamic characteristics of normotensive (NORM) and spontaneously hypertensive rats (SHR)

	Females 6 months NORM	SHR	18 months NORM	SHR	Males 18 months NORM	SHR
Arterial pressures						
(mm Hg) Systolic	139 ± 4	173 ± 1[a]	140 ± 4	176 ± 14[c]	137 ± 4	181 ± 17[c]
Mean	120 ± 4	149 ± 2[a]	119 ± 4	145 ± 10[c]	119 ± 4	158 ± 14[c]
Diastolic	99 ± 4	125 ± 2[a]	98 ± 4	123 ± 9[c]	101 ± 3	134 ± 14[c]
Left ventricular end-diastolic pressure (mm Hg)	3.6 ± 0.5	3.7 ± 0.5	4.2 ± 0.5	3.8 ± 0.3	3.9 ± 0.5	5.7 ± 0.5[c]
+ dP/dt (mm Hg/s)	18165 ± 1239	20122 ± 732	17074 ± 1494	15976 ± 1152	17074 ± 1494	16009 ± 1034
−dP/dt	11082 ± 787	14638 ± 570[b]	11405 ± 1143	9398 ± 844	10607 ± 650	10033 ± 1379
Mean right atrial pressure (mm Hg)	− 0.2 ± 0.5	− 0.2 ± 0.2	0.4 ± 0.4	0.1 ± 0.8	0.3 ± 0.4	1.7 ± 1.1
Heart rate (beats/min)	428 ± 8	424 ± 7	419 ± 15	411 ± 11	407 ± 7	406 ± 10

[a] $P <^{0}_{1} .001$
[b] $P <^{0}_{1} .01$
[c] $P <^{0}_{1} .05$

significantly, increased in 18-month-old male SHR. Despite differences in arterial blood pressures between SHR and NORM, no differences in maximum positive or negative dP/dt occurred, except in the young female SHR with a greater negative dP/dt. There were no differences in heart rate or mean right atrial pressure between SHR or NORM for any group examined.

The passive pressure-volume relations of 6- and 18-month-old female SHR were similar to those of age-matched female NORM (Fig. 2). In fact, the volumes at 10, 15, 20, and 30 mm Hg in the 18-month-old SHR were significantly greater than those of age-matched NORM (Fig. 2).

The ejection phase characteristics of 6-month-old female SHR were similar to those of age-matched NORM (Table 2). These young SHR ejected the same peak stroke volumes from equivalent end-diastolic volumes at equal rates of acceleration as did the normotensives, yet did so with a 31% greater cardiac mass. However, in both 18-month-old female and male SHR, peak pumping ability was significantly reduced, despite a greater than 50% increase in ventricular mass. A reduced peak stroke volume was delivered from a normal

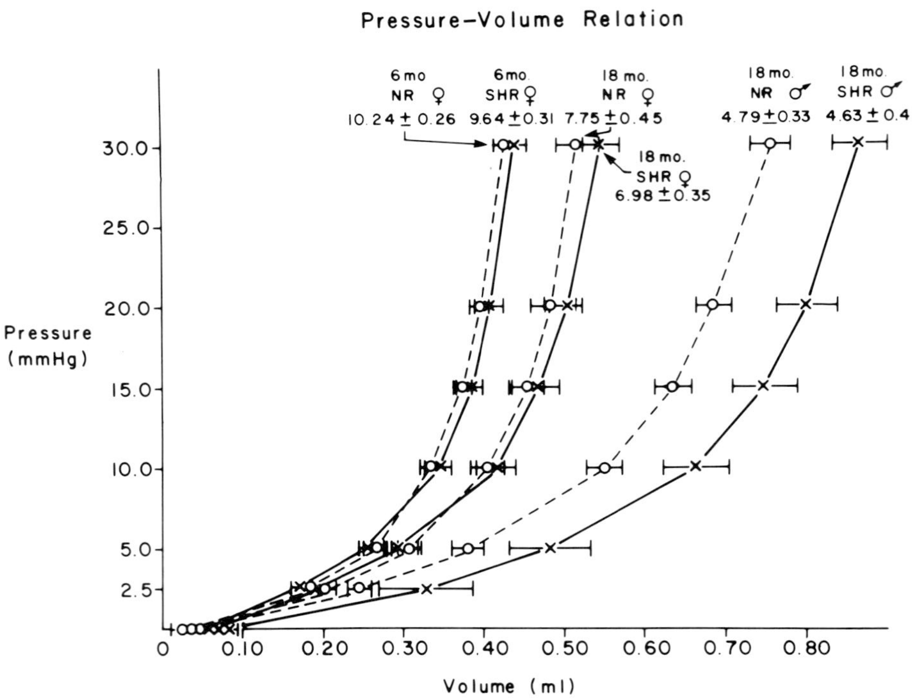

Fig. 2. Pressure-volume relations of male and female spontaneously hypertensive (SHR) and normotensive rats (NR). Presented are the means ± SEM. The *numbers* appearing under each group are the slopes of the pressure-volume curves calculated over pressure range of 2.5 to 30 mm Hg. There were no statistical differences between the slopes of age- and sex-matched SHR and NR

Table 2. Peak pumping and pressure generating ability of normotensive (NORM) and spontaneously hypertensive rats (SHR)

	Females 6 Months NORM	SHR	18 Months NORM	SHR	Males 18 Months NORM	SHR
Peak stroke volume (ml)	0.30 ± 0.01	0.31 ± 0.11	0.35 ± 0.02	0.30 ± 0.02[b]	0.50 ± 0.03	0.35 ± 0.01[c]
Ejection fraction index (%)	76 ± 3	76 ± 3	75 ± 7	61 ± 3[b]	73 ± 4	44 ± 2[a]
Maximum acceleration of aortic blood flow (g)	21.8 ± 0.4	20.7 ± 1.7	17.9 ± 1.6	14.1 ± 0.7[b]	19.4 ± 0.7	12.7 ± 0.9[a]
Peak developed pressure (mm Hg)	222 ± 4	273 ± 4[a]	215 ± 8	291 ± 9[a]	212 ± 4	260 ± 23[a]

[a] $P <^{0}_{1} .001$
[b] $P <^{0}_{1} .05$
[c] $P <^{0}_{1} .01$

end-diastolic volume in 18-month-old female SHR, so that the ejection fraction index was only moderately reduced, and from a dilated ventricle in old SHR, so that the ejection fraction index was substantially reduced. Similarly, maximum acceleration of aortic blood flow was significantly decreased in 18-month-old female SHR and even more so in 18-month-old male SHR. Maximum developed pressure was significantly greater in every SHR group (Table 2).

Discussion

When subjected to a sustained augmented load, the heart responds by increasing its mass in an attempt to maintain functional capacity. If this challenge is a pressure overload, the ventricular wall thickens to reduce wall tension [7], permitting the ejection of a normal stroke volume against the increased resistance. However, a pressure load of long-standing duration may eventuate in impaired ventricular pumping performance despite increases in cardiac mass. In our previous studies of peak pumping ability of male SHR, the peak stroke volume and cardiac output of 11-, 24-, and 52-week-old SHR were similar to those for age-matched NORM despite the elevated arterial pressures of the SHR [1, 3]. Even though these arterial pressures did not increase further, 19-month-old SHR were unable to eject the same stroke and minute volumes as the young SHR and age-matched NORM.

In the present study, an impairment of cardiac pumping ability also was demonstrated in 18-month-old SHR. The reduction in stroke volume could be explained by a reduced ventricular volume at any given end-diastolic pressure in the SHR. Averill et al. found that renal hypertensive rats, when compared to NORM, had a reduced stroke volume and cardiac output at left ventricular end-diastolic pressures greater than 10 mm Hg [8]. They suggested that the two-fold increase in hydroxyproline content found in the hearts of the hypertensive rats implicated a decreased ventricular compliance as possibly accounting for the stroke volume. Using an isolated working heart preparation, Hallback, Isaksson, and Noresson demonstrated a reduced stroke volume at normal ventricular diastolic pressures in 6- and 30-week-old SHR when compared to age-matched normotensive rats [9]. However, the passive pressure-volume relations determined in our study do not show a decreased compliance in either 6- or 18-month-old SHR. However, passive pressure-volume relations determined in vitro may not be representative of compliance characteristics existing in vivo, and it is possible that, in the latter circumstance and at the rapid heart rate of the rat, incomplete ventricular relaxation may reduce ventricular compliance. Nonetheless, we measured negative dP/dt as an indicator of ventricular relaxation and found it not to be reduced in any group of SHR.

An index of the ejection fraction was obtained by dividing peak stroke volume by the maximum end-diastolic volume attained during volume loading. Although this index was normal in six-month-old female SHR, it was impaired in 18-month-old male and female SHR. This reduced index of the ejection fraction was not related to an increase in blood pressure, for arterial pressures did not increase further from 6 to 18 months in our SHR.

Both a compensated and a decompensated phase of cardiac performance has been found in hypertensive man. In patients with essential hypertension and left ventricular hypertrophy without coronary artery disease, Strauer has shown ventricular function at rest and during exercise to be normal [10]. Using echocardiographic techniques, Karliner et al. found end-diastolic diameters and ejection fraction to be normal in patients with systemic arterial hypertension and left ventricular hypertrophy and without clinical evidence of coronary artery disease [11]. Savage et al. also found ejection fraction and end-diastolic transverse diameters to be within normal limits in 234 subjects with mild to moderate hypertension and left ventricular hypertrophy when compared to 124 normotensive subjects [12]. A reduction in the ejection fraction was found by Toshima et al. only in hypertensive patients considered to be in congestive heart failure [13]. A decrease in ejection fraction with an increase in severity of hypertension has been shown in other echocardiographic studies [14, 15].

The reduced ejection of blood from a normal end-diastolic volume suggests that impaired cardiac performance in SHR is not a result of inadequate filling, but is a consequence of systolic dysfunction. The maximum acceleration of aortic blood flow has been shown to be a valid index of the initial phase of ventricular ejection [16, 17]. To eliminate possible differences in preload, maximum acceleration of aortic blood flow was measured at the peak of volume loading. In old female and male SHR with reduced indexes of ejection fraction, this additional index of ventricular ejection was significantly decreased, and in young female SHR whose index of ejection fraction was comparable to that of NORM, it was normal.

The increased left ventricular mass of young SHR permits a normal ejection of blood in the face of an increased afterload. With increasing duration of this afterload and further growth of cardiac mass, the capacity of the left ventricle to develop sufficient tension for the ejection of blood is maintained, but the ability to eject this blood is impaired. To assess the ability of the left ventricle to generate pressure, isovolumic contractions were produced by aortic occlusion and developed pressure then was calculated from measurements of peak systolic and end-diastolic pressures. We have found this measurement to be unaltered by the animal's sex [5]. All groups of SHR developed significantly more pressure than did the NORM. Thus, the pressure-generating capacity of the hypertrophied left ventricle of all groups of SHR was greater than that of normotensive rats. However, the 18-month-old SHR did not develop higher pressures than did the 6-month-old SHR, even though their left ventricular weights were greater, suggesting that even this aspect of ventricular performance might have declined with age.

In summary, cardiac mass increases with age in SHR despite the maintenance of a stable elevation of systemic arterial pressures. This hypertrophic growth of the left ventricle is associated with both a compensated and a depressed phase of cardiac performance. Young SHR with moderate left ventricular hypertrophy eject a normal stroke volume from a normal end-diastolic volume in the face of an increased afterload. With time and a marked increase in cardiac mass, the ejection process is significantly impaired.

Acknowledgments. The authors wish to express their appreciation to Cynthia Steinberg, Penny Wiltz, and Carol Hackett for their fine technical assistance and to Dolores Koedyker for her secretarial assistance.

References

1. Pfeffer MA, Pfeffer JM, Frohlich ED (1976) Pumping ability of the hypertrophying left ventricle of the spontaneously hypertensive rat. Circ Res 38 : 423–429
2. Pfeffer MA, Frohlich ED (1973) Hemodynamic and myocardial function in young and old normotensive and spontaneously hypertensive rats. Circ Res [Suppl I] 32/33 : 28–38
3. Pfeffer JM, Pfeffer MA, Fishbein MC, Frohlich ED (1979) Cardiac function and morphology with aging in the spontaneously hypertensive rat. Am J Physiol : H461–H468
4. Pfeffer MA, Frohlich ED (1972) Electromagnetic flowmetry in anesthetized rats. J Appl Physiol 33 : 137–140
5. Pfeffer MA, Pfeffer JM, Fishbein MC, Fletcher PJ, Spadaro J, Kloner RA, Braunwald EB (1979) Myocardial infarct size and ventricular function in rats. Circ Res 44 : 503–512
6. Snedecor GW, Cochran WG (1967) Statistical methods, 6th edn Iowa State University Press, Ames, Iowa
7. Grossman W, Jones D, McLaurin L (1975) Wall stress and patterns of hypertrophy in the human left ventricle. J Clin Invest 56 : 56–64
8. Averill DB, Ferrario CM, Tarazi RC, Sen S, Bajbus R (1976) Cardiac performance in rats with renal hypertension. Circ Res 38 : 280–288
9. Hallbäck M, Isaksson O, Noresson E (1975) Consequences of myocardial structural adaptation of left ventricular compliance and the Frank-Starling relationship in spontaneously hypertensive rats. Acta Physiol Scand 94 : 259–270
10. Strauer BE (1978) The heart in hypertension. I. Left ventricular function at rest and during exercise. Z Kardiol 67 : 375–383
11. Karliner JS, Williams D, Gorwit J, Crawford MH, O'Rourke RA (1977) Left ventricular performance in patients with left ventricular hypertrophy caused by systemic arterial hypertension. Br Heart J 39 : 1239–1245
12. Savage DD, Drayer JIM, Henry WL, Mathews EC, Ware JH, Gardin JM, Cohen ER, Epstein SE, Laragh JH (1979) Echocardiographic assessment of cardiac anatomy and function in hypertensive subjects. Circulation 59 : 623–632

13. Toshima H, Koga Y, Toshioka H, Akiyoshi T, Kimura N (1975) Echocardiographic classification of hypertensive heart disease. A correlative study with clinical features. Jpn Heart J 16 : 377—393
14. Dunn FG, Chandraratna P, deCarvalho JGR, Basta LL, Frohlich ED (1977) Pathophysiologic assessment of hypertensive heart disease with echocardiography. Am J Cardiol 39 : 789—795
15. Schlant RC, Felner JM, Heymsfield SB, Gilbert CA, Shulman NB, Tuttle EP, Blumenstein BA (1977) Echocardiographic studies of left ventricular anatomy and function in essential hypertension. Cardiovasc Med 2 : 477—491
16. Noble MIM, Trenchard A, Guz A (1966) Left ventricular ejection in conscious dogs: I. Measurement and significance of the maximum acceleration of blood from the left ventricle. Circ Res 19 : 139—147
17. Nutter DO, Noble RJ, Hurst VM (1971) Peak aortic flow and acceleration as indices of ventricular performance in the dog. J Lab Clin Med 77 : 307—318

Pathophysiologic Basis of Antihypertensive Therapy in Man

K.A. MEURER, H. FELTKAMP, G. BÖNNER, A. KONRADS, R. LANG, A. HELBER AND W. KAUFMANN

Regarding different theories on the pathogenesis of arterial hypertension, for instance, Page's mosaic theory, the concept of Helmer, or Guyton's analysis of circulation [16], it becomes obvious that arterial hypertension has a multifactorial etiology.

According to Guyton's hypothesis [15, 16], renal sodium and water excretion, influenced by other control systems, seems to play a dominant role in blood pressure homeostasis.

In the various forms of arterial hypertension these factors show more or less variations but, besides pheochromocytoma and primary aldosteronism, always more than one factor or system is altered, leading at least to elevated blood pressure.

Therefore, antihypertensive drug therapy will not be able to correct hypertension in a causative way, but with the drugs now available, it is possible to influence these pathopysiologic abnormalities. This possibility will be discussed in brief.

For a long time a major role has been accepted for a disturbed sodium and volume homeostasis in the pathogenesis of hypertension [7, 32]. Relations between sodium and hypertension become clear by the fact that in human as well as in animal experiments it is possible to induce hypertension by a high salt intake. Moreover, sodium content of arterial vessel walls and in red blood cells is elevated in various forms of experimental hypertension and in patients with primary hypertension [7, 32].

High sodium intake causes hypertension if it is followed by expansion of extracellular volume and an increase of effective blood volume [15]. This can be derived from an increased activity or administration of mineralocorticoid hormones and occurs when an impaired kidney is unable to excrete a high sodium load. Together with an increase of central venous pressure and cardiac output, blood pressure increases as much as is necessary to excrete sodium and water. At this point, fluid balance is positive. According to Guyton's hypothesis, an autoregulatory process is established, leading to an increase in peripheral resistance and normalization of cardiac output but also to an elevated blood pressure [15]. This mechanism may play a role in the pathogenesis of human arterial hypertension, because in early states of primary hypertension kidney function already seems to be impaired, as was shown by Hollenberg et al. [20]. Moreover, the relations between sodium and water balance and other control systems may be disturbed.

Sodium content and extracellular volume differ in various forms of hypertension and are dependent on the state of hypertension [9]. In mineralocorticoid-dependent hypertension and in patients with terminal renal failure or after nephrectomy, sodium and fluid volume is elevated, whereas it is normal or even reduced in uncomplicated primary or renal parenchymatous hypertension and in malignant hypertension. Fluid volume, however, may be inappropriately high as far as the corresponding blood pressure is concerned.

On the basis of various studies in animals, the central and peripheral autonomous nervous system takes part in maintenance of hypertension, although it has not been possible until now to quantify this [2]. This results from methodological difficulties as well as from interactions between autonomous nervous system and the renin-angiotensin system and their combined influence on renal functions.

Altered concentrations of enzymes involved in catecholamine biosynthesis and elevated concentrations of epinephrine and norepinephrine could be found in peripheral blood and in various cerebral regions, especially the medulla, brain, stem, locus ceruleus, and hypothalamus. These adrenergic centers are linked with each other and with the vasomotor center. They also receive impulses from the baroreceptors, whereas inhibitory neurons arise from the vagus nucleus. Inhibitory neurons from the nucleus tractus solitarii influence the vasomotor center. By influencing each other, these centers regulate peripheral sympathetic activity [6].

Excessive sympathetic nervous activity, especially in human borderline hypertension, may play a pathophysiologic role, whereas in established hypertension elevated levels of plasma catecholamines in age-matched patients could not be found [2]. However, plasma catecholamines do not necessarily represent increased sympathetic overactivity.

As far as the renin-angiotensin system is concerned, a pathogenetic role in human arterial hypertension is accepted in unilateral renal artery stenosis, in renin secreting tumors, in malignant hypertension, and in some cases of hypertension in terminal renal failure [14]. But very recently there have been some hints indicating a participation of the renin-angiotensin system in the maintenance of human primary hypertension.

The renin-angiotensin system could well be able to play a key role in hypertension because its components influence a variety of other control systems. Recently, connections to the prostaglandins and to the kinin-kallikrein system, with the discovery that angiotensin I converting enzyme and the kininase II are identical, became obvious, indicating interactions between a pressor and a depressor system [1, 11, 17, 18, 25, 27, 29, 33].

The kallikrein-kinin system takes part in the regulation of renal blood flow and exerts diuretic and vasodepressor properties [17, 18]. Connections to the renin-angiotensin system have already been mentioned; in addition kinins and sodium ions promote prostaglandin formation, and the effects of the kallikrein-kinin system are modified or mediated by prostaglandins [1, 17, 18, 27].

In spontaneously hypertensive rats and rats with unilateral renal artery stenosis as well as in human primary hypertension, urinary kallikrein excretion is reduced, while it is enhanced in secondary hypertension, pheochromocytoma, and primary aldosteronism [17, 18, 25, 29]. It seems possible that the kallikrein-kinin system protects the renal vessels against the vasoconstrictive properties of the renin-angiotensin system.

Furthermore, exogenous bradykinin enhances and aprotinin (Trasylol) decreases prostaglandin release, whereas desoxycorticosterone (DOCA) augments kallikrein as well as prostaglandin excretion [25, 29].

Thus, both systems induce a diuresis and natriuresis which counteracts the sodium-retaining effects of mineralocorticoid hormones in positive sodium and fluid balance. From the prostaglandins, the E and A series have vasodilating properties with reflectory increase of heart rate and cardiac output [18]. By infusion into isolated vascular beds, blood flow increases but mostly without a fall in blood pressure. Infusion into the renal artery leads to osmotic diuresis by increased sodium and potassium excretion [18]. Norepinephrine release during stimulation of sympathetic nerves is diminished under the influence of PG_E. On the other hand, angiotensin increases renal prostaglandin release.

Whereas these findings mentioned above are of minor degree in primary and in most forms of secondary hypertension, there are clear-cut abnormalities in endocrine hypertension, for instance, primary aldosteronism, Cushing's syndrome, and pheochromocytoma. These abnormalities, however, may cause secondardy alterations, for instance, in blood volume, cardiac output, peripheral vascular resistance, and electrolyte balance.

Besides these changes, hemodynamic alterations can be measured in all forms of hypertension. In primary hypertension, these hemodynamic alterations are dependent on the degree of severity of the hypertension [9, 23, 24]. With increasing severity of hypertension, cardiac index and cardiac output decrease, whereas heart rate and peripheral resistance increase. In renovascular hypertension, cardiac output is higher and peripheral resistance lower than in patients with primary hypertension of the same degree. In renoparenchymal hypertension, usually opposite findings can be obtained. Hypertension in patients with chronic renal failure is characterized by increased plasma and extracellular volume, increased cardiac output, and peripheral resistance. Initially, Cushing's syndrome and Conn's syndrome show an elevated cardiac output, whereas an increase in peripheral resistance later occurs [8, 9].

Dependent on the excretion of epinephrine or norepinephrine, pheochromocytoma is characterized by an elevated cardiac output or an elevated peripheral vascular resistance. Plasma volume is markedly decreased [9].

Thus, there are multiple pathophysiologic changes in nearly all forms of arterial hypertension, and it is difficult to decide which one is responsible for the development or maintenance of hypertension and which is an accompanying secondary phenomenon. On the other hand, by antihypertensive drug therapy in most cases one or more of the above-mentioned variables also will be affected, depending on the severity of hypertension and especially on the mechanism of drug action, as is observed, for instance, in the case of sympatholytic and diuretic agents.

Though the mechanism of action of the diuretics is not yet fully understood, it seems clear that their acute antihypertensive effect is due to a reduction of extracellular fluid volume with a consequent decrease in cardiac output [10, 12, 13]. In addition to volume contraction, there seems to be an attenuated response of the vessels to naturally occuring pressure substances or neural stimuli [10, 31].

A depressed peripheral resistance accounts for chronic antihypertensive action of diuretics, though cardiac output may remain reduced as was shown by Tarazi et al [31]. It is assumed that vasodilation induced by the diuretics has its cause in mobilization of sodium from the arterial walls of hypertensive patients [10, 32]. Probably, the diuretics have a direct relaxing effect on arterial smooth muscles, as is known in the case of diazoxide, the nondiuretic benzothiadiazine derivative [10].

The importance of the saluretic action of the diuretic compounds becomes clear by the fact that the antihypertensive effect can be attenuated by a high sodium load, whereas it is potentiated by sodium restriction [10, 12]. These observations also point to the importance of increased volume and sodium retention in the maintenance of hypertension.

Furthermore, the volume-depleting effects of diuretics are responsible for their potentiation of other antihypertensive agents which except for the β-receptor blockers, induce sodium retention [10]. This effect accounts for the decreased efficacy of these agents with time.

A second class of widely used and very potent antihypertensive agents is the sympatholytic drugs which influence sympathetic tone at various levels. There are the centrally acting α-receptor agonistic drugs, i.e., clonidine and α-methyldopa, the peripheral postsynaptic α-receptor blockers, the β-receptor blocking agents, the ganglion-blocking drugs, and the postganglionic depletors of norepinephrine.

Especially the mechanism of action of α-methyldopa and clonidine, which stimulate central α-adrenoceptors in the lower brain stem and, consequently, inhibitory neurons, thereby diminishing peripheral sympathetic activity [19, 35], points to the importance and to the participation of the sympathetic nervous system in the pathogenesis of arterial hypertension. A decrease of arteriolar restistance is the consequence of this mechanism. Methyldopa may also act as a false transmitter [22]: the drug is converted to α-methylnoradrenaline, which binds to α-adrenergic receptors that compete with norepinephrine.

The peripheral α-receptor blocking agents phentolamine and especially phenoxybenzamine have only limited usefulness in the treatment of primary hypertension, but act promptly in patients with pheochromocytoma during a pheochromocytoma crisis, in preoperative treatment of these patients, and in the long-term treatment of patients with malignant pheochromocytoma.

Prazosin, a recently marketed postsynaptic α-receptor blocking agent, has a more pronounced vasodilating effect, more often causing orthostatic hypotension [13]. In this way it resembles the combined α- and β-receptor blocking drug labetalol. Both drugs are indicated in patients with mild to moderate hypertension. Because of their sodium retaining effect, they should be combined with diuretic agents [10, 12].

The other sympatholytic agents, i.e., the ganglion and postganglion blocking drugs, now have very limited use in treatment of uncomplicated hypertension, where they are replaced by vasodilators, for instance, dihydralazine, minoxidil, and in the case of hypertensive emergencies, diazoxide and sodium nitroprusside. Furthermore, vasodilators are widely used in combination with β-adrenergic blocking drugs, the role of which will be discussed in two following articles.

The vasodilating drugs lower peripheral resistance by decreasing directly smooth muscle tone in the arterioles [10, 12]. As a consequence of the fall of vascular resistance and blood pressure, a reflectory tachycardia results. Furthermore, these drugs cause sodium retention, so that it is recommended that they should be used in combination with a diuretic and a β-blocker.

This triple therapy is highly effective, causes only a few side-effects, and influences three of the major abnormalities in arterial hypertension: sodium and water balance, sympathetic nervous tone, and peripheral resistance. In 1972, Zacest et al. [34] showed that additive effects of a β-blocker and hydralazine when given together with a diuretic.

Using minoxidil, the most potent vasodilator now available, a combination with a diuretic and a β-blocker is essential to prevent tachycardia and edema formation. Furthermore, administration of these therapeutic regimens makes antihypertensive therapy more convenient to the patient, because a reduction of the tablet quantity is possible (Fig. 1).

Recently, drugs have become available which, in contrast to the diuretic and sympatholytic agents, affect the renin-angiotensin system directly. These are saralasin, the competetive antagonist of angiotensin II, and captopril and teprotide, the peptidic inhibitors of the angiotensin I converting enzymes. Administration of these drugs should provide some insight into the mechanism by which the renin-angiotensin system affects blood pressure regulation.

Thus, these agents should lower blood pressure in those forms of hypertension in which high levels of renin or angiotensin II can be measured, as is the case in

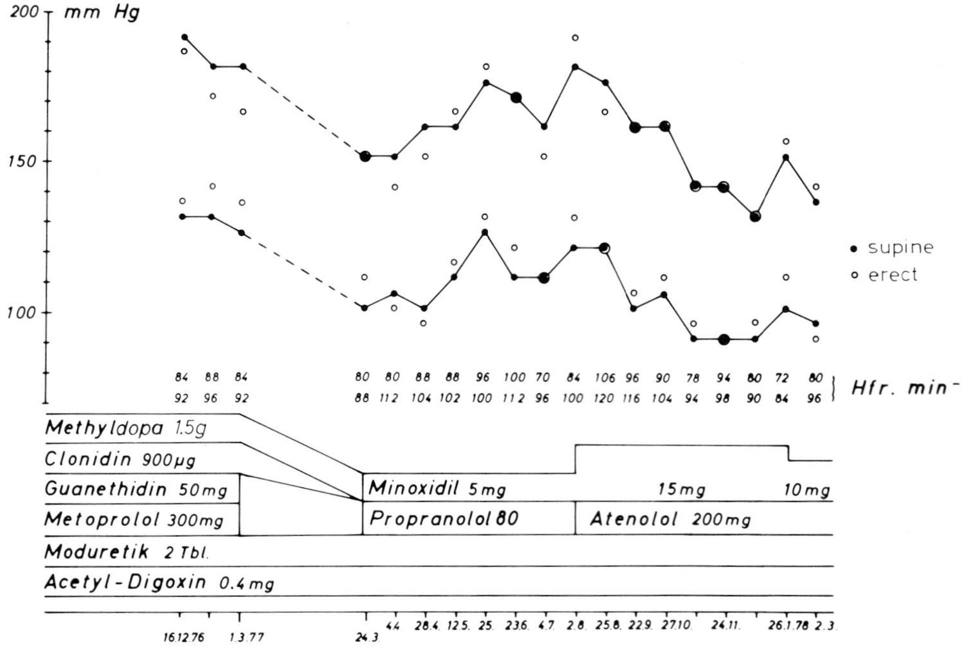

Fig. 1. Minoxidil therapy in a 52-year-old male patient with accelerated primary hypertension

proven renovascular hypertension, in malignant hypertension, and in some cases of hypertension in terminal renal failure. Intravenous infusion of saralasin in a constant dose of 10 µg/min per kilogram body weight in a patient with renovascular hypertension (Fig. 2) during salt depletion induced a pronounced fall in systolic and diastolic blood pressure, which in this patient continued after cessation of drug administration. Plasma-renin concentration rose significantly. After the patient was salt repleted, the same maneuver caused an increase in blood pressure, due to the agonistic activity of saralasin, whereas plasma-renin concentration did not change. In additional studies performed by our group [5], no blood pressure lowering effect could be observed in patients with primary hypertension, whether they were salt depleted or not (Fig. 3). In salt-loaded patients, a blood pressure response could be seen. However, others observed a fall in blood pressure in a small number of patients with primary hypertension [21]. Patients with renoparenchymal hypertension, without or with only moderate impaired renal function, showed significant blood pressure responses (Fig. 3).

Fig. 3. Effects of sodium balance on saralasin responsiveness in patients with primary, renoparenchymal, and renovascular hypertension (acc. to 5) ▸

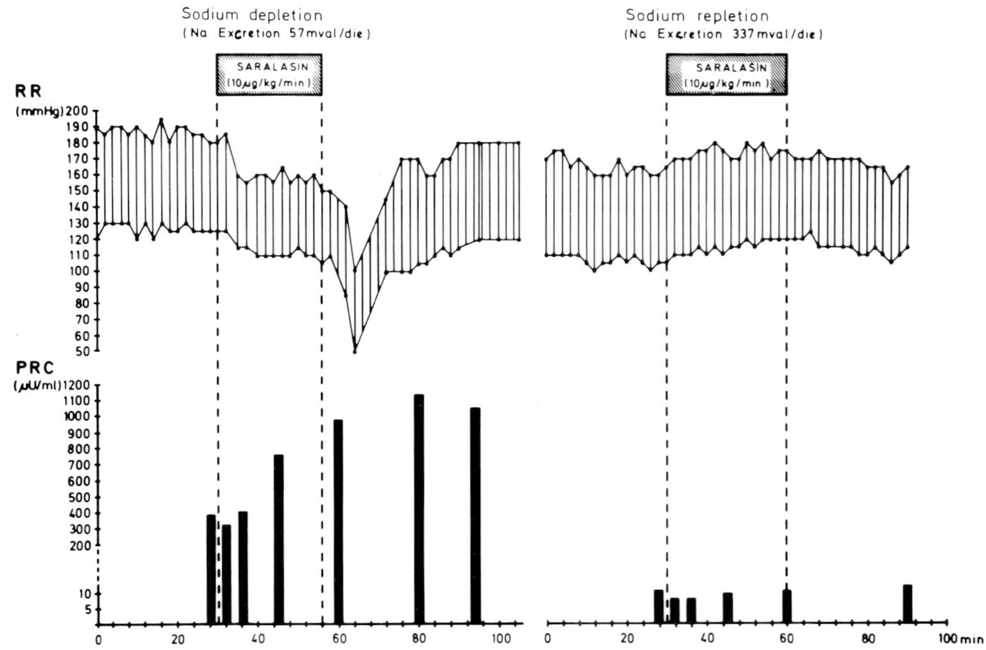

Fig.2. Effects of saralasin on blood pressure and plasma-renin concentration in a patient with renovascular hypertension. *Left*, saralasin test was performed after sodium depletion; *right*, after sodium repletion (acc. to 5)

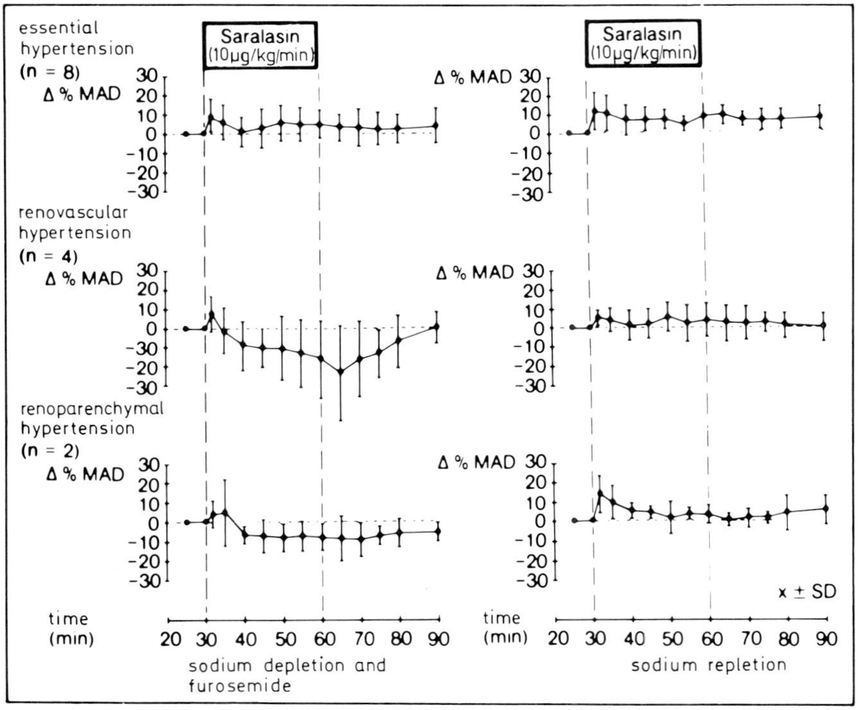

As can be seen, the blood pressure response during administration of saralasin is greatly dependent on sodium balance, consequently, on circulating levels of renin or angiotensin.

The depressor response to angiotensin II blockade is correlated inversely with the rise of plasma-renin activity, as was shown by Baer et al. [3] and Bönner et al. [5]. These findings suggest that during angiotensin II blockade the control of renin release is not mediated by a baroreceptor-sensitive mechanism is due to blockade of the short feedback loop [5].

Coincidentally with the fall in blood pressure, a decrease in peripheral resistance can be measured in patients responding to saralasin application, indicating that the vasoconstrictive effect of angiotensin II is, indeed, blocked (Fig. 4 according to [4]).

Unfortunately, saralasin is not suitable for chronic therapy, because it must be given intravenously. Therefore, it mainly serves to detect angiotensin-dependent, surgically curable forms of hypertension.

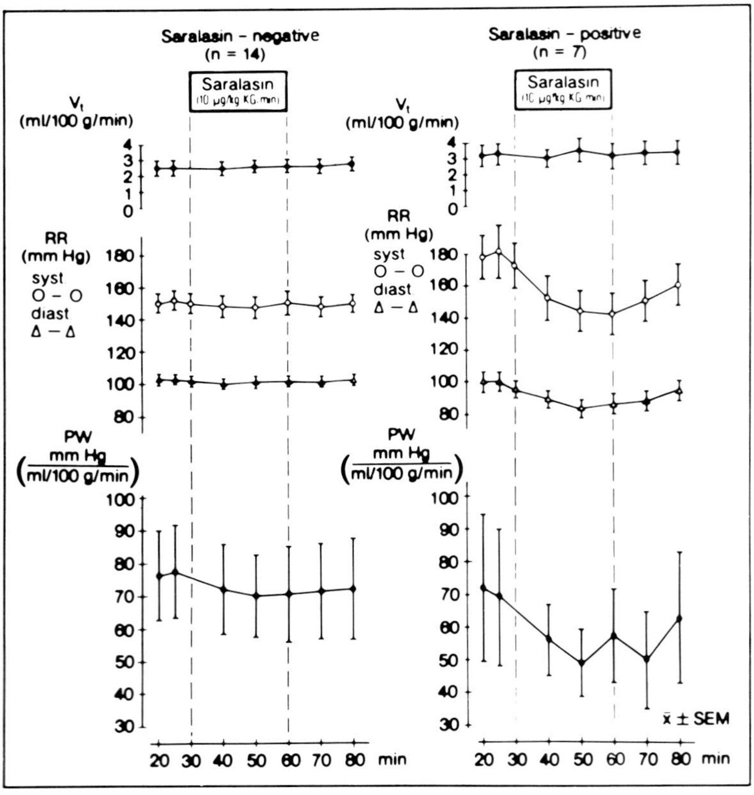

Fig. 4. Changes of central and peripheral hemodynamics in hypertensive patients during the administration of saralasin according to the test results (acc. to 4)

However, another approach to investigate angiotensin dependence of hypertension is possible by the use of captopril (SQ 14, 225), the orally acitve inhibitor of the conversion of angiotensin I to angiotensin II. But in addition, this compound potentiates the action of bradykinin. As already mentioned, converting enzyme and kininase II, the bradykinin-degrading enzyme, are identical [17]. The antihypertensive activity of captopril is also dependent on the levels of circulating renin or on the sodium balance, but probably to a minor degree. Thus in contrast to saralasin, captopril lowers blood pressure in a higher percentage of patients with primary hypertension [21].

An example of the properties of captopril is demonstrated in Fig. 5 in a female patient with moderate primary hypertension on liberal salt intake. In a moderate dosage, captopril reduced both systolic and diastolic blood pressure to normal values. Besides renin activity, kallikrein excretion increased after the beginning of therapy, and then, after one week, declined to pretreatment values. This also could be observed in animal experiments by McCaa et al. [26], who also measured an increase in blood kinin concentration, which may be due to decreased degradation of kinins. Similar observations are reported by Swartz et al. [30] in patients with primary hypertension under treatment with teprotide, the intravenously active converting enzyme inhibitor.

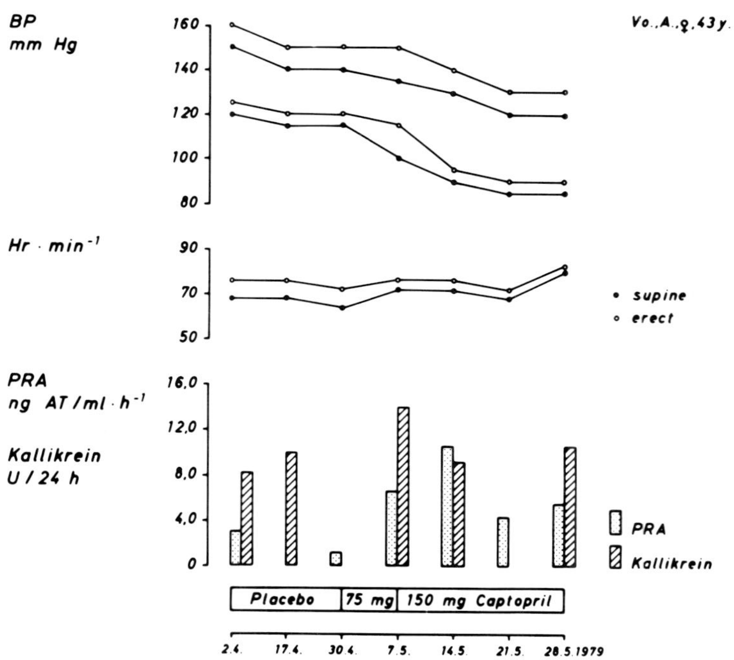

Fig. 5. Effect of captopril (SQ 14.225) on blood pressure (*BP*), heart rate (*Hr*), plasma-renin acitvity (*PRA*), and kallikrein excretion in a female patient with moderate primary hypertension

These findings, together with the above-mentioned difference between the hypotensive activity of converting enzyme inhibitors versus saralasin, make it possible that other factors, possibly bradykinin, may attribute to the hypotensive potency of these compounds. In addition with activation of phospholipase A by bradykinin, an increased release of arachidonic acid, the precursor for prostaglandins, occurs; consequently, prostaglandins also may be involved in the hypotensive action of converting enzyme inhibitors [17, 28].

Thus, these observations made during administration of saralasin and the converting enzyme inhibitors suggest that the vasoconstrictor action of angiotensin II is required for the maintenance of blood pressure in the salt-depleted subject who is standing upright, but not in the salt-replete supine subject [12].

In summary, with the present state of knowledge of the pathophysiologic abnormalities in human arterial hypertension, it is quite possible to influence the various pathophysiologic abnormalities involved in hypertension by various drugs. However, because a single abnormality is not known in most forms of hypertension, combined drug therapy is necessary to achieve adequate blood pressure control, whereas a specific therapeutic approach by surgical means is possible in renal artery stenosis, one-sided shrunken kidneys, primary aldosteronism, Cushing's syndrome, and pheochromocytoma.

References

1. Abe K, Irokawa N, Yasujima M, Seino M, Chiba S, Sakurai Y, Yoshinaga K, Saito T (1978) The kallikrein-kinin system and prostaglandins in the kidney. Their relation to furosemide-induced diuresis and to the renin-angiotensin-aldosterone system in man. Circ Res 43 : 254
2. Axelrod J (1976) Catecholamines and hypertension. Clin Sci Mol Med 51 : 415
3. Baer L, Parra-Carrillo JZ, Radichevich I (1979) Angiotensin II blockade: Evidence for baroreceptor-mediated renin release and the role of sodium balance. Kidney Int [Suppl] 15 : 60
4. Bönner G, Saborowski F, Caesar K, Helber A, Hummerich W, Wambach G, Kaufmann W (1978) Wirkung von 1-Sar-8-Ala-Angiotensin II (Saralasin) auf die periphere und zentrale Hämodynamik bei Hypertonikern. Herz Kreislauf 10 : 239
5. Bönner G, Helber A, Meurer KA, Hummerich W, Wambach G, Kaufmann W (1978) Methodische Probleme des Saralasin-Infusions-Testes in der Diagnostik der Hypertonie. Int Welt 1 : 267
6. Chalmers JP (1975) Brain amines and models of experimental hypertension. Circ Res 36 : 469
7. Dahl LK (1977) Salt intake in hypertension. In: Genest J, Koiw E, Kuchel O (eds) Hypertension. McGraw-Hill, New York pp 548–559
8. Distler AH, Just J, Philipp T (1973) Studies on the mechanism of aldosterone-induced hypertension in man. Clin Sci Mol Med 45 : 743

9. Frohlich ED (1977) Hemodynamics in hypertension. In: Genest J, Koiw E, Kuchel O (eds) Hypertension. McGraw-Hill, New York pp 15–49
10. Frohlich ED (1978) Newer concepts in antihypertensive drugs. Prog Cardiovasc Dis 20 : 385
11. Gerber JG, Branch RA, Nies AS, Gerkens JF, Shand DG, Hollifield J, Oates JA (1978) Prostaglandins and renin release. II. Assessment of renin secretion following infusion of PGI_2, E_2 and D_2 into the renal artery of anesthetized dogs. Prostaglandins 15 : 81
12. Goldberg LI, Rick JH, Oparil S (1977) Pharmacology of antihypertensive agents. In: Genest J, Koiw E, Kuchel O (eds) Hypertension. McGraw-Hill, New York pp 990–1024
13. Graham RM, Pettinger WA (1979) Prazosin. N Engl J Med 300 : 232
14. Gross F, Dietz R, Haebara H, Lüth JB, Mann JFE (1977) Spielt Renin eine Rolle in der Pathogenese des Hochdrucks? In: Dietz R, Ganten D, Hofbauer KG, Lüth JB (eds) Essentielle Hypertonie und ihre Behandlung. Schattauer, Stuttgart, p 54
15. Guyton AC (1977) Personal views on mechanism of hypertension. In: Genest J, Koiw E, Kuchel O (eds) Hypertension. McGraw-Hill, New York, pp 566–575
16. Guyton AC, Coleman TG, Cowley AW, Scheel KW, Manning RD Jr, Norman RA Jr (1972) Arterial pressure regulation. Overriding dominance of the kidneys in long-term regulation and in hypertension. Am J Med 52 : 584
17. Haberland GL (1978) Gewerbshormone der gesunden und der kranken Niere. Renin-Angiotensin-System, Kallikrein-Kinin-System. Prostaglandine. Med Welt 29 : 1844
18. Heinemann HO, Lee JB (1976) Prostaglandins and blood pressure control. Am J Med 61 : 681
19. Heise A (1976) Hypotensive action by central alpha-adrenergic and dopaminergic receptor stimulation. In: Scriabine AC, Sweet CS (eds) New antihypertensive drugs. Spectrum, Holliswood, p 135
20. Hollenberg NK, Adams DF (1976) The renal circulation in hypertensive disease. Am J Med 60 : 773
21. Hollenberg NK, Williams GH (1979) Angiotensin as a renal, adrenal, and cardiovascular hormone: Responses to saralasin in normal man and in essential and secondary hypertension. Kidney Int [Suppl] 15 : 29
22. Kopin IJ (1968) False adrenergic transmitters. Ann Rev Pharmacol 8 : 377
23. Lund-Johansen P (1977) Hemodynamic alterations in hypertension — spontaneous changes and effects of drug therapy. A review. Acta Med Scand [Suppl] 603 : 1
24. Lund-Johansen P (1977) Central hemodynamics in essential hypertension. Acta Med Scand [Suppl] 606 : 35
25. Margolius HS, Horwitz D, Pisano JJ, Keiser HR (1976) Relationship among urinary kallikrein, mineralocorticoids and hypertensive disease. Fed Proc 35 : 203
26. McCaa RE, Hall JE, McCaa CS (1978) The effects of angiotensin I-converting enzyme inhibitors on arterial blood pressure and urinary sodium excretion. Cirs Res [Suppl] 43 : 32

27. McGiff JC, Itskowitz HD, Terraqano A, Y-Kwong P (1976) Modulation and mediation of the action of the renal kallikrein-kinin system by prostaglandins. Fed Proc 35 : 175
28. Murthy VS, Waldron TL, Goldberg ME (1978) The mechanism of bradykinin potentation after inhibition of angiotensin-converting enzyme by SQ 14, 225 in conscious rabbits. Circ Res [Suppl] 43 : 40
29. Nasjletti A, Colina-Chourio J (1976) Interaction of mineralocortidoids, renal prostaglandins and the renal kallikrein-kinin system. Fed Proc 35 :189
30. Swartz SL, Williams GH, Hollenberg NK, Moore TJ, Dluhy RG (1979) Converting enzyme inhibition in essential hypertension: The hypotensive response does not reflect only reduced angiotensin II formation. Hypertension 1 : 106
31. Tarazi RC, Frohlich ED, Dustan HP (1970) Long-term thiazide therapy in hypertension. Evidence for persistent alteration of plasma volume and renin acitivity. Circulation 41 : 709
32. Tobian L (1977) Salt and hypertension. In: Genest J, Koiw E, Kuchel O (eds) Hypertension. McGraw-Hill, New York pp 423—433
33. Vinci JM, Zusman RM, Izzo JL Jr, Bowden RE, Horwitz D, Pisano JJ, Keiser HR (1979) Human urinary and plasma kinins. Relationship to sodium-retaining steroids and plasma renin acitvity. Circ Res 44 : 228
34. Zacest R, Gilmore E, Koch-Weser J (1972) Antihypertensive therapy with combination of propranolol and hydralazine. N Engl J Med 286 : 617
35. Van Zwieten PA (1975) Antihypertensive drugs with a central action. Prog Pharmacol 1 : 1

Central Hemodynamics at Rest and During Exercise Following Intravenous Digoxin in Hypertension

W. DOERING, E. KÖNIG, W. NECHWATAL, H. GREDING AND J. ISBARY

Chronic pressure overload of the left ventricle due to hypertensive cardiovascular disease (HCD) is the predominant etiological precursor of congestive heart failure [10]. At this end stage of HCD treatment with cardiac glycosides is well established.

However, during the long period between the onset of hypertension and the development of clinical heart failure, the heart adjusts to the chronic pressure overload by a series of compensatory mechanisms, the most obvious of which is ventricular hypertrophy. Despite numerous investigations in man and experimental animals, the question is still unresolved whether — or at what stage — this compensatory ventricular hypertrophy is accompanied by impaired ventricular performance [4, 17, 22]. Our studies over the last years have concentrated on the cardiac performance of hypertensive patients without a history or signs of heart failure and also on the role of digitalis in the treatment of these patients.

Central Hemodynamics of Hypertensive Patients Without Clinical Evidence of Heart Failure

For detection of depressed cardiac function at an early stage, exercise testing is crucial. Cardiac performance of our patients was, therefore evaluated during supine bicycle exercise using a flow-directed Swan-Ganz-catheter combined with a thermodilution cardiac output computer (for methodological details see [14]).

In 91 patients with untreated, mild to moderate hypertension and without symptoms and signs of cardiac failure, central hemodynamics were evaluated at rest and during submaximal exercise. Sixteen normotensive age-matched patients with no evidence of cardiovascular disease served as a control group.

At rest and during exercise the two groups of patients did not differ significantly in heart rate (78.1 vs. 78.3 and 120.0 vs. 128.8 min^{-1}) and in cardiac output (11.6 vs. 11.1 l/min). The mean systolic and diastolic blood pressures of the hypertensive patients were, of course, elevated (209/106 vs. 172/84 mm Hg, exercise values).

At rest the indexes of mean right and left ventricular filling pressures, that is, right atrial (RAM) and pulmonary capillary pressures (PCP), were identical for both groups, but they were considerably elevated for the hypertensive patients during exercise (RAM 8.5 vs. 3.5 mm Hg and PCP 20.0 vs. 12.0 mm Hg, exercise values).

Now, may I draw your attention to a point raised by Dr. Frohlich earlier during this symposium (see session E, Part II). That is, his very interesting finding that in the spontaneous hypertensive rats (SHR) early in the development of systemic hypertension right ventricular hypertrophy also occurs. The reason for this is yet unknown, but I would like to point out that throughout our studies on patients with systemic hypertension right atrial pressure always behaved similarly to left atrial pressure.

Fig. 1 gives the individual data for PCP and exercise tolerance of the 91 patients and demonstrates that PCP rose to abnormal values in almost half of the patients. Similar results were obtained earlier by Taylor and colleagues [24] in a small group of patients. However, Strauer [20] recently found no pathological elevation of filling pressures during exercise in a similar group of 14 patients.

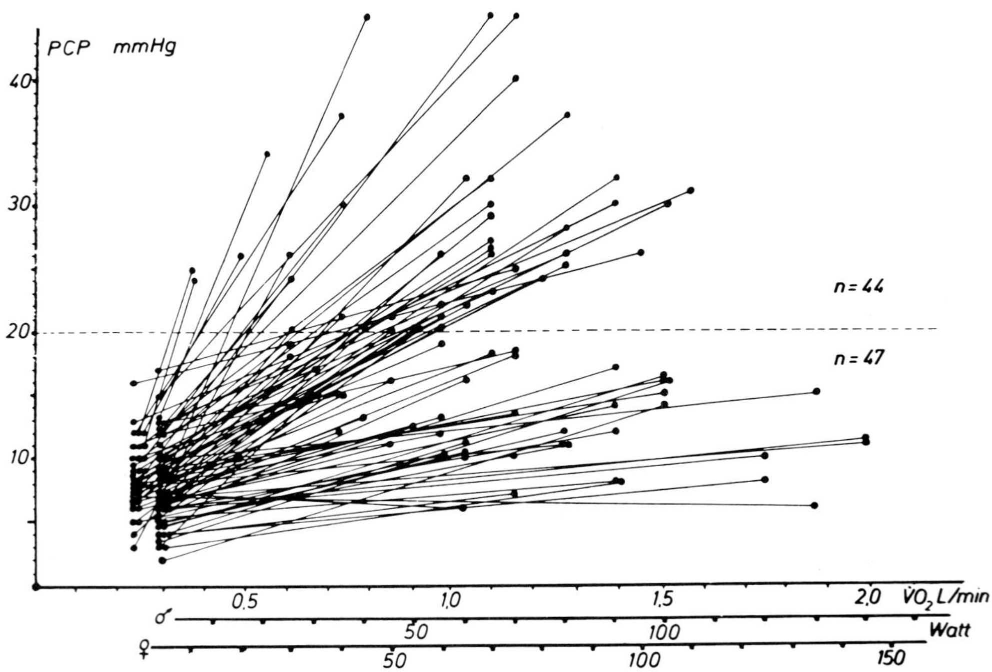

Fig. 1. Pulmonary artery wedge pressure (*PCP*) at rest and during exercise in 91 hypertensive patients without clinical signs of cardiac insufficiency. The increase in PCP for each patient is compared to the work lead achieved. The *dotted line* indicates the upper limit of normal PCP increase during exercise . From [11]

But, in contrast to our patients, his patients on the average were 10 years younger and were exposed to approximately half the work load as indicated by the rise in tension-time index.

The abnormal left ventricular filling pressures seen in half of our patients during exercise in the presence of a normal cardiac output indicates abnormal left ventricular dynamics, the pumping performance of the heart not being yet depressed. The fact that flow increases normally, even though there may be a rise in filling pressures, allows for at least two different explanations. First, a normal cardiac output in the presence of elevated filling pressures is seen in the early stage of cardiac insufficiency according to the classification by Roskamm and co-workers [16]. However, an alternate explanation is possible. The hypertrophied myocardium contains excess collagen [22], and the increased stiffness of the ventricular wall may well account for the elevated filling pressures.

Inotropic Stimulation

In this situation the administration of a positive inotropic agent should be of discriminating value. Inotropic stimulation will lower the elevated filling pres-

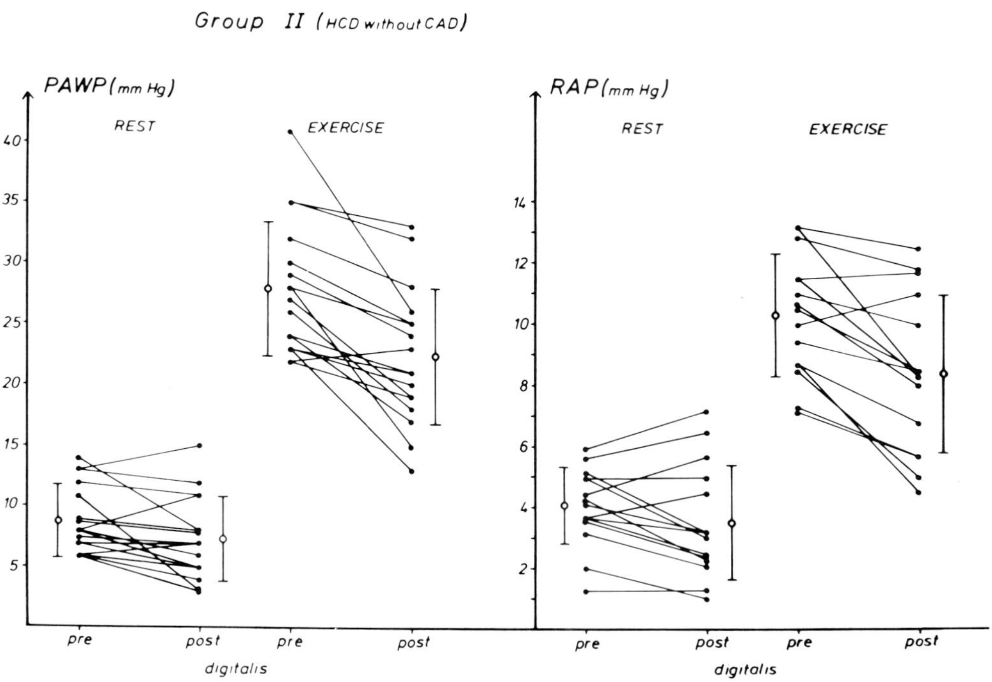

Fig. 2. Pulmonary artery wedge pressure (*PAWP*) and right atrial pressure (*RAP*) at rest and during exercise in 17 patients with hypertensive cardiovascular disease (*HCD*) and without coronary artery disease (*CAD*) before and after administration of 0.6 mg β-methyl-digoxin. From [12]

sure caused by impaired contractility while the elevated filling pressures due to reduced ventricular compliance will not be affected.

Therefore, 41 patients with elevated filling pressures (PCP more than 20 mm Hg) during exercise were re-examined after acute digitalis administration. However, not all of them responded favorably to inotropic stimulation. Close analysis of the results revealed that only those patients without concomitant coronary artery disease (CAD) showed an almost uniform and significant reduction of PCP and right atrial pressure (Fig. 2).

In contrast, those hypertensive patients with documented CAD demonstrated a varying reaction to digitalis, resulting in no significant improvement of either PCP or RAM (Fig. 3). As expected, cardiac output was unaltered by digitalis administration, since both groups of patients had normal cardiac output during exercise before glycosides were administred.

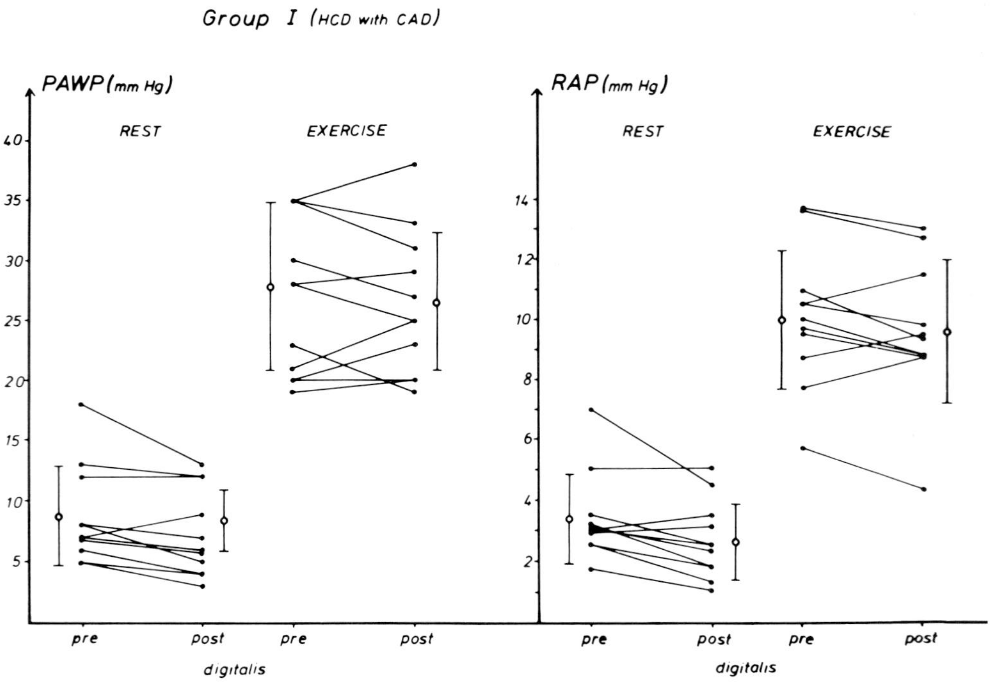

Fig. 3. Pulmonary artery wedge pressure (*PAWP*) and right atrial pressure (*RAP*) at rest and during exercise in 11 patients with hypertensive cardiovascular disease (*HCD*) and coronary artery disease (*CAD*) before and after administration of 0.6 mg β-methyl-digoxin. From [12]

Effect of Chronic Digitalis Administration

To our knowledge hemodynamic studies on the effect of chronic glycoside administration in hypertensive patients have not yet been published. In order to evaluate this long-term effect, 13 patients were re-examined after 8 weeks of digitalis treatment with 0.2 mg β-methyldigoxin per day [15].

In seven patients with a significant decrease of PCP during acute inotropic stimulation — here referred to as "responders" — chronic digitalis administration resulted in a further significant decrease of PCP (from 27.3 without digitalis to 23.7 after acute digitalis administration and to 21.5 mm Hg after chronic administration; see Fig. 4, upper panel). In the six nonresponders chronic glycoside administration resulted in no significant change of left ventricular filling pressures (25.3 vs. 27.6 vs. 28.1 mm Hg; Fig. 1, lower panel).

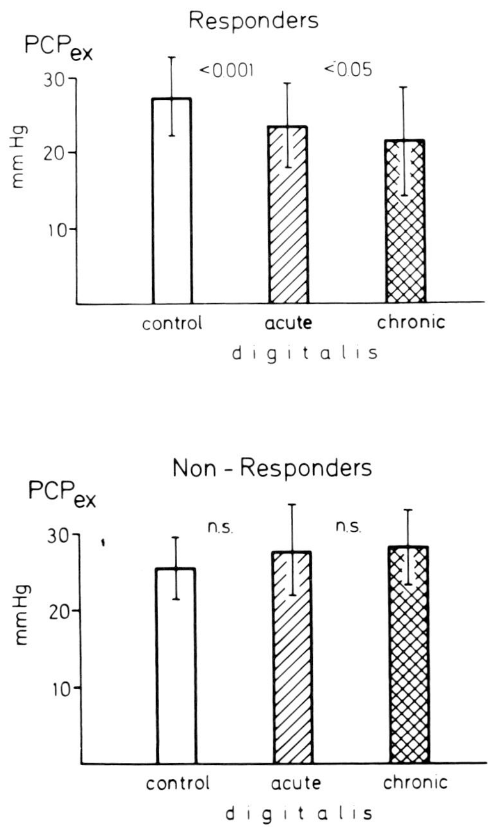

Fig. 4. In seven patients who responded favorably to acute digitalis administration, chronic administration resulted in a further decrease of pulmonary artery wedge pressure (PCP_{ex}) at the same work load (*upper panel*). Those six patients who did not respond to acute digitalis administration also showed no decrease of PCP after chronic administration (*lower panel*)

Again, cardiac output was not significantly altered by digitalis adiministration. These results document that in a considerable percentage of hypertensive patients the abnormal flow-pressure relation during exercise is due to impaired contracitlity which responds favorably to acute and chronic digitalis administration.

Results concerning the contractility and the performance of the hypertrophied ventricle in man are conflicting: Dr Just reported (see session D), as have others [20], an increased contractility in mild to moderate hypertension, while the groups of Spann [19], Krayenbühl [8], Alicandri [1] and Frohlich [5] all reported depressed performance of the human heart in hypertension, sometimes even before the more obvious signs of hypertrophy were apparent and well before signs of heart failure had developed. And I think the echocardiographic findings under stress conditions reported by Kment et al. (see session D, Part II) underline this notion.

Results of animal studies give a more uniform picture, and this has been emphasized by the papers presented earlier during this symposium: Although a slight increase in contractility during the very early phase of hypertension was reported by some authors like Hawthorne [7], thereafter no investigator found evidence that the animal heart with ventricular hypertrophy was able to perform better than the normal heart [4], and depressed cardiac performance occurred sooner or later during the course of hypertension [22].

Tarazi in a recent review explained the discrepancies between the results obtained in man and in the experimental animal as resulting mainly from a wider spectrum of adrenergic acitvity in man which allows him to adjust to chronic pressure overload by a varying degree of increased sympathetic acitvity [22]. Our results in hypertensive patients without other organic heart disease point in the same direction: During submaximal exercise the differences in adrenergic activity become negligible and digitalis exerts an almost uniform benificial effect on the depressed cardiac performance. At rest such a constant beneficial effect of digitalis did not always occur. On the contrary, at rest acute intravenous digitalis administration may result in the untoward effect, first described by Mason and Braunwald [9] and termed *Luxusinotropie* by Strauer [21].

Our results in hypertensive patients with documented CAD are in agreement with the literature, demonstrating that the ventricular compliance of these patients is considerably reduced. Furthermore, the cardiac performance of these patients is impaired by regional contraction abnormalities and changes in ventricular geometry. These factors limit any possible favorable effect of digitalis on the remaining nonischemic myocardium and explain clearly why digitalis administration in this particular group of patients results in such a varying effect.

Beta-Blocker Treatment and Digitalis

As mentioned before, increased sympathetic activity in hypertensive patients may help the heart to maintain its normal function. Thus it seems logical that deprivation of this adrenergic drive as induced by β-blockade may result in a further impairment of cardiac performance. Although there are not many reports in the literature indicating that β-blockade results in cardiac insufficiency in hypertensive patients, heart failure may occur [2, 23], especially if additional organic heart disease is present.

At least in our country (Federal Republic of Germany), physicians are greatly aware of this problem [18], and there is a tendency in everyday medical practice to counteract the β-blocker-induced reduction of cardiac performance by coadministration of cardiac glycosides. On the other hand, there are relevant theoretical objections against the simultaneous administration of two agents which exert opposing effects on cardiac inotropy. The combined use of β-blocker and a positive inotropic substance could endanger one of the supposed mechanisms by which the β-blockers exert their hypotensive effect, that is, the reduction in cardiac output which will eventually result in a readjustment of total peripheral resistance [23].

This question has prompted us to investigate the influence of digitalis on the β-blocker-induced changes of central hemodynamics [14]. Twelve hypertensive patients underwent exercise testing and were reexamined at the same work load 20 min after intravenous injection of 5 mg propranolol and again 30 min after 0.6 mg β-methyldigoxin (IV).

At rest β-blocker administration resulted in an insignificant rise in PCP which was counteracted by coadministration of digitalis. Again, right atrial pressure behaved similarly to PCP. During exercise these changes in filling pressures are markedly pronounced. After propranolol the mean PCP rises by 10 mm Hg compared to control values (28.0 vs. 18.0 mm Hg) and the mean RAM by 6 mm Hg (12.2 vs. 6.3 mm Hg).

Fig. 5 gives the individual PCP values during exercise and demonstrates clearly the uniform reaction to this type of pharmacological intervention. All patients reacted with an increase of PCP after β-blockade and again with a decrease after glycoside administration (from 28.0 to 22.8 mmHg), and the same holds true for the right atrial pressure (12.2 vs. 9.8 mm Hg).

Cardiac output reacted, however, quite differently. After β-blockade it was already significantly reduced at rest and even more so during exercise (13.6 vs. 11.5 l/min, exercise values). Acute digitalis administration, however, exerted no significant effect on this β-blocker-induced decrease of cardiac output, neither at rest nor during exercise (11.5 vs. 11.9 l/min, exercise values). This is due mainly to the fact that the decreased cardiac output during β-blockade is chiefly an effect of the strongly reduced heart rate [6] and, therefore, cannot be compensated for by glycoside administration.

Our results thus demonstrate that the β-blocker-induced elevation of filling pressure is uniformly and significantly reduced by glycoside administration. Moreover, coadministration of cardiac glycosides will not endanger the hypotensive effect of β-blocker treatment. This notion is substantiated by results of Crawford

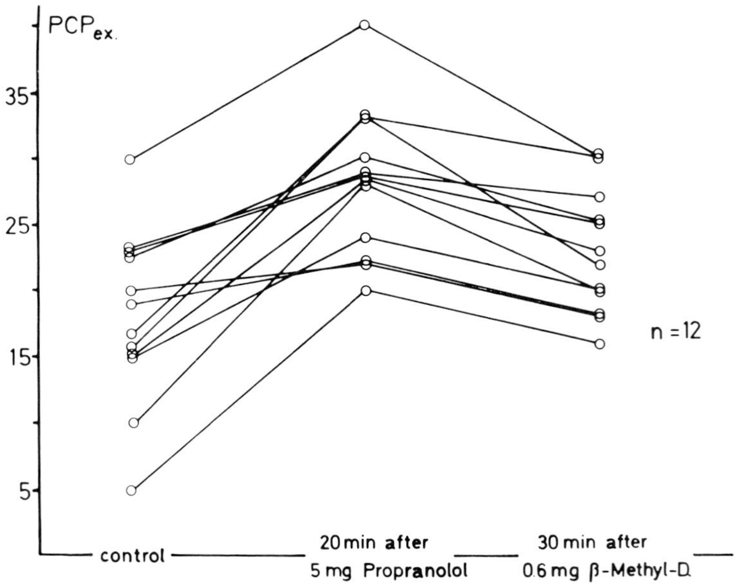

Fig. 5. The influence on hypertensive patients of propranolol and β-methyl-digoxin on the pulmonary artery wedge pressure (PCP_{ex}) during exercise. From [14]

et al., [3], who demonstrated that the β-blocker-induced reduction of blood pressure is also maintained when digitalis is added to treatment.

Conclusion

In conclusion, exercise testing of hypertensive patients without clinical signs of cardiac insufficiency revealed abnormal hemodynamics in almost half of them. However, only patients without concomitant CAD benefit from digitalis administration, while the effect of cardiac glycosides is not uniform in the group with CAD. These results of acute digitalization were confirmed by reexamination during chronic administration.

The β-blocker-induced elevation of filling pressures is uniformly decreased by cardiac glycosides, while the β-blocker-induced reduction of cardiac output remains unaltered. However, longitudinal observations of patients with elevated filling pressures during exercise will have to demonstrate whether early administration of digitalis exerts a protective effect on the heart in hypertension.

References

1. Alicandri CM, Fouad FM, Tarazi RC, Bravo EL, Dustan HP (1977) Cardiac performance in hypertension. Circulation [Suppl III] 55/56 : 29

2. Bühler FR, Laragh JH, Baer L (1972) Propranolol inhibition of renin secretion. N Engl J Med 287 : 1209
3. Crawford MH, Winter MM, O'Rouke RA, Karliner JS, Ross J Jr (1975) Combined propranolol and digoxin therapy in angina pectoris. Ann Intern Med 83 : 449
4. Frohlich ED (1977) Hemodynamics of hypertension. In: Genest J, Koiw E, Kuchel O (eds) Hypertension, McGraw-Hill, New York, pp 15—49
5. Frohlich ED, Tarazi RC, Dustan HP (1971) Clinical-physiological correlations in the development of hypertensive heart disease. Circulation 44 : 446—455
6. Hansson L, Zweifler AJ, Julius S, Hunyor SN (1974) Hemodynamic effects of acute and prolonged β-adrenergic blockade in essential hypertension. Acta Med Scand 196 : 27—34
7. Hawthorne EW, Hinds JE, Crawford WJ, Tearneg RJ (1974) Left ventricular myocardial contractility during the first week of renal hypertension in conscious instrumented dogs. Circ Res [Suppl I] 34 : 223
8. Krayenbühl HP (1972) Die Bedeutung der Myokardhypertrophie für die Dynamik und Kontraktilität des Herzens.Verh Dtsch Ges Kreislaufforsch 38 : 65
9. Mason DT, Braunwald E (1963) Studies on digitalis. IX. Effects of ouabain on the nonfailing human heart. J Clin Invest 42 : 1105
10. McKee PA, Castelli WP, McNamara PM, Kannel WB (1971) The natural history of heart failure. The Framingham study. N Engl Med 285 : 1441
11. Nechwatal W, König E, Eversmann A, Saltner K (1975) Untersuchungen zur Frage der Belastungsherzinsuffizienz bei Hypertonie. Z Kardiol 64 : 375
12. Nechwatal W, König E, Kronski D, Eversmann A, Eversmann T (1976) Hemodynamic response to digitalisation in patients with hypertensive cardiovascular disease. Basic Res Cardiol 71 : 553
13. Nechwatal W, König E, Eversmann A, Lehnert J (1977) Zur Frage der Frühdigitalisierung bei Patienten mit arterieller Hypertonie. Dtsch Med Wochenschr 102 : 989
14. Nechwatal W, König E, Isbary J, Greding H (1977) Hämodynamische Interaktion von Propranolol und Digitalis bei Patienten mit Hypertonie. Z Kardiol 66 : 572—577
15. Palos K (to be published) Disseration, University of Munich
16. Roskamm H, Weidemann H, Meinecke B, Petersen J, Reindell H (1969) Die Diagnostik einer beginnenden Herzinsuffizienz mit Hilfe eines Einschwemmkatheterverfahrens. Z Kreislaufforsch 59 : 119
17. Ross J Jr, Sobel BE (1972) Regulation of cardiac contraction. Ann Rev Physiol 34 : 47
18. Simon H (1978) Herzwirksame Pharmaka. Urban & Schwarzenberg, München, p 116
19. Spann JF, Buccino RA, Sonnenblick EH, Braunwald E (1966) Contractile state of myocardium in ventricular hypertrophy and heart failure. Circulation [Suppl III] 34 : 222
20. Strauer BE (1979) Das Hochdruckherz. Springer, Berlin Heidelberg New York, p 12

21. Strauer BE (1979) Das Hochdruckherz. Springer, Berlin Heidelberg New York, p 71
22. Tarazi RC (1979) Effect of hypertension on the heart. In: Onesti G, Klimt CR (eds) Hypertension: Determinants, complications and intervention. Grune & Stratton, pp 211—227
23. Tarazi RC, Dustan HP (1972) Beta-adrenergic blockade in hypertension. Am J Cardiol 29 : 633
24. Taylor SH, Donald KW, Bishop JB (1957) Circulatory studies in hypertensive patients at rest and during exercise. Clin Sci 16 : 351

Part II: Use of Beta-Receptor Blocking Agents

Beta-Adrenergic Receptor Blockade in the Treatment of Essential Hypertension

E.D. FROHLICH

Introduction

Well over 15 years have elapsed since beta-adrenergic receptor blocking therapy was introduced for the treatment of hypertension [1, 2]. Since this time over a score of different beta-adrenergic receptor blocking compounds have been introduced commercially worldwide; this class of antihypertensive therapy has, indeed, gained tremendous popularity (Table 1). Although the United States was late in accepting the beta-blocking drugs as a class of legitimate hypotensive agents, two have been approved by our Food and Drug Administration, and a dozen or more others are undergoing active clinical investigation. It is anticipated that some others will gain approval in the near future. Clearly, this group of antihypertensive drugs must no longer be considered as "stepchild" therapy just because its mechanism of antihypertensive action escapes full elucidation.

Table 1. Characteristics of the major beta-adrenergic receptor blocking drugs that have been shown to reduce arterial pressure[a]

Generic name	Membrane stabilizing activity	Cardio-selectiv	Partial agonist activity
Acebutolol	+	+	+
Alprenolol	+	0	+
Atenolol	0	+	0
Metoprolol	±	+	0
Oxprenolol	+	0	+
Penbutolol	+	+	0
Pindolol	+	0	+
Practolol	+	+	+
Propranolol	+	0	0
Sotalol	0	0	0
Timolol	0	0	±
Tolamolol	0	+	0

[a] + = pressent; 0 = not present; ± = present or not present

For the oral diuretics were introduced well before the beta-adrenergic blocking drugs, and we still fall short of a total understanding for the explanation of their antihypertensive action.

In the United States and certain other countries, beta-adrenergic receptor blocking drugs have been classified as one of the "step 2" group of hypotensive agents after initially introducing the thiazide diuretic as a "step 1" modality [3]. Recently, the World Health Organization, in its Expert Committee on Hypertension's report on arterial hypertension recommended that as the first step of antihypertensive therapy a therapeutic alternative between the thiazide diuretic and a beta-adrenergic blocking drug could be made [4]. Inherent in this latter decision is the concept that a certain number of patients with hypertension will respond to beta-adrenergic blocking drugs alone; in those who do not, the thiazide drug may then be added. Thus, at the completion of "step 2", it is generally held that the combination of a beta-blocking drug and diuretic makes the most sense for antihypertensive therapy on a mass population treatment basis.

In reality there are certain criteria that may permit the selection of a diuretic first for the patient with essential hypertension. It has been shown that there are certain patients with essential hypertension who may be more volume responsive [5]. These individuals may include groups primarily comprised of women, black patients, older individuals, and patients with essential hypertension who are volume-dependent or who have low plasma renin activity. In contrast, criteria may be developed that will permit the selection of beta-adrenergic receptor blocking drug first. These individuals might be comprised primarily of men, younger patients, white individuals, and patients who are volume-contracted; perhaps as a result of the reduced plasma volume, they may also have high plasma renin acitvity [6]. Thus, selection of patients on pure algorithm or empirical basis for a particular course of antihypertensive therapy is to beg but a major question — one that is fundamental to a quest to learn more about the clinical nature and improved rational treatment of essential hypertension.

Hemodynamic Effects

Systemic Hemodynamics. We have studied the systemic hemodynamic effects of a variety of beta-adrenergic receptor blocking drugs [7—14]. Initially, we observed that following the intravenous administration of propranolol to patients with hypertension, there is a reduction in heart rate and cardiac output and a rise in total peripheral resistance unassociated with a change in arterial pressure [7]. However, if these patients are treated for a prolonged period of time with oral therapy, arterial pressure will soon fall and this fall in pressure is associated with a maintained reduction in cardiac output and a total peripheral resistance that is not significantly lower than pretreatment levels [8]. It has been argued by some that because output remained reduced at the same level while arterial pressure fell, there must be at least some fall in total peripheral resistance and vasodilation must occur in time [15—19]. The explanations for this phenomenon have been varied and included resetting of arterial baroreceptors [20] or in the carotid sinus [21], or a "readjustment" or adaptation of the circulation to the persistent reduction in cardiac output [15], much the same as if total body autoregulation that might occur in the genesis of hypertension may be associated with an adapted circulation to a high cardiac output, resulting in a consequent increased total peripheral resistance [22]. Nevertheless, in time most patients who have been followed with these beta-adrenergic blocking agents alone seem to demonstrate a reduced cardiac output unassociated with a significant reduction in total peripheral resistance from pretreatment levels [8, 10, 14, 18, 19, 23].

We have compared the systemic hemodynamic effects of a number of beta-adrenergic receptor blocking drugs and have found that whether these agents are cardioselective (e.g., practolol, tolamolol, atenolol, or acebutolol) or whether they had greater or lesser degrees of nonspecific cardiac effects (e.g., propranolol, sotalol, or timolol), each seems to be associated with greater or lesser degrees of cardiac output reduction [24]. However, each drug must be associated with some form of circulatory adaptation in order to provide a hemodynamic explanation for the maintained reduced cardiac output which is coincident with an eventual pressure fall [8, 15–19, 23]. Propranolol and timolol both demonstrate a reduced arterial pressure associated with unchanged or a contracted plasma volume [9, 14], a reduced cardiac output and an elevated total peripheral resistance [8, 14]. This unchanged plasma volume is an unusual finding when an antihypertensive drug is administerd to inhibit adrenergic function [6, 25]. It is not known why fluid volume does not expand — whether it is a result of inhibited plasma renin acitivity and consequent aldosterone generation from the adrenal cortex, whether there are differential effects of this anithypertensive agent on different regional circulations or on the arteriolar and venular limbs of the circulation, or whether there are direct renal effects of these agents that do not favor the retention of sodium and water in the face of arterial pressure reduction. Certainly, these questions merit intensive investigation.

Regional Hemodynamics. Because measurements of each of the organ blood flows have not been possible in intact man treated(or not treated, for that matter) with beta-adrenergic receptor blocking drugs, we have studied spontaneously hypertensive and normotensive Wistar-Kyoto rats with either propranolol or timolol [26]. In these studies, although arterial pressure was not reduced with either agent (it seems that prolonged treatment with beta-adrenergic blocking drugs has not been particularly effective in this genetic strain of hypertension), we did observe the same magnitude of reduction of cardiac output with these drugs (approximately 25%). Nevertheless, our results indicated that renal blood flow remained either unchanged or increased. Similarly, there was little change in blood flow to the brain, liver, adrenals, and testes, but skeletal muscle and cardiac muscle blood flows were significantly reduced (Table 2). Therefore, the significant reduction in systemic blood flow (i.e., cardiac output) can be explained by a large reduction in blood flow to the major mass of the body (i.e., skeletal muscle) and by the fact that blood flow to the vital organs seems to be preserved [26].

Table 2. Circulatory redistribution associated with an approximate 25% to 30% reduction in cardiac output produced by either propranolol or timolol in spontaneously hypertensive (SHR) or normotensive (WKY) rats treated from conception until 11 weeks of age. [26][a]

Blood flow	Tap water		Propranolol		Timolol	
(ml/min/kg)	WKY	SHR	WKY	SHR	WKY	SHR
Cardiac output	302	318	221^{+}	197^{++}	218^{+}	237^{+}
Skeletal muscle	0.5	0.3	0.1^{+}	0.1^{+}	0.1^{+}	0.1^{+}
Heart	6.0	8.2*	3.7^{+}	5.0^{+}	4.5^{+}	5.6^{+}
Brain	1.6	1.9	1.6	1.4	1.4	1.6
Kidneys	3.0	3.1	3.6	4.2	4.6^{+}	4.5^{+}
Lungs	1.6	2.3	2.3	1.7	2.2	2.7
Liver	1.2	1.0	1.6^{+}	1.2*	1.4	1.2
Adrenals	5.4	7.6	7.7^{+}	8.1	7.4	8.7
Testes	0.2	0.3	0.3^{+}	0.2	0.4^{+}	0.3

[a] + = $P < 0.05$; ++ = $P < 0.02$; * = $P < 0.01$

Ventricular Hypertrophy. In addition to the above hemodynamic effects of beta-adrenergic blocking drugs, these compounds have also been shown to reduce cardiac mass significantly in normotensive rabbits [27] and in rats with renal hypertension [28]. However, perhaps because arterial pressure was not reduced in the genetically spontaneously hypertensive rats (Okamoto-Aoki strain), this might explain the absence of a significant reduction of cardiac mass [29]. However, in the foregoing study when we compared the changes in cardiac weight of male and female rats who were treated from conception with either propranolol or timolol therapy, we found that the female rats seemed to demonstrate some slight reduction in cardiac mass which was independent of any change in arterial pressure; this was not observed in the male rats [29]. These data underscore the contention that other factors in addition to reduction in arterial pressure may be associated with reduced cardiac mass or, conversely, with ventricular hypertrophy [30].

Antihypertensive Mechanisms

Several mechanisms have been postulated to explain the antihypertensive action of the beta-adrenergic receptor blocking drugs (Table 3).

These mechanisms have included a reduced cardiac output, adaptations of the peripheral circulation, initiation of either central or peripheral reflex adjustments, modification of the biosyhthesis of catecholamines, reduced plasma renin acitvity, and perhaps even direct or indirect actions of metabolites of the administered beta-blocking drugs.

Table 3. Possible antihypertensive mechanisms of the beta-adrenergic receptor blocking drugs

1. Hemodynamic mechanisms
   a. Reduced cardiac output
   b. Different responses of the component peripheral circulations
   c. Total body autoregulation ("reverse Guyton")
   d. Reduced vessel distention ("reverse Bayliss")
2. Neural mechanisms
   a. Induction of central or peripheral reflex adjustments (including baroreceptor "resetting")
   b. Inhibition of central (brain) beta-receptors
   c. Modified catecholamine biosynthesis
   d. Central action of an active metabolite
3. Reduction of plasma renin activity

Reduced Cardiac Output. It was probably because the long-term antihypertensive effects of propranolol therapy were associated with a reduced cardiac output, but not total peripheral resistance, that we suggested that the paradoxical hemodynamic antihypertensive effects of this beta-blocking drug could be explained by a reduced cardiac output [8]. However, it subsequently became clear that not all beta-adrenergic blocking drugs reduced cardiac output to the equivalent degrees [24], although in these studies involving the same patients, arterial pressure was similarly reduced. Moreover, these studies fail to explain why arterial pressure was reduced subsequent to a maintained similar reduction of cardiac output in the chronic and acute phases of drug administration. Clearly, an alternative hypothesis must be considered.

Circulatory Readjustments. One appealing hypothesis could be that of a readjustment of the circulation similar to the concept offered for the total body autoregulation associated with the development of hypertension in many forms of experimental hypertension [21]. Thus, these workers have suggested that sustained arterial hypertension may follow a total body autoregulation which would be initiated by an expansion of intravascular volume, thereby increasing cardiac output and associated with a normal vascular resistance. With time, they believe, there is an adaptation of the circulation (i.e., autoregulation), which permits a reduction of the intravascular volume and a consequent reduced cardiac output to normal levels, but also then an associated elevated total peripheral resistance and high arterial pressure [21]. Alternatively, this phenomenon might also be similar to a reverse of the Bayliss mechanism [31] in which there was a postulated adaptation of distended vessels resulting from an increased flow leading to a consequently reduced flow associated with increased vascular resistance and pressure [32]. Unfortunately, these concepts still remain highly theoretical and have not been shown to occur in many experimental hypertensive models [29, 33] or in man with essential hypertension [34]. Nevertheless, it is intriguing that the reverse of these theoretical autoregulatory hemodynamic phenomena seems also to be associated with the reduction of arterial pressure which is related to a variety of antihypertensive medications, including the seemingly disparate actions of the beta-receptor blocking drugs and oral diuretics (e.g., thiazides).

A third postulated circulatory adaptation may occur by a preferential redistribution of blood flow to specific organs, while other organs may not demonstrate this redistributed flow. The net result might be no actual change in total peripheral resistance, whereas the arterial pressure may become reduced. Previous studies using in vivo as well as mathematical models have shown that changes (such as those already described) in regional or organ blood flows and blood flow distribution could have profound effects on cardiac output [35, 36]. Thus, redistribution of blood flow from the peripheral (e.g., skeletal muscle) to the splanchnic (or renal) circulations could reduce arterial pressure while decreasing cardiac output. It, therefore, is not unrealistic to conceive that the modest arteriolar dilation in the splanchnic and renal circulations associated with constriction in the skeletal muscle vasculature, which results from beta-adrenergic receptor inhibition, might reduce arterial pressure and coincide with a fall in cardiac output.

Neural Readjustments. One of the first mechanisms suggested for the reduction of arterial pressure was that of a "resetting of baroreceptors" [20]. While attractive in concept and, indeed, in phraseology, this resetting has not been demonstrated, although the sequence is appealing. However, since baroreceptors respond primarily to changes in pressure, there should be a secondary fall in total peripheral resistance. It seems, then, hardly possible that baroreceptor resetting could be the major mechanism for the antihypertensive action of the beta-adrenergic blocking drug. Alternative possibilities might be offered by altered function of volume (or "low pressure") receptors, thereby producing adaptations reflexively initiated from the central circulation. Volume receptors are present in the cardiopulmonary area, and it would seem that coincident with cardiac output reduction, there could be possible readjustments in peripheral blood flow distribution initiated through these reflexes. If this is so, then this concept would be consonant with the studies cited previously [35, 36] suggesting that a reduced cardiac output associated with altered peripheral blood flow distributions might provide the hemodynamic explanation for the anithypertensive action of the beta-blockers.

Alpha-adrenotropic receptors have been demonstrated in the brain in specific cardiovascular centers. These central alpha receptors, in contrast to alpha receptors in the periphery, when stimulated reduce arterial pressure by decreasing central adenergic outflow to the cardiovascular system [6, 37, 38]. Conversely, alpha-adrenergic inhibition in the brain serves to increase adrenergic outflow from the brain. While knowledge of beta-adrenoreceptor localization in the brain is more controversial, it seems at least possible at this time that beta-adrenergic receptor stimulation should raise arterial pressure through an increased adrenergic outflow from the brain. Conversely, beta-adrenergic receptor inhibition should reduce adrenergic outflow to the cardiovascular system from the brain and thereby reduce arterial pressure. This concept is indeed appealing; however, the problem is that several beta-adrenergic receptor blocking drugs that reduce arterial pressure do not seem to pass the blood-brain barrier to gain entrance to the brain. While this does not definitely exclude a central action of all beta-adrenergic blocking drugs, it has been used by many to exclude this antihypertensive action. An alternative explanation might be that certain vasoactive metabolites of these administered beta-adrenergic blocking drugs pass the blood-brain barriers and then exert their central antihypertensive effect, even though the administered compound may not gain entrance to the brain. Finally, it has been suggested by some that beta-adrenergic blocking drugs may modify the biosynthesis of catecholamines, either in the peripheral sympathetic nerve endings, the adrenal gland, or centrally in the brain, thereby modifying the neurohumoral mechanisms serving to control arterial pressure.

Plasma Renin Activity. Several mechanisms have been offered to explain the release of renin from the kidney. Included among these are a sodium-sensitive locus in the macula densa; an intrarenal angiotensin-mediated negative feedback suppression mechanism; an intrarenal baroreceptor mechanism; direct responses by the juxtaglomerular apparatus to changing concentrations of plasma electrolytes (specifically, the potassium and calcium ions), vasopressin, prostaglandins, and the kallikrein-kinin system; and the adrenergic nervous system [5]. With respect to the latter meachanism, renal sympathetic nerve stimulation and synthetic sympathomimetic drugs, as well as naturally occurring sympathomimetic agents (i.e., norepinephrine, epinephrine), will promote release of renin form the kidney. Conversely, nerve block to the kidney and beta-adrenergic blockade will inhibit the release of renin from kidney and shift a dose-response curve of adrenergic agonist drugs to the left [39]. Utilizing this concept, Laragh and his associates have popularized a concept whereby patients having high pretreatment plasma renin activity seem to be more responsive to the antihypertensive effects of beta-adrenergic blocking drugs [40, 41]. In contrast, patients with low plasma renin activity seem to have less responsiveness to these drugs but will respond better to diuretic therapy [42]. This has prompted Laragh and his co-workers to suggest classifying that patients according to high, normal, or low plasma renin activity might provide a means of selection for beta-adrenergic receptor blocking therapy [43]. Although this concept remains controversial, it has provided the genesis of much work concerning the role of the renin-angiotensin-aldosterone system in the pathogenesis and therapeutics of essential hypertension. Nevertheless, with respect to beta-adrenergic receptor blocking therapy, the same drawbacks that one finds with cardiac output reduction seem also to be present with the concept of plasma renin activity. Reports have indicated that not all beta-adrenergic blocking drugs seem to reduce plasma renin acitvity, while, nevertheless, they do reduce arterial pressure [44].

Therapeutic Concepts

It is clear that beta-adrenergic receptor blocking therapy has gained a real place in the treatment of hypertension [3, 4]. Much is known about the hemodynamic and specific local organ effects of these beta-blocking drugs. Nevertheless, our thinking at present is in a state of flux and concepts concerning how arterials pressure is reduced with these drugs remain controversial [45]. This, however, should not be disturbing. One may ask, even at this late date after the introduction of oral diuretic agents, how total peripheral resistance is actually reduced with prolonged thiazide therapy. There have been many speculations concerning the mechanism of this class of drugs: reduced total body sodium and water: decreased sodium and water content in the arteriolar walls; altered transmembrane ionic gradients; or reduced responsiveness to circulating naturally occurring pressor substances.

It is clear, however, that there are certain patients who may respond with a significant reduction in arterial pressure to a beta-adrenergic blocking drug itself. And in those patients who have a minimal response to this form of therapy, a more dramatic antihypertensive effect will be demonstrated when a diuretic agent is added to this treatment program. In a still more severe group of hypertensive patients in whom a vasodilating agent is necessary to further reduce arterial pressure through a fall in total peripheral resistance, the beta-adrenergic blocking drug provides a useful adjunct to this form of therapy [46, 47]. Under these circumstances the beta-blocker will prevent the reflexive chronotropic and inotropic stimulation of the heart induced by the vasodilating drug. This concept has been offered and used effectively for the treatment of severe essential hypertension.

In addition, other major questions to the beta-blockers are currently being raised. Does beta-adrenergic receptor blocking therapy provide regression of ventricular hypertrophy? Does beta-adrenergic blocking therapy for patients with hypertension alter the development of atherosclerotic coronary arterial disease? Certain multicenter clinical trials have already suggested that the number of sudden deaths in patients with previous myocardial infarctions can be reduced with beta-adrenergic receptor blocking drug therapy [48]. If these findings and others relating to hypertension and coronary heart disease are corroborated, then a new and exciting future of clinical investigations can be expected.

References

1. Prichard BNC (1964) Hypertensive action of pronethalol. Br Med J 1 : 1227
2. Prichard BNC, Gillam PMS (1964) The use of propranolol in the treatment of hypertension. Br Med J 2 : 725
3. Joint National Committee on Detection, Evaluation, and Treatment of High Blood Pressure (1980) Report of the Joint National Committee on Detection, Evaluation, and Treatment of High Blood Pressure. Arch Intern Med 140 : 1280

4. World Health Oragnization (1978) Arterial Hypertension. Report of a WHO Expert Committee. WHO Tech Rep Ser 628
5. Dustan HP, Tarazi RC, Hinshaw LB (1976) Mechanisms controlling arterial pressure. In: Frohlich ED (ed) Pathophysiology: Altered regulatory mechanisms in disease, 2nd edn. Lippincott, Philadelphia, p 49
6. Frohlich ED (1978) Newer concepts in antihypertensive drugs. Prog Cardiovasc Dis 20/5 : 385
7. Ulrych M, Frohlich ED, Dustan HP, Page IH (1968) Immediate hemodynamic effects of beta-adrenergic blockade with propranolol in normotensive and hypertensive man. Circulation 37 : 411
8. Frohlich ED, Tarazi RC, Dustan HP, Page IH (1968) The paradox of beta-adrenergic blockade in hypertension. Circulation 37 : 417
9. Tarazi RC, Frohlich ED, Dustan HP (1971) Plasma volume changes with long-term beta-adrenergic blockade. Am Heart J 82 : 770
10. Frohlich ED (1973) The use of beta-adrenergic blockade in hypertension. In: Onesti G, Kim KE, Moyer JH (eds) Hypertension: Mechanisms and management. Grune & Stratton, New York, p 333
11. Pfeffer MA, Frohlich ED, Pfeffer JM, Weiss AK (1974) Pathophysiological implications of the increased cardiac output of young spontaneously hypertensive rats. Circ Res 34/I : 235
12. Frohlich ED (1975) Dissimilar hemodynamic effects of propranolol, practolol, and sotalol in hypertensive man with a discussion of antihypertensive mechanisms. In: Dengler HJ (ed) Kardiale Sympathikolyse als therapeutisches Prinzip. Thieme, Stuttgart, p 205
13. Frohlich ED, Dunn FG, Chrysant SG (1975) Beta-blocking agents: Nonessentiality of cardiac output in antihypertensive action. Circulation 52/II : 184
14. Dunn FG, de Carvalho JGR, Frohlich ED (1978) Hemodynamic, reflexive, and metabolic alterations induced by acute and chronic timolol therapy in hypertensive man. Circulation 57 : 140
15. Frohlich ED, Page IH (1966) The clinical meaning of cardiovascular beta-adrenergic receptors. Physiol Pharmacol Pyhsicians 1/11
16. Frohlich ED (1971) Beta-adrenergic blockade in the circulatory regulation of hyperkinetic states. Am J Cardiol 27 : 195
17. Frohlich ED (1972) Mechanism of beta-blockade hypertension. N Engl J Med 287 : 1247
18. Tarazi RC, Dustan HP (1972) Beta-adrenergic blockade in hypertension: Pracital and theoretical implications of long-term hemodynamic variations. Am J Cardiol 29 : 633
19. Hansson L, Zweifler AJ, Julius S, Hunyor SN (1974) Hemodynamic effects of acute and prolonged beta-adrenergic blockade in essential hypertension. Acta Med Scand 196 : 633
20. Prichard BNC, Gillam PMS (1966) Propranolol in hypertension. Am J Cardiol 18 : 387
21. Coleman TG, Granger HJ, Guyton AC (1971) Whole-body circulatory autoregulation and hypertension. Circ Res 28/I : 76

22. Tuttle RS, McCleary M (1978) A mechanism to explain the antihypertensive action of propranolol. J Pharm Exp Ter 207 : 56
23. Lund-Johansen P (1977) Hemodynamic alterations in hypertension — spontaneous changes and effects of drug therapy. A review. Acta Med Scand 603 : 1
24. Frohlich ED (1978) Concepts of pressor mechanisms in hypertension evolved through clinical experience with beta-adrenergic receptor blocking drugs. In: Braunwald E (ed) Beta-adrenergic blockade: A new era in cardiovascular medicine, Excerpta Medica, Amsterdam Princeton, p 225
25. Frohlich ED (1974) Inhibition of adrenergic function in the treatment of hypertension. Arch Intern Med 133 : 1033
26. Nishiyama K, Nishiyama A, Pfeffer MA, Frohlich ED (1978) Systemic and regional blood flow distribution in normotensive and spontaneously hypertensive young rats subjected to lifetime beta-adrenergic receptor blockade. Blood Vessels 15 : 333
27. Vaughan-Williams EM, Raine N (1974) Effect of prolonged beta-receptor blockade on dry weight and electrophysiological responses of rabbit hearts. Lancet II : 1048
28. Fernandes M, Onesti G, Fiorentini R, Kim DE, Schwartz C (1976) Effect of chronic administration of propranolol on the blood pressure and heart weight in experimental renal hypertension. Life Sci 18 : 967
29. Pfeffer MA, Pfeffer JM, Weiss AK, Frohlich ED (1977) Development of SHR hypertension and cardiac hypertrophy during prolonged beta-blocking therapy. Am J Physiol 232 : H639
30. Frohlich ED, Tarazi RC (1979) Are pressure and afterload the sole factors responsible for hypertensive cardiac hypertrophy? Am J Cardiol 44 : 959
31. Bayliss WM (1902) On the local reactions of the arterial wall to changes of internal pressure. J Physiol (Lond) 28 : 220
32. Ledingham JM, Cohen RD (1963) The role of the heart in the pathogenesis of renal hypertension. Lancet II : 979
33. Trippodo NC, Walsh GM, Ferrone RA, Dugan RC (to be published) Fluid partitions and cardiac output in volume-depleted Goldblatt hypertensive rats. Am J Physiol
34. Frohlich ED (1977) Haemodynamics of hypertension. In: Genest J, Koiw E, Kuchel O (eds) Hypertension: Physiopathology and treatment, McGraw-Hill, New York, p 15
35. Caldini P, Permutt S, Waddell JA, Riley RL (1974) Effect of epinephrine on pressure, flow, and volume relationships in the systemic circulation of dogs. Circ Res 34 : 606
36. Coleman TG, Manning RD, Norman RA, Guyton AC (1974) Control of cardiac output by regional blood flow distribution. Ann Biomed Eng 2 : 149
37. Frohlich ED (1980) Metyldopa: Mechanisms and treatment: 25 years later. Arch Intern Med 140 : 954
38. Frohlich ED (1980) Adrenergic inhibiting drugs. In: Hunt JC (ed) Hypertension update: Mechanisms, epidemiology, evaluation, and management. Health Learning Systems, Philadelphia, pp 226—235

39. Davis JO, Freeman RH (1976) Mechanisms regulating renin release. Physiol Rev 56 : 1
40. Bühler FR, Laragh JH, Baer L, Vaughan ED Jr, Brunner HR (1972) Propranolol inhibition of renin secretion. N Engl J Med 287 : 1209
41. Bühler FR, Laragh JH, Vaughan ED Jr, Brunner HR, Gavras H, Baer L (1973) Antihypertensive action of propranolol. Am J Cardiol 32 : 511
42. Vaughan ED Jr, Laragh JH, Gavras I, Bühler FR, Gavras H, Brunner HR, Baer L (1973) The volume factor in low and normal renin essential hypertension: Its treatment with either spironolactone or chlorthalidone. Am J Cardiol 32 : 523
43. Laragh JH (1976) Modern system for treating high blood pressure based on renin-profiling and vasoconstriction-volume analysis: A primary role for beta blocking drugs such as propranolol. Am J Med 61 : 797
44. Stokes GS, Weber MA, Thornell JR (1974) B-blockers and plasma renin activity in hypertension. Br Med J I : 60
45. Frohlich ED (1980) Are beta-blockers too dangerous for general clinical use? In: Lasagna L (ed) Controversies in therapeutics. Saunders, Philadelphia, pp 347—357
46. Gilmore W, Weil J, Chidsey C (1970) Treatment of essential hypertension with a new vasodilator in combination with beta-adrenergic blockade. N Engl J Med 282 : 521
47. Zacest R, Gilmore E, Koch-Weser J (1972) Treatment of essential hypertension with combined vasodilation and beta-adrenergic blockade. N Engl J Med 286 : 617
48. Wilhelmsson C, Vedin A, Wilhelmsen L, Tibblin G, Werkö L (1974) Reduction of sudden deaths after myocardial infarction by treatment with alprenolol. Lancet II : 1157

Beta-Receptor Blockade in the Treatment of Renal Hypertension

J. GIRNDT

In earlier studies we showed that an application of β-blocking agents is a successful antihypertensive treatment in more than one-third of patients suffering from primary hypertension, whereas the hypotensive effect is poor in renal hypertension, unless these agents are given in combination with diuretic agents [5]. On the other hand, some authors found that the therapeutic effect of β-blocking agents was related to a stimulated renin secretion of the kidney [1]. These conflicting results provided a reason to test β-receptor blockade in experimental renal hypertension.

Experiments were performed in two types of hypertension in the rat (see Fig. 1).

Goldblatt-II kidney hypertension — in a rather simplified manner, of course — may be supposed to depend on a stimulated renin secretion, whereas the increase in blood pressure in Goldblatt-I kindney hypertension could be due to an extension of the extracellulary fluid volume, the plasma renin acitvity in this type being low or suppressed.

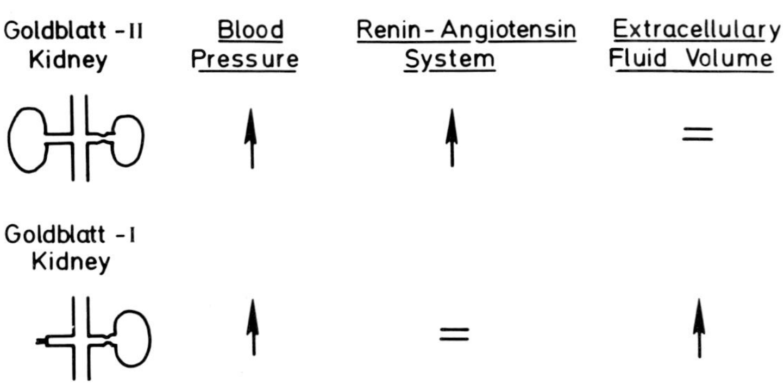

Fig. 1. Types of hypertension in the rat

Methods

Female Wistar rats with body weights from 140 to 160 g were clamped at one renal artery. The contralateral kidney was left in situ (Goldblatt-II hypertension) or was extirpated (Goldblatt-I hypertension). Some groups of animals were fed with Altromin C 1036, a sodium-restricted diet containing only 0.03% sodium. Other groups were fed with the sodium-unrestricted diet Altromin C 1000. In earlier studies we found that β-blocking agents were effective in Wistar rats only in a rather high dosage. Pindolol in doses ranging from 0.2 to 2.0 mg/kg and propranolol in doses ranging from 2.0 to 50.0 mg/kg per day did not alter the blood pressure [4]. Thus, in the following study propranolol was given in daily doses of 100 mg/kg and pindolol in daily doses of 10 mg/kg. The drugs were given together with the drinking water, so that perhaps they were only partially ingested. In summary, the following experimental groups of animals were used: Goldblatt-1 type, Goldblatt-2 type, sodium restriction, no sodium restriction, propranolol, pindolol, and controls. Each group comprised 20 animals, which were distributed equally in each group with respect to body weight and blood pressure readings were done in weekly intervals. The handling of the experimental groups was conducted over a 6-week period as described. After this time the animals were killed, the plasma renin activity was measured, and the left ventricular heart weight was determined.

Results

In rats with Goldblatt hypertension the blood pressure is altered by β-blocking agents only when these are given in rather high daily doses. Pindolol in doses of 10 mg/kg per day increases the blood pressure in both Goldblatt-I and Goldblatt-II hypertension, the pressor reaction being more prominent in experimental groups without sodium restriction. Propranolol lowers the blood pressure in Goldblatt-II hypertensive rats which had no sodium restriction. In Goldblatt-II

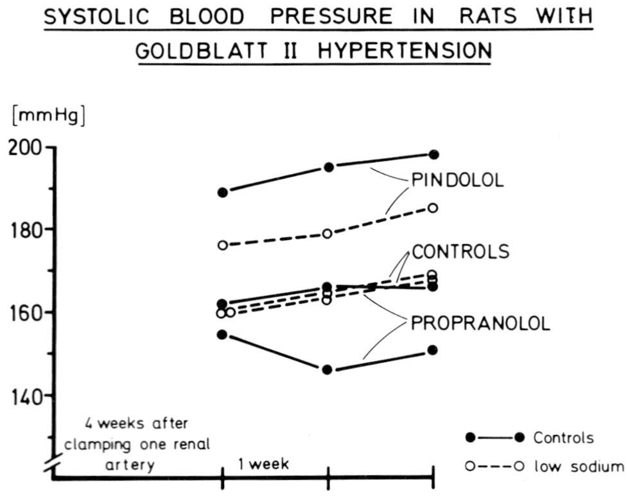

Fig. 2. Blood pressure values in rats 4, 5, and 6 weeks after clamping one renal artery

hypertensive rats fed a sodium-restricted diet, propranolol does not alter the blodd pressure (Fig. 2).

In Goldblatt-I type hypertension there is no hypotensive effect of propranolol. This holds true for animals either on a sodium-restricted diet or without sodium restriction (Fig. 3). Plasma renin activity in Goldblatt-II hypertension is slightly elevated. Animals with sodium restriction show an additional stimulation of the renin-angiotensin syste. This stimulation is diminished by propranolol or by pindolol, the former being more effective in this respect.

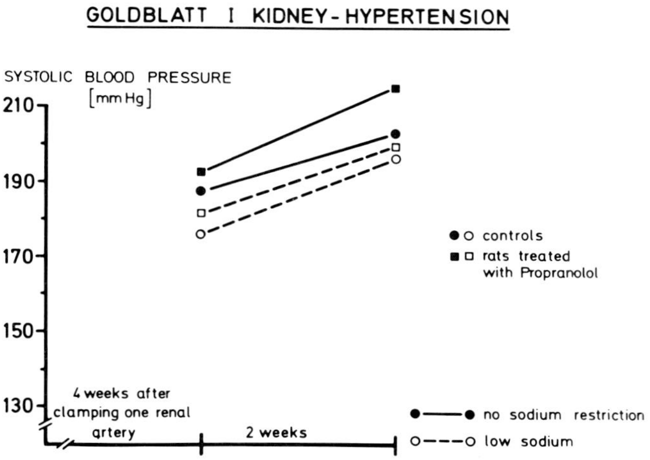

Fig. 3. Blood pressure values in rats 4 and 6 weeks after clamping one renal artery and removing the contralateral kidney

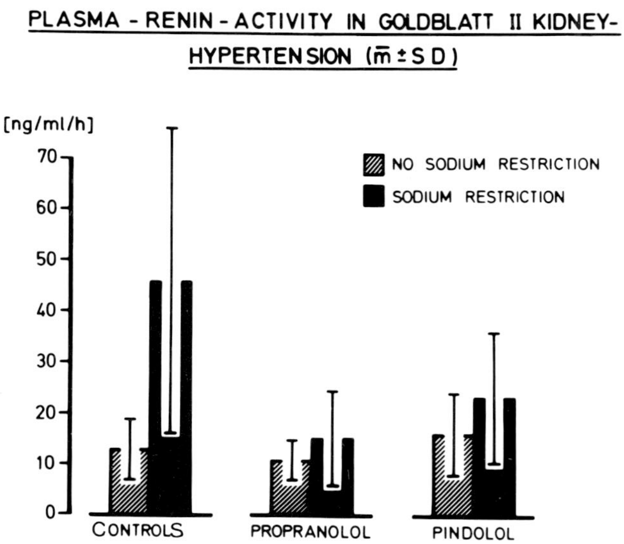

Fig. 4. Plasma renin activity in rats 6 weeks after clamping one renal artery

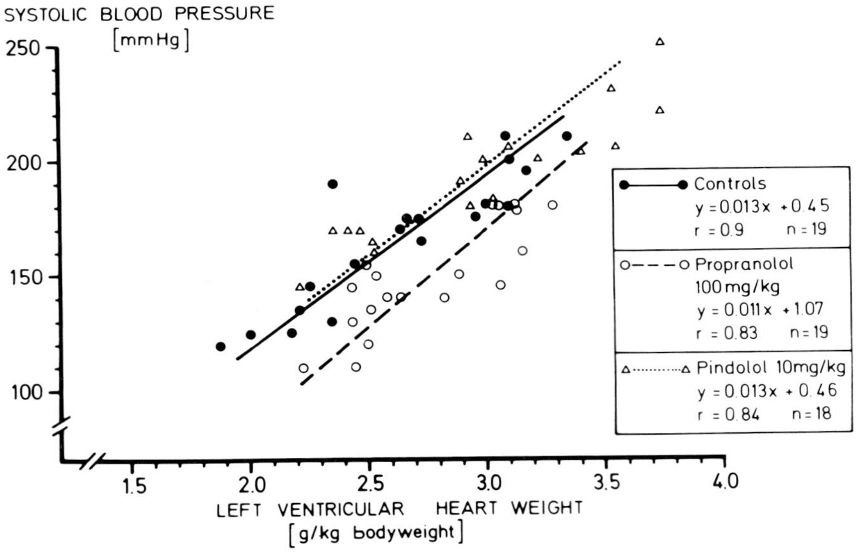

Fig. 5. Correlation between the systolic blood pressure at the end of the study and the left ventricular heart weight in those animals with Goldblatt-II hypertension and no sodium restriction

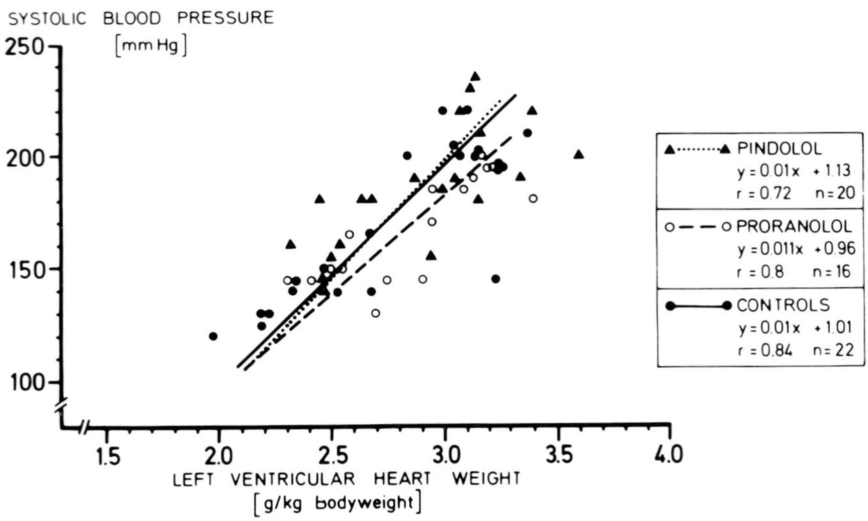

Fig. 6. Correlation between the systolic blood pressure at the end of the study and the left ventricular heart weight in animals with Goldblatt-II hypertension fed a sodium-restricted diet

In Goldblatt-I hypertension plasma renin activity is normal or low. The effect of β-blocking agents equals the effect in Goldblatt-II hypertension, all values moving at a lower level in Goldblatt-I hypertension (Fig. 4). The systolic blood pressure measured at the end of the study is correlated linearly with the left ventricular heart weight. In Goldblatt-II hypertension the same correlation holds true for controls and rats treated with pindolol. Figure 5 shows that in rats without sodium restriction the group of animals treated with propranolol shows an increase in left ventricular heart weight despite the lowered blood pressure values.

This difference is reveresed in those animals which were fed a sodium-restricted diet (Fig. 6). In all the groups with sodium restriction the same correlation holds true between systolic blood pressure value and left ventricular heart weight.

In Goldblatt-I hypertension, which in no situation was reversed by β-blocking agents, there is no influence by either drug on left ventricular heart weight. We found the following correlations:

1. Controls: $y = 0.011x + 1.05$, $r = 0.7$, $n = 19$;
2. Pindolol: $y = 0.011x + 0.62$, $r = 0.82$, $n = 19$;
3. Propranolol: $y = 0.011x + 0.99$, $r = 0.88$, $n = 18$.

Discussion

Beta-blocking agents are well proved in antihypertensive treatment. Some authors believe that these drugs are most effective in those kinds of hypertension which depend on a stimulation of the renin-angiotensin system [1, 2, 6]. We found in an earlier study that β-blocking agents had a rather poor hypotensive effect in renal hypertension [5]. The current experimental study was done to clarify the mode of action of β-blockers in renal hypertension. Some years ago we had already found that only rather high doses of the drugs are able to influence Goldblatt hypertension of Wistar rats [4]. This corresponds to the findings of other authors, who found that β-blocking agents in low dosage were without hypotensive effectiveness [7, 8, 10]. On the other hand, some β-blockers given in high doses are known to cause pressor reactions [9, 11].

We found in this study a pressor reaction of pindolol in Goldblatt-I as well as in Goldblatt-II hypertension. This pressor reaction is demonstrated in rats fed a sodium-restricted diet as well as in rats fed the control diet. Pindolol is known to possess high intrinsic sympathomimetic activity, and the pressor reaction may easily be related to this intrinsic activity when the drug is given in high doses. Pindilol does not alter the blood-pressure-dependent weight gain of the left heart ventricle.

Propranolol was of hypotensive effect only in Goldblatt-II hypertension and only in those animals which had no sodium restriction. Goldblatt-II hypertension may be supposed to be related to a stimulated renin-angiotensin system, whereas Goldblatt-I hypertension may be volume dependent. At least 6 weeks after inducing the pressor mechanism the plasma renin activity is elevated in Goldblatt-II and low or suppressed in Goldblatt-I hypertensive rats. So, this finding may be interpreted as a relation of a hypotensive effect of propranolol to an activation of renin secretion.

In those animals which showed the depressor effect of propranolol, we found significantly higher weights of the left heart ventricle with respect to the systolic blood pressure values. The depressor reaction as well as the left ventricular weight gain were reversed by sodium restriction. So, it may be supposed that the blood pressure lowering effect of propranolol could be due to a cardiodepressor reaction.

Summary

Wistar rats with Goldblatt-II and Goldblatt-I hypertension were treated with propranolol 100 mg/kg per day or pindolol 10 mg/kg per day. Pindolol increased the blood pressure in all experimental groups. Propranolol showed an antihypertensive effect in Goldblatt-II hypertension in animals which had no sodium restriction. In Goldblatt-I hypertension and in Goldblatt-II hypertension of animals fed a sodium-restricted diet, propranolol did not alter the blood pressure. A linear correlation between the weight of the left heart ventricle and the systolic blood pressure was found in animals treated with pindolol as well as in untreated Goldblatt rats. On the contrary, the weights of the left heart ventricle were significantly higher in those animals which showed a hypotensive reaction after treatment with propranolol. The pressor reaction after application of pindolol may be due to the intrinsic sympathomimetic activity of the drug. Propranolol, possibly because of a cardiodepressor effect, leads to a decrease in blood pressure in renin-dependent hypertension, the decrease being reversed by sodium restriction.

References

1. Bühler FR (1976) Antihypertensive Wirkung von β-Blockern in Abhängigkeit von Reninaktivität und Alter bei essentiellem Hochdruck. In: Ganten D, Dietz R, Lüth B, Gross F (eds) β-adrenerge Blocker und Hochdruck. Thieme, Stuttgart, p 88
2. Drayer JIM, Weber MA, Longworth DL, Laragh JH (1978) The possible importance of aldosterone as well as renin in the long-term antihypertensive action of propranolol. Am J Med 64 : 187
3. Girndt J (1979) Hochdosierte Anwendung von β-Rezeptorenblockern bei experimenteller renaler Hypertonie. Klin Wochenschr 57 : 793—795
4. Girndt J, Kramer A, Scheler F (1977) Der Einfluß des β-Rezeptorenblockers Pindolol auf Blutdruck und Herzgewicht bei Ratten mit Goldblatt-Hypertonie. Klin Wochenschr 55 : 349

5. Girndt J, Matthaei D, Scheler F (1978) Die Bedeutung von β-Rezeptorenblockern in der Hochdrucktherapie. Therapiewoche 28 : 8713
6. Karlberg BE, Tolagen K (1976) Different antihypertensive effect of β-blocking drugs in a low and normal-high renin hypertension. Am J Med 60 : 891
7. Karppanen H (1974) Effect of propranolol on the blood pressure of normotensive and pinealectomized hypertensive rats. Nauyn Schmiedebergs Arch Pharmacol 281 : 1
8. Menard J, Alexandre JM, Guideceilli JF, Auzan C, Chevillard C (1973) Lack of antihypertensive effects of chronic administration of DL-propanolol in Grollman rats. Arch Int Pharmacodyn Ther 202 : 298
9. Regoli D (1970) Pressor action of β-blocking agents in rats. Can J Physiol Pharmacol 48 : 481
10. Takeda K, Sakurai H, Imai S (1975) Antihypertensive effects of β-blockers in hypertensive rats. Jph J Pharmacol 25 : 8
11. Yamamoto U, Sekiya A (1972) Further studies on the pressure action of propranolol in the rat. Arch Int Pharmacodyn Ther 189 : 347

Left Ventricular and Coronary Response to Beta Receptor Blockade in Essential Hypertension[1]

A. KMENT, S.B. BÜRGER AND B.E. STRAUER

The aim of β-blocking drugs is the treatment of essential hypertension and angina pectoris in coronary artery disease. Inhibitions of β-receptor mediated stimulation of heart rate and myocardial contractility as well as lowering of blood pressure is believed to result in an improved energy demand of the myocardium. Investigations of the relationship between left ventricular function, coronary response, and myocardial oxygen consumption in essential hypertension during β-receptor blockade have not yet been published. In this paper, therefore, the acute effect of β_1-selective-receptor blocker (atenolol) on left ventricular function and coronary hemodynamics will be investigated.

Material and Methods

Studies were carried out on 11 patients who had low and normal stress hypertrophy and no signs of heart failure. At the time of diagnostic cardiac catheterization, quantaitative left ventriculography and coronary arteriography were accomplished. Drug therapy was discontinued 8—10 days before the study. Patients were studied in the fasting state and under local anesthesia (1% xylocaine). Catheters were placed according to the technique of Seldinger into the left ventricle, aorta, right atrium, arteria pulmonalis, and the sinus coronarius for hemodynamic measurements.

Patients were kept 30 min under resting conditions. Hemodynamic measurements were taken after 20 and 25 min [1]. After 25 min the total coronary blood flow was also determined. The method used was the argon inert gas method with gas chromatographic analysis in arterial and coronary venous blood [2].

Details as well as the accuracy of coronary blood flow determinations up to 400—450 (ml/min x 100 g), coronary resistance, and arterial-coronary venous oxygen difference have been described in detail [3]. Left ventricular oxygen consumption was calculated as the product of coronary flow and the arterial-coronary venous oxygen difference.

---

1 Supported by the Deutsche Forschungsgemeinschaft

Subsequently, atenolol (Tenormin) in a dosage of 5 mg was given intravenously over a period of 5 min. Thirty minutes after administration of the drug, hemodynamic measurements of left ventricular coronary blood flow as well as left ventricular oxygen consumption were repeated. Statistical comparisons were made using the t-test for paired observations, and differences were considered significant when $P < 0.05$.

Results

Patients

Case histories are represented in Table 1. No asynchronous contraction or paradoxical motion of the ventricular wall was present in any of the patients. However, one patient showed asymmetric hypertrophy without left ventricular obstruction. Mean left ventricular mass was increased to 148 g/m^2. According to a normal end-diastolic volume of 91 ml/m^2, the mass to volume ration was increased to 1.64 (normals: 1.21).

Table 1. Case histories of patients involved in the study

Number of patients	11	Left ventricle hypertrophy	
Average age (years)	37	(chest X-ray)	11
Degree (WHO report)	II	(ECG)	10
Duration of hypertension		Left atrial hypertrophy	
(years)	2	(ECG)	8
		Coronary disease	3
		Irregular wall contraction	—
Angina pectoris	7	Asymmetric hypertrophy	1
Dyspnea at rest	—	Left ventricle mass	148 m^2
Dyspnea on exertion	2	End-diastolic volume	91 ml/m^2
Myocardial infarction	1	Mass to volume ratio	1.64

Ventricular Function

Thirty minutes after administration of atenolol an evident decrease of heart rate by 13.8% could be observed (Fig. 1, Table 2). Because stroke volume index was nearly unchanged (+1.2%), the diminution of cardiac index by 11.5% was heart ratte dependent. Left ventricular systolic pressure (Fig. 2) was lowered only by 5.4% without significant alteration of left ventricular end-diastolic pressure (—2.4%). The maximum rate of left ventricular pressure development decreased by 7.5%. The decrease of systolic pressure, cardiac index, and heart rate caused a decrease of external cardiac work by 14.3% and of the tension-time index by 19.2% (Fig. 3).

Table 2. Ventricular function and coronary hemodynamics before and 30 min after atenolol (5 mg IV) [a]

		Before	After Atenolol	*P*	%
P_{LV}	(mm Hg)	189 ± 20	179 ± 17	0.001	− 5.4
P_{LVED}	(mm Hg)	15.4 ± 2.5	15 ± 14	n.s.	− 2.4
Peak dp/dt	(mm Hg/s)	2260 ± 470	2090 ± 359	0.01	− 7.5
HR	(1/min)	80 ± 9	69 ± 9	0.001	−13.8
CI	($l/min \cdot m^2$)	3.43 ± 0.45	3.03 ± 0.32	0.001	−11.5
SVI	($ml/beat \cdot m^2$)	43.3 ± 4.12	43.8 ± 5.31	n.s.	+ 1.2
ECW	($mm\ Hg \cdot ml \cdot min \cdot m^2$)	612 ± 84	524 ± 61	0.001	−14.3
~TTI	($P_{syst} \cdot bpm$)	14481 ± 2539	11713 ± 1699	0.001	−19.2
V_{cor}	($ml/min \cdot 100\ g$)	86.4 ± 9.8	73.9 ± 12.5	0.005	−14.5
R_{cor}	($mm\ Hg \cdot min \cdot 100\ g \cdot ml^{-1}$)	1.57 ± 0.32	1.76 ± 0.32	0.005	+12.5
$avDO_2$	(Vol%)	12.26 ± 1.01	12.20 ± 0.95	n.s.	−0.44
MVO_2	($ml/min \cdot 100\ g$)	10.43 ± 1.23	9.01 ± 1.4	0.005	−13.6

[a] Abbreviatians: P_{LV} = left ventricular systolic pressure; P_{LVED} = left ventricular end-diastolic pressure; Peak dp/dt = maximum rate of left ventricular pressure development; HR = heart rate; CI = cardiac index; SVI = stroke volume index; ECW = external cardiac work; ~TTI = tension-time index; V_{cor} = coronary blood flow; R_{cor} = coronary resistance; $avDO_2$ = arterial-coronary venous oxygen difference; and MVO_2 = left ventricular oxygen consumption. Values are mean ± SE

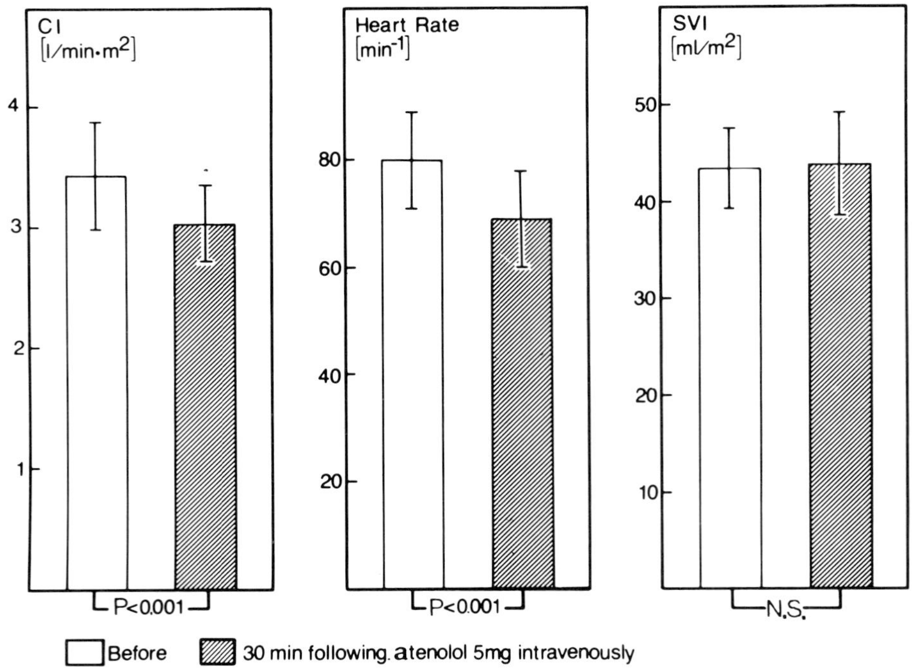

Fig. 1. Cardiac index (*CI*), heart rate (*HR*), and stroke volume index (*SVI*) before and after atenolol

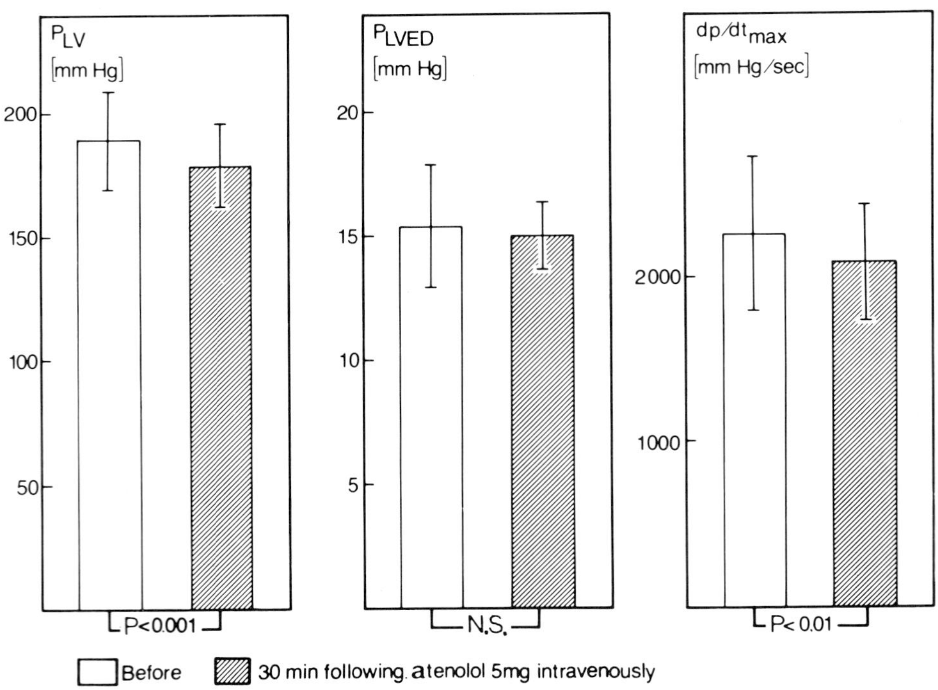

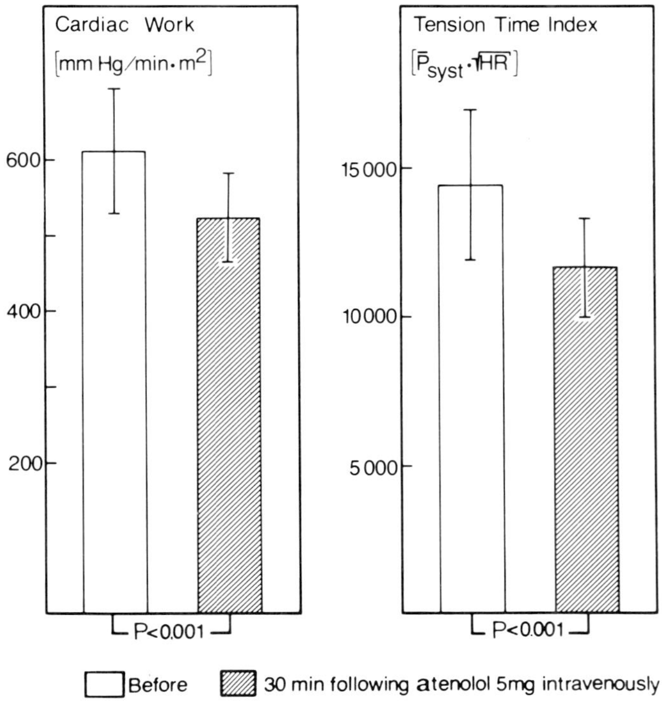

Fig. 3. Cardiac work and tension-time index before and after atenolol

Coronary Hemodynamics and Myocardial Oxygen Consumption

Coronary blood flow decreased by 14.5% (Fig. 4; Table 2). While coronary perfusion pressure did not change significantly, coronary resistance did increase by 12.7%. The decrease of coronary blood flow was accompanied by a decrease of myocardial oxygen consumption by 13.6%. Arterial-coronary oxygen difference was not changed significantly.

Coronary Vascular Reserve

In addition, coronary vascular reserve (R_{cor}/R^{+}_{cor}) was determined in five patients without coronary artery disease after administration of atenolol. Coronary vascular reserve is defined as the ratio between coronary resistance in the resting state and under maximum coronary vasodilation with dipyridamole

◄ Fig.2. Left ventricular pressure (P_{LV}), left ventricular end-diastolic pressure (P_{LVED}), and maximum rate of left ventricular pressure development before and after atenolol

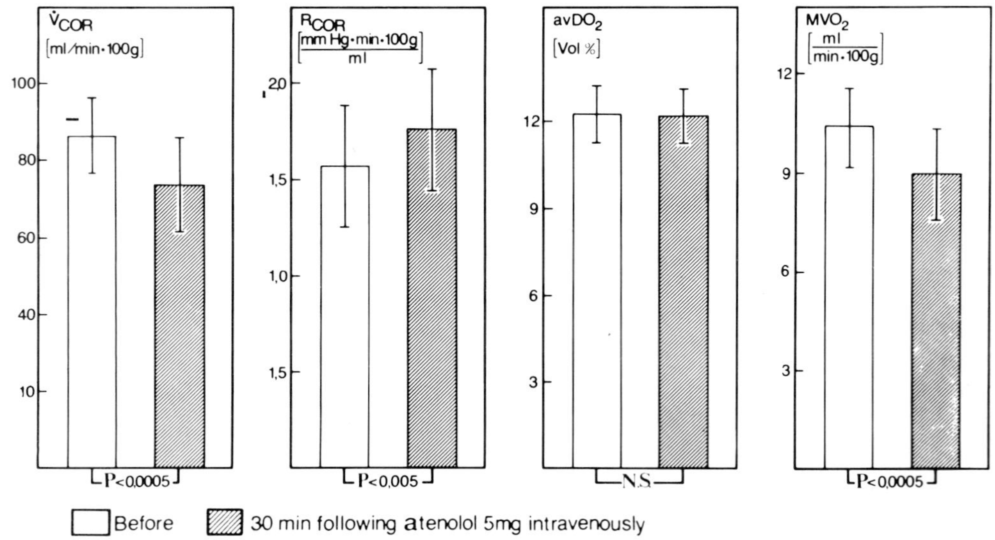

Fig. 4. Coronary blood flow of the left ventricle (V_{cor}), coronary resistance (R_{cor}), arterial-coronary venous oxygen difference ($avDO_2$), and left ventricular oxygen consumption (MVO_2) before and after atenolol

Table 3. Coronary vascular reserve before and after atenolol (5 mg IV) [a]

	V_{cor} (ml/min·100 g)	R_{cor} (mm Hg·min·100 g·ml^{-1})	R^*_{cor}	Coronary reserve (R_{cor}/R^*_{cor})
Control	89.2	1.61	0.53	3.03
Atenolol	74.8	1.79	0.49	3.66

[a] Abbreviations: R^*_{cor} = coronary vascular resistance with dipyridamol 0.5 mg/kg IV; V_{cor} = coronary blood flow; and R_{cor} = coronary resistance

(0.5 mg/kg IV). Coronary reserve of these patients was compared to the coronary reserve of 21 patients with essential hypertension and comparable systolic wall stress. Atenolol (Table 3) augmented coronary vascular reserve from 3.03 to 3.66 in essential hypertension.

Calculation of Myocardial Oxygen Consumption by the Bretschneider Method

In order to evaluate the relationship between myocardial oxygen consumption (argon method) and single hemodynamic determinatns of myocardial oxygen consumption, left ventricular oxygen consumption was claculated by the formu-

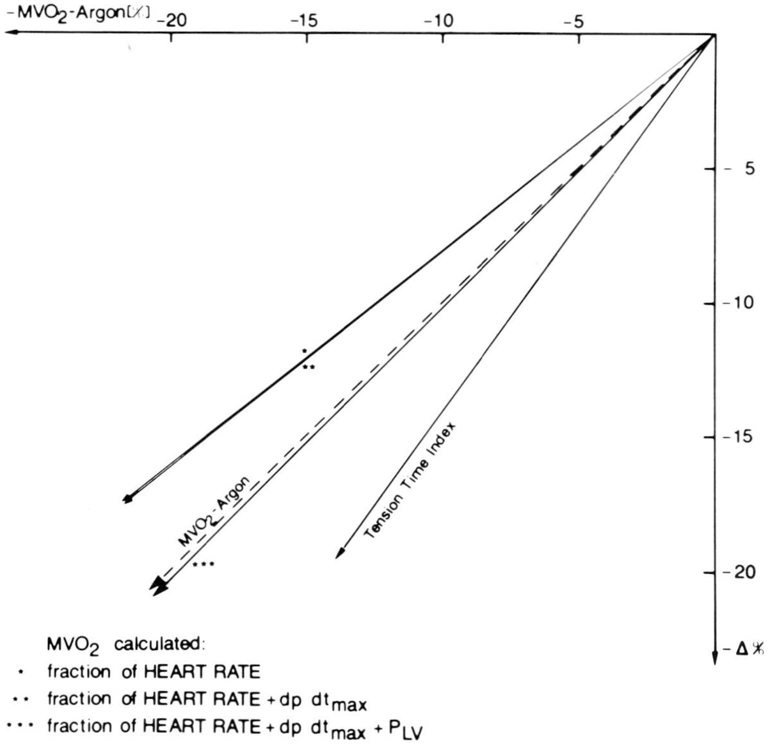

Fig. 5. Relationship between relative change of myocardial oxygen consumption (argon method) and single hemodynamic determinants of myocardial oxygen consumption calculated as the sum of three energy-equivalent links. Note that tension-time index overestimates myocardial oxygen consumption (argon method). MVO_2, left ventricular oxygen consumption; P_{LV}, left ventricular systolic pressure

Table 4. Myocardial oxygen consumption calculated by the hemodynamic parameter of Bretschneider (1976) before and after atenolol (5 mg IV)

	MVO_2 before A	Fraction of HR	Fraction of peak dp/dt	Fraction of P_{LV}	MVO_2 after A
MVO_2 (ml/min·100 g)	8.97	0.81	0.003	0.44	7.72

Abbreviations: A = atenolol; Peak dp/dt = maximum rate of left ventricular pressure development; HR = heart rate; P_{LV} = left ventricular systolic pressure; and MVO_2 = left ventricular oxygen consumption la of Bretschneider [4], which consists of three energy-equivalent links (E_1, E_2, E_3). When control values were set at 100%, a decrease of 13.6% in left ventricular oxygen consumption (argon method) was found and similarly a decrease of 14% (Bretschneider formula) was found (fig. 5; Table 4).

Furthermore, it could be shown that the decrease of heart rate contributed to the calculated myocardial oxygen consumption by 9.05% while the rate of left ventricular systolic pressure development contributed 0.033% and the left ventricular systolic pressure contributed 4.91%. The tension-time index used in this paper decreased by 19.2%, which would overestimate the myocardial oxyten consumption by 5.6% (argon method) and 5.2% (Bretschneider formula), respectively.

Discussion

This study has shown that the acute effects of atenolol are characterized by an effective lowering of left ventricular load with significant decrease of heart rate, left ventricular systolic pressure, and maximum rate of left ventricular systolic pressure development. The decrease of maximum rate of left ventricular pressure. development could also be caused indirectly by decreasing systolic pressure. The diminution of external cardiac work and tension-time index is dependent on the marked decrease of heart rate and systolic blood pressure. The decrease in myocardial energy requirements was followed by a decrease in coronary blood flow. There was no significant change shown in arterial-coronary oxygen difference after atenolol, while myocardial oxygen consumption was decreased. Since the coronary venous oxygen saturation remained unchanged, the increase of coronary resistance must be considered as metabolically induced. Therefore a direct coronary vasoconstrictive effect by alpha-receptor activity, for instance, is unlikely. It may be reasonable to assume that chronic administration of atenolol leads to further decrease of systolic pressure (15%—18%), thereby still more effectively lowering myocardial energy demand [5, 6].

Total myocardial oxygen consumption also could be calculated by the hemodynamic parameter of Bretschneider. The result is almost identical to that of the argon method. Lowering of the heart rate by 13.8% contributes to fractional decrease of myocardial oxygen consumption by 64%, whereas lowering of the fractions of maximum rate of left ventricular pressure development and left ventricular systolic pressure contribute 0.9% and 35%, respectively.

It may be assumed that an antihypertensive regimen with chronic administration of atenolol will not only decrease heart rate, but in additon will further decrease systolic blood pressure. As a consequence, the fraction of blood-pressure-dependent myocardial oxygen consumption is expected to increase further.

Indirect assessment of myocardial oxygen consumption, such as several heart rate-blood pressure products [7, 8], are regarded to be useful methods in bedside techniques, since heart rate and blood pressure can be readily determined.

However, it must be emphasized that pressure-heart rate products do not take into account the contracile state of the myocardium, changes in ventricular volume, or left ventricular wall thickness [9]. So our calculations show that there is a limitation in the validity of investigation of tension-time index, because true myocardial oxygen consumption was clearly overestimated.

In addition, coronary vascular reserve was determined in five patients without coronary artery disease after administration of atenolol. β-Blockade augmented coronary vascular reserve in chronic hypertensive heart disease by 21%. This augmentation was due to an increase in coronary resistance under atenolol, whereas minimal coronary resistance was nearly the same in both groups, with and without β-blockade. The reason for this is thought to be a decreasing energy demand after β-blockade and consecutive increase of coronary resistance. Thus, augmented coronary reserve may have its clinical equivalent in an enhanced metabolic working capacity in patients with coronary artery disease with an improvement in the ventricle's ability to adjust to increased metabolic requirements.

References

1. Strauer BE (1978) Das Hochdruckherz. VII. Die Wirkung von Atenolol auf Funktion, koronare Hämodynamik und Sauerstoffverbrauch des linken Ventrikels. Dtsch Med Wochenschr 45 : 1785
2. Bretschneider HJ, Cott L, Hilgert C, Probst R, Rau G (1966) Gaschromatographische Trennung und Analyse von Argon als Basis einer neuen Fremdgasmethode zur Durchblutungsmessung von Organen. Verh Dtsch Ges Kreislaufforsch 32 : 267
3. Strauer BE (1977) Die quantitative Bestimmung der Koronarreserve in der Diagnostik koronarer Durchblutungsstörungen. Internist (Berlin) 18 : 579
4. Bretschneider HJ (1976) Pathophysiologie der Ventrikelkontraktion-Kontraktilität, Inotropie, Suffizienzgrad und Arbeitsökonomie des Herzens. Verh Dtsch Ges Kreislaufforsch 42 : 14
5. Amery H, Billiert L, Boel A, Fagard R, Reybrouck T, Willems J (1976) Mechanism of hypotensive effect during beta-adrenergic blockade in hypertensive patients. Am Heart J 91 : 364
6. Sannerstedt R (1975) Auswahl von Hypertonikern für die alleinige oder kombinierte Behandlung mit Betablockern. Therapiewoche 33 : 64
7. Katz LN, Feinberg H (1958) The relation of cardiac effort to myocardial oxygen consumption and coronary flow. Circ Res 6 : 656
8. Neill WA, Levine HJ, Wagman RJ, Gorlin R (1963) Left ventricular oxygen utilization in intact dogs, effect of systemic hemodynamic factors. Circ Res 12 : 163
9. Amsterdam EA, Hughes IL, de Maria AN, Zelis R, Mason DT (1974) Indirect assessment of myocardial oxygen consumption in the evaluation of mechamisms and therapy of angina pectoris. Am J Cardiol 33 : 737

Subject Index

Evaluation of Cardiac Function by Echocardiography

Editors: W. Bleifeld, S. Effert, P. Hanrath, D. Mathey
1980. 160 figures, 17 tables. IX, 198 pages
ISBN 3-540-10045-8

Hypertension: Mechanisms and Management

Editors: T. Philipp, A. Distler
1980. 72 figures, 17 tables. XVII, 279 pages
(International Boehringer Mannheim Symposium)
ISBN 3-540-10171-3

Hypertension and the Kidney

Proceedings of a Symposium on 'Hypertension and the Kidney', Milan, Italy, September 28–29, 1974
Guest Editors: B. Kincaid-Smith, M. H. Maxwell
1975. 26 tables. I, 140 pages
(Kidney International Supplement 5 to Volume 8)
ISBN 3-540-90146-9

Myocardial Failure

Editors: G. Rieker, A. Weber, J. Goodwin
Co-Editors: H.-D. Bolte, B. Lüderitz, B. E. Strauer, E. Erdmann
1977. 172 figures, 52 tables. XII, 374 pages
(International Boehringer Mannheim Symposia)
ISBN 3-540-08225-5
Distribution rights for Japan: Nankodo Co. Ltd., Tokyo

B. E. Strauer

Hypertensive Heart Disease

Translated from the German
1980. 65 figures, 19 tables. VII, 105 pages
ISBN 3-540-10041-5

Systolic Time Intervals

Editors: W. F. List, J. S. Gravenstein, D. H. Spodick
Editorial Consultant: J. Barden
1980. 159 figures, 46 tables. XV, 303 pages
(International Boehringer Mannheim Symposia)
ISBN 3-540-09871-2

Springer-Verlag
Berlin
Heidelberg
New York